MCQs in Spine Surgery

Cristian Gragnaniello •
Gabriel Tender • Kevin Phan •
Ralph Mobbs • Remi Nader
Editors

MCQs in Spine Surgery

Springer

Editors
Cristian Gragnaniello
The University of Texas Health Science
Center at San Antonio
San Antonio, TX, USA

Kevin Phan
School of Clinical Medicine
University of New South Wales (Sydney)
Randwick, NSW, Australia

Remi Nader
University of Texas Medical Branch
Galveston, TX, USA

Gabriel Tender
Louisiana State University
New Orleans, LA, USA

Ralph Mobbs
Prince of Wales Hospital
Randwick, NSW, Australia

ISBN 978-3-031-69331-1 ISBN 978-3-031-69332-8 (eBook)
https://doi.org/10.1007/978-3-031-69332-8

This Springer imprint is published by the registered company Springer Nature Switzerland AG
The registered company address is: Gewerbestrasse 11, 6330 Cham, Switzerland

Contents

Anatomy, Embryology, Examination and Imaging of the Spine

1

Zayed Almadidy, Darius Ansari, and Saavan Patel

1. A 73-year-old woman is being evaluated in the emergency department due to acute-onset back pain. Past medical history is significant for osteoporosis diagnosed via dual-energy x-ray absorptiometry (DEXA) 10 years ago. Imaging reveals compression fractures of T10 and T11. Given these findings, which portion of the vertebrae is most likely to be fractured in this patient?
   a. Intervertebral disc
   b. Transverse process
   c. Superior articular process
   d. Vertebral body
   e. Lateral mass

Preferred Response: (d) Vertebral body. Vertebral compression fractures, which most commonly occur in the setting of osteoporosis, are typically anterior column injuries resulting from compression with flexion. The transverse and superior articular processes can be injured during trauma, but are more likely to occur due to oblique, transverse, or comminuted fractures. The intervertebral discs are not associated with compression fractures. The lateral mass is a structure present in the cervical spine [1].

2. An individual is being evaluated in the emergency department after major trauma. Upon evaluation, the patient is intubated, holding their arms in pronation and extension, and extending their lower extremities. Damage to which of the following structures is most likely responsible for this type of positioning in this patient?
   a. Rubrospinal tract
   b. Dorsal column-medial lemniscus pathway
   c. Spinothalamic tract
   d. Vestibulospinal tract
   e. Pontine reticulospinal tract

Preferred Response: (a) Rubrospinal tract. The patient described is in decerebrate posturing. Lesions that interrupt fibers of the red nucleus lead to inhibition of the rubrospinal tract and constant excitation of the vestibulospinal and pontine reticulospinal tracts. The unopposed, continuous excitation results in extensor posturing when stimulation is applied. The spinothalamic tract is also typically injured in such lesions but continues to give off reticular fibers below the lesion to the reticular formation and other pontine nuclei and is not responsible for the maintenance of flexion [2].

3. In the evaluation of a patient complaining of radicular pain, the attending radiologist read of an MRI notes disc herniation at L4-L5. An extreme lateral disc herniation involving the foraminal zone at the level of L4-L5 is most likely to affect which of the following nerve roots?
   a. L3
   b. L4
   c. L5
   d. S1
   e. None

Preferred Response: (b) L4. While central and paramedian disc herniations typically involve the traversing nerve root and therefore usually 1 level below (in this case, the L5 nerve root), far lateral disc herniations involving the foraminal zone involve the nerve root exiting at that level (in this case, the L4 nerve root). The L3 nerve root is unlikely to be affected by such a lesion as it has already exited the spinal canal. Similarly, an L4-L5 far lateral disc herniation is unlikely to produce symptomatic compression of the S1 nerve root.

Z. Almadidy (✉) · D. Ansari · S. Patel
Department of Neurosurgery, University of Illinois at Chicago, Chicago, USA
e-mail: zalmad3@uic.edu

D. Ansari
e-mail: dansari2@uic.edu

S. Patel
e-mail: spate327@uic.edu

C. Gragnaniello et al. (eds.), *MCQs in Spine Surgery*,
https://doi.org/10.1007/978-3-031-69332-8_1

4. Which of the following is the most appropriate noninvasive imaging technique to order to differentiate spinal abscess from primary tumor?
   a. CT without contrast
   b. CT with and without contrast
   c. MRI without contrast
   d. MRI with and without contrast

Preferred Response: (d) MRI with and without contrast. Although distinguishing infectious from neoplastic processes can be challenging based on imaging data alone, MRI is the investigation of choice for differentiating several spinal pathologies. On MRI scan, abscesses appear iso-intense or hypo-intense on T1-weighted images and hyperintense on T2-weighted images. Contrast studies show a peripheral rim of enhancement. Conversely, contrast MRI studies of ependymomas and meningiomas typically enhance homogeneously. MRI scan without contrast would provide less discriminatory capability as tumors such as ependymomas may appear iso-intense on T1 and hyperintense on T2-weighted images, similar to abscesses [3].

5. A 59-year-old man presents to the office with complaints of low back pain and weakness in his left leg. MRI demonstrates compression of the exiting nerve root between L4 and L5 vertebrae. Which of the following structures is most likely responsible for producing this lesion?
   a. Posterior longitudinal ligament
   b. Annulus fibrosus
   c. Interspinous ligament
   d. Ligamentum flavum
   e. Nucleus pulposus

Preferred Response: (e) Nucleus pulposus. Nerve compression at the intervertebral foramen is most commonly caused by a disc herniation. Disc herniation is caused by herniation of the nucleus pulposus through the annulus fibrosus, which can affect the spinal canal or the intervertebral foramen. The posterior longitudinal ligament is located posterior to the disc space, but symptomatic disc herniations generally are the result of posterolateral herniation of the nucleus pulposus. The interspinous ligament is located in the posterior column and would not be responsible for the described MRI findings. The ligamentum flavum may become hypertrophied, causing symptoms of canal stenosis, but unilateral compression at the intervertebral foramen is more likely to be caused by herniated nucleus pulposus [1].

6. A 79-year-old man experiences cramping pain in his low back and bilateral legs while walking. He states that this has gradually progressed over several months. His pain is worsened while walking downhill, and relieved by resting or bending forwards while walking. On examination, peripheral pulses are intact. MRI of the lumbar spine reveals non-displaced intervertebral discs and increased thickening of the posterior spinal canal with compression of the posterior thecal sac. Which of the following structures is most likely responsible for this patient's symptoms?
   a. Posterior longitudinal ligament
   b. Annulus fibrosus
   c. Interspinous ligament
   d. Ligamentum flavum
   e. Nucleus pulposus

Preferred Response: (d) Ligamentum flavum. Hypertrophy of the ligamentum flavum can cause symptoms of lumbar spinal stenosis, as observed in this elderly gentleman with cramping pain while walking ("neurogenic claudication").

7. A patient with a history of advanced renal cell carcinoma undergoes elective commissural myelotomy. As part of the procedure, an incision is made through the fibers of the anterior white commissure of the spinal cord. Deficits in which of the following would be expected as a result of this injury? There may be multiple correct answers.
   a. Proprioception
   b. Pain sensation
   c. Vibratory sensation
   d. Temperature sensation
   e. Fine touch discrimination
   f. a + b
   g. b + c
   h. b + d
   i. b + d + e

Preferred Response: (h) Pain sensation and Temperature sensation. A lesion affecting the anterior white commissure of the spinal cord would affect the second-order neurons of the spinothalamic tract, resulting in deficits of pain, temperature, pressure, and crude (rather than fine) touch. Following decussation of the second-order neurons in the spinothalamic tract, these fibers ascend and synapse in the ventral posterolateral nucleus of the thalamus. Additionally, up to 15% of corticospinal tract fibers cross at the anterior white commissure. Proprioception, fine touch, and vibration are primarily governed by the dorsal column medial lemniscus tract, which would be spared in an isolated lesion to the anterior white commissure [4].

8. Which of the following is the correct sequence of structures of the spinothalamic tract from distal to proximal?

a. Sensory nerve ending > ipsilateral gray matter of spinal cord > anterior white commissure > VPL nucleus of the thalamus > 1° somatosensory cortex
b. Sensory nerve ending > ventral horn of spinal cord > anterior white commissure > VPL nucleus of the thalamus > 1° somatosensory cortex
c. Sensory nerve ending > nucleus gracilis/cuneatus > medial lemniscus > VPL nucleus of the thalamus > 1° somatosensory cortex
d. Sensory nerve ending > ipsilateral gray matter of spinal cord > anterior white commissure > VPM nucleus of the thalamus > 1° somatosensory cortex

Preferred Response: (a) Sensory nerve ending > ipsilateral gray matter of spinal cord > anterior white commissure > VPL nucleus of the thalamus > 1° somatosensory cortex. The nucleus gracilis and medial lemniscus are involved in the dorsal-column medial lemniscus tract. The ventral horn of the spinal cord contains cell bodies involved in the descending corticospinal tract. The ventral posteromedial nucleus of the thalamus is involved in facial sensation [5].

9. A child with history of neurofibromatosis type 2 is undergoing an anterolateral cordotomy for intractable pain secondary to a sciatic nerve tumor. Preoperatively, the patient undergoes high-resolution MRI to locate the dentate ligament. The dentate ligament serves as an important intraoperative landmark between two spinal cord structures, which ones?
   a. Lateral corticospinal tract and dorsal columns
   b. Anterior corticospinal tract and lateral spinothalamic tract
   c. Lateral spinothalamic tract and anterior spinocerebellar tract
   d. Lateral corticospinal tract and lateral spinothalamic tract
   e. Anterior spinocerebellar tract and anterior corticospinal tract

Preferred Response: (d) Lateral corticospinal tract and lateral spinothalamic tract. The dentate ligament is located immediately ventral to the lateral corticospinal tract and dorsal to the spinothalamic tract. Identification of this ligament preoperatively (if possible) and intraoperatively during an anterolateral chordotomy is critical for definition of the desired lesion [6].

10. A patient with longstanding history of alcoholism presents to the office with progressive fatigue, gait ataxia, and bilateral lower extremity paresthesias. Physical examination discloses diminished sensation to light touch and vibration over the bilateral lower extremities, with positive Romberg sign. Complete blood count reveals macrocytic anemia. Which of the following findings confers the highest sensitivity for the patient's suspected condition?
    a. Decreased serum cobalamin levels
    b. Peripheral blood smear with hyper segmented neutrophils
    c. Increased serum methylmalonic acid and homocysteine
    d. Decreased cobalamin on Schilling test
    e. Increased serum anti-Intrinsic factor levels

Preferred Response: (c) Increased serum methylmalonic acid and homocysteine. This patient is presenting with symptoms of subacute combined degeneration, a demyelinating disorder as a result of low levels of cobalamin (vitamin B12). High serum concentrations of methylmalonic acid and homocysteine (metabolites of cobalamin) are the most sensitive indicators of intracellular cobalamin deficiency. Their levels are high in more than 90% of patients with cobalamin deficiency and are elevated before serum levels of cobalamin fall below normal limits [7].

11. A 63-year-old woman is diagnosed with herpes zoster virus infection after presenting to the office with painful rash in a T6 distribution on the left side. In which of the following structures did the virus proliferate to cause the patient's symptoms?
    a. Lateral horn of the T6 spinal cord segment
    b. Posterior cutaneous branch of the dorsal ramus of T6
    c. Ventral horn of the T6 spinal cord segment
    d. Dorsal root ganglion of the T6 spinal nerve
    e. Greater chain ganglion of the sympathetic plexus

Preferred Response: (d) Dorsal root ganglion of the T6 spinal nerve. Herpes zoster virus infection ("shingles") remains latent in the dorsal root ganglia of sensory nerves. Upon reactivation, symptoms include painful skin rash in a dermatomal distribution of the affected nerve. Affected patients may develop postherpetic neuralgia (PHN), a condition characterized by residual pain following the disappearance of the primary rash. PHN refractory to medical management may be the target of neurosurgical intervention with procedures such as spinal cord stimulation, dorsal root ganglion stimulation, dorsal root entry zone lesioning, subcutaneous peripheral nerve stimulation, among others [8].

12. Which of the following ligaments provides the majority of the strength to the atlantoaxial joint, considered the strongest ligament of the craniocervical junction?
    a. Alar ligament
    b. Transverse atlantal ligament

c. Cruciate ligament, descending band
d. Apical odontoid ligament

Preferred Response: (b) Transverse atlantal ligament (TAL). The TAL attaches at the medial tubercles of the atlas and secures the dens against the anterior arch of the atlas. Several cadaveric studies have demonstrated that the TAL can sustain the most force of any ligament prior to rupture. The atlanto-alar portion of the alar ligament and the cruciate ligament also secure the axis to the atlas, but do not contribute as much strength as the TAL. The apical odontoid ligament is a weak structure that originates at the tip of the dens and attaches to the foramen magnum [9].

13. Which of the following combinations of ligaments are considered most crucial for maintaining atlantooccipital stability?
    a. Tectorial membrane and alar ligament
    b. Tectorial membrane and cruciate ligament
    c. Cruciate ligament and alar ligament
    d. Apical dentate ligament and tectorial membrane
    e. Cruciate ligament and apical dentate ligament

Preferred Response: (a) Tectorial membrane and alar ligament. The tectorial membrane, alar ligament, cruciate ligament, and apical dentate ligament all secure the atlantoaxial region to the occiput. However, violation of the tectorial membrane and alar ligament are more likely to cause atlantooccipital instability than the cruciate ligament and apical dentate ligament [10].

14. A 32-year-old female athlete presents to the office with a 1-month history of pain, weakness, and numbness in her right arm. She undergoes MRI which demonstrates posterolateral herniation of a cervical vertebral disc. She undergoes anterior cervical discectomy and fusion with intraoperative findings of severely damaged nucleus pulposus and annulus fibrosus. What are the embryologic origins of the nucleus pulposus and annulus fibrosus, respectively?
    a. Neural crest cells and endoderm
    b. Notochord and ectoderm
    c. Mesenchymal cells from sclerotome and notochord
    d. Notochord and neural crest cells
    e. Notochord and mesenchymal cells from sclerotome

Preferred Response: (e) Notochord and sclerotome. The nucleus pulposus is formed by the remnant of the notochord and the annulus fibrosus is derived from surrounding sclerotome mesenchyme. The ectoderm and endoderm are not involved in the formation of the intervertebral disc structures. The neural crest cells give rise to several diverse lineages of cells including smooth muscle, peripheral enteric neurons, glial cells and melanocytes, but not the nucleus pulposus or annulus fibrosus [11].

15. A 6-month-old male is brought to the office for a routine well-child visit. The child appears and feels normal except for an isolated tuft of hair growing over the midline of the lumbar region with a shallow dimple. There is no evidence of skin thinning or open defects. This finding is most likely attributable to which of the following embryological phenomena?
    a. Normal neurological development
    b. Failure of the caudal neuropore to close without herniation
    c. Failure of the caudal neuropore to close with meningeal herniation
    d. Herniation of cauda equina through a bony defect
    e. Failure of the rostral neuropore to close without herniation
    f. Failure of the rostral neuropore to close with meningeal herniation

Preferred Response: (b) Failure of the caudal neuropore to close without herniation. The condition described is most likely spina bifida occulta, which typically manifests as a dimple with a tuft of hair over the bony defect. Failure of the caudal neuropore to close with meningeal herniation describes a meningocele. Herniation of the cauda equina would be seen in a myelomeningocele (both neural tissue and meninges). Failure of the rostral neuropore to close results in anencephaly.

16. A newborn is diagnosed with myelomeningocele. Which of the following weeks of gestational development did this occur?
    a. Week 2
    b. Week 3
    c. Week 4
    d. Week 6
    e. Week 8

Preferred Response: (c) Week 4. Neural tube defects such as myelomeningocele are the result of failure of the caudal neuropore to close in week 4 during the process of neurulation.

17. What carotid-vertebrobasilar anastomoses may be present at the craniovertebral junction?
    a. Proatlanto intersegmental artery and transverse cervical artery
    b. Sternocleidomastoid branch of occipital artery and persistent hypoglossal artery

c. Transverse cervical artery and persistent hypoglossal artery
d. Proatlanto intersegmental artery and persistent hypoglossal artery

Preferred Response: (d) Proatlanto intersegmental artery and persistent hypoglossal artery. These anastomoses may be encountered at the approach to the craniovertebral junction. Thin-cut CT angiography may be useful preoperatively to evaluate the patency of the vertebral arteries and to localize any aberrant vascular anatomy. The sternocleidomastoid branch of the occipital artery is located anterior to the spine and is not in the craniovertebral junction area. The transverse cervical artery is the middle branch of the thyrocervical trunk, from the subclavian artery [12].

18. A 41-year-old male is evaluated in the emergency department following a motor vehicle collision in which he was an unrestrained driver. Among other injuries, non-contrast CT scan of the cervical spine reveals a fracture of the transverse process of the C4 vertebrae on the left with surrounding hyperdensity. Given this finding, which artery is most likely to be damaged?
    a. Inferior thyroid artery
    b. Anterior spinal artery
    c. Posterior spinal arteries
    d. Vertebral artery

Preferred Response (d) Vertebral artery. An injury to the transverse process is most likely to damage the vertebral artery, which courses through the transverse foramina of C6 to C1. The inferior thyroid artery and anterior spinal artery are located anteriorly and are not likely to be damaged in direct association with a transverse process fracture. The posterior spinal arteries are adherent to the posterior aspect of the spinal cord and are not directly associated with the transverse processes.

19. Which of the following is not an element of the National Emergency X-Radiography Utilization Study (NEXUS) criteria that must be present to determine that a trauma patient does not require cervical spine imaging?
    a. Alert and stable
    b. Absence of focal neurological deficit
    c. Presence of witness at time of injury
    d. Lack of intoxication
    e. Lack of midline spinal tenderness

Preferred Response: (c) Presence of witness at time of injury. The NEXUS criteria have a sensitivity of 99.6% for ruling out cervical spine injury when all elements are present. These include alert and stable, lack of the following: focal neurological deficit, altered consciousness, neurological deficit, midline spinal tenderness, and distracting injury [13].

20. A patient is being evaluated in the emergency department following a motor vehicle collision. Past medical history significant for atrial fibrillation for which the patient takes Warfarin. Imaging reveals bleeding from Batson's venous plexus, with adjacent hematoma. In which space has the blood most likely accumulated to produce this finding?
    a. Superficial subcutaneous tissue
    b. Epidural space
    c. Subdural space
    d. Subarachnoid space
    e. Central canal
    f. Lumbar cistern

Preferred Response: (b) Epidural space. The internal vertebral plexus (Batson's venous plexus) is located within the epidural space and surrounds the dura mater. Bleeding from the plexus would therefore cause accumulation of blood in the epidural space. Spinal epidural hematomas are rare, but the primary risk factor is anticoagulation. The most common cause of subarachnoid blood accumulation are subarachnoid hemorrhages. Subdural hematoma is more commonly encountered as an intracranial venous bleed as a result of injury to the cerebral veins. The lumbar cistern is a continuation of the subarachnoid space between the caudal conus medullaris and caudal end of the subarachnoid space. The central canal is located within the spinal cord and does not contain the Batson's venous plexus.

21. Which of the following structures is primarily responsible for maintaining the midline position of the spinal cord?
    a. Denticulate ligaments
    b. Posterior longitudinal ligament
    c. Ligamentum flavum
    d. Nuchal ligament
    e. Transverse ligament of the atlas

Preferred Response: (a) Denticulate ligaments. The denticulate ligaments are extensions of the pia mater that attach to the dura between the dorsal and ventral roots of the spinal nerves. The function of these ligaments is to maintain the midline position of the spinal cord within the canal. The posterior longitudinal ligament courses along the posterior aspect of the vertebral bodies within the canal and functions to limit spinal flexion. The ligamentum flavum is the connecting ligament between the laminae of vertebrae. The nuchal ligament is an extension of the supraspinous ligaments from the cervical vertebrae to the occiput. The transverse ligament of the atlas functions to limit posterior translation of the odontoid process.

22. In the thoracolumbar spine, the posterior radicular arteries branch directly off of which vessels?
    a. Posterior spinal arteries
    b. Anterior spinal artery
    c. Segmental spinal arteries
    d. Posterior intercostal arteries
    e. Aorta

Preferred Response: (c) Segmental spinal arteries. The spinal cord is supplied by both longitudinal and segmental vessels. The anterior and posterior spinal arteries are longitudinal vessels that originate within the cranial cavity. Feeder arteries, or segmental spinal arteries, enter the intervertebral foramina at each level. After entering the intervertebral foramina, the segmental spinal arteries branch into anterior and posterior radicular arteries. At various vertebral levels, these segmental spinal arteries also branch into segmental medullary arteries that course longitudinally.

23. Which of the following statements regarding the artery of Adamkiewicz is false?
    a. It joins the anterior spinal artery
    b. It is the largest anterior segmental artery
    c. It arises from the right side of the aorta in most individuals
    d. It arises between T8 and L2 in most individuals
    e. It shares collateral circulation with the lumbar arteries

Preferred Response: (c) It arises from the right side of the aorta in most individuals. The artery of Adamkiewicz arises from the left side in 75% of individuals. It is known as the largest anterior segmental artery and joins the anterior spinal artery. This vessel supplies the "watershed" zone between T8 and L2 in most individuals, but in up to 25% of individuals it can arise above T8. Caudal collateral circulation with the lumbar arteries are common.

24. At how many years of age does the secondary ossification center of the odontoid process (ossiculum terminale) normally fuse?
    a. 1 year
    b. 3 years
    c. 6 years
    d. 12 years
    e. 18 years

Preferred Response: (d) 12 years. The axis has several secondary ossification centers, the latest of which to mature in normal humans being that of the odontoid process. In some patients, the ossiculum terminale fails to fuse by 12 years—this is known as "ossiculum terminale persistens" or "Bergman's ossicle." This is typically a benign condition that is incidentally noted on imaging; rarely, it may present with symptoms such as neck pain and neurological signs [14].

25. How many primary ossification centers are typically present in the subaxial spine in a developing human?
    a. One
    b. Two
    c. Three
    d. Four
    e. Five

Preferred Response: (c) Three. The C3-L5 vertebrae have three primary ossification centers that appear in the 9th or 10th week in utero and finish primary ossification by one year. One of these ossification centers is in the center of the vertebral body; the other two are located on either half of the neural arch. These ossification centers hold clinical relevance in that they may be mistaken for fractures on radiologic studies in young individuals.

26. In the evaluation of a patient with spinal trauma, what is the imaging modality of choice to evaluate the integrity of the ligamentous complex?
    a. Plain radiographs
    b. Flexion–extension radiographs
    c. CT
    d. MRI

Preferred Response: (d) MRI. In a patient with questioned or suspected soft tissue damage or ligamentous injury, MRI is the imaging study of choice. Radiographs and CT scans are useful in the evaluation of bony injury and are relatively quick imaging methods that can rule out various acute neurosurgical indications. Flexion–extension radiographs may provide evidence of spinal instability, but direct evaluation of the ligaments is best achieved with MRI.

27. What is the MRI imaging sequence of choice in evaluating a patient with suspected spinal cord hemorrhage?
    a. T1 weighted
    b. T2 weighted
    c. Short tau inversion recovery (STIR)
    d. Gradient recalled echo (GRE)

Preferred Response: (d) Gradient recalled echo (GRE). GRE sequences carry the most specificity in identifying blood products as a result of spinal cord hemorrhage, compared to the T1, T2, and STIR sequences [15].

28. What is the MRI sequence of choice in evaluating a patient with suspected spinal cord ligamentous injury?
    a. T1 weighted
    b. T2 weighted
    c. Short tau inversion recovery (STIR)
    d. Gradient recalled echo (GRE)

Preferred Response: (c) Short tau inversion recovery. Presence of significant edema or obvious disruption of the ligamentous complex on STIR is sensitive for injury to the ligaments. In patients with suspected injury to the odontoid process, STIR sequence is commonly used to evaluate the integrity of the transverse atlantal ligament [15].

29. The presence of which of the following on imaging of the spine is most indicative of poor prognosis in a patient with spinal cord trauma?
    a. Presence of cord hemorrhage on MRI
    b. Acute fracture of the lumbar transverse process
    c. Disruption of the anterior longitudinal ligament
    d. Paraspinal muscle hyperintensity on MRI STIR sequence

Preferred Response: (a) Presence of cord hemorrhage. Presence of cord hemorrhage is the most important prognostic indicator in a patient with spinal cord injury18.

30. What is the diagnostic study of choice to distinguish an acute from chronic fracture of the vertebrae?
    a. CT scan without contrast
    b. CT scan with contrast
    c. MRI
    d. Lumbar puncture
    e. Plain radiograph

Preferred Response: (c) MRI. Presence of marrow edema on MRI is associated with acute fracture and can be of particular use when CT or plain radiograph identifies an age-indeterminate fracture [15].

31. A 4-month-old boy is admitted to the hospital with E. Coli meningitis. During workup for underlying causes, the patient undergoes MRI of the lumbosacral spine which demonstrates a hypointense tract with communication between the spinal canal and the skin. This finding most likely attributable to which of the following?
    a. Incomplete separation of endoderm and ectoderm during gastrulation
    b. Incomplete closure of the caudal neuropore without herniation of neural tissue
    c. Incomplete closure of the caudal neuropore with herniation of neural tissue
    d. Premature separation of the neural tube prior to complete closure
    e. Failure of surface ectoderm to separate from neuroectoderm

Preferred Response: (e) Failure of surface ectoderm to separate from neuroectoderm. The patient in the vignette described has a dermal sinus tract, an abnormal epithelium-lined communication between the spinal canal and the skin, resulting from a primary defect in neurulation. This condition affects an estimated 1 in 2500 live births and clinical presentation can range from lack of symptoms to significant disease, including infectious complications. Incomplete separation of the endoderm and ectoderm during gastrulation results in diastematomyelia, a rare condition marked by sagittal splitting of the notochord. Incomplete closure of the caudal neuropore with/without herniation of neural tissue describes spina bifida occulta or myelomeningocele, in which tracts between the skin and spinal canal are not present. Premature separation of the neural tube prior to closure results in intradural lipoma, which appears on MRI as fat-appearing tissue [16].

32. A 6-year-old child exhibits progressive bladder incontinence, bilateral lower extremity weakness, and paresthesias. MRI of the lumbosacral spine reveals a thickened filum with low-lying conus medullaris. Which of the following are potential causes of tethered cord syndrome?
    a. Prior infection
    b. Impaired neural canalization
    c. Lipoma
    d. Meningocele
    e. All of the above
    f. (b) and (c)
    g. (b) and (d)
    h. (a), (c), and (d)

Preferred Response: (e) All of the above. Tethered cord syndrome most commonly presents in the first months of life up until the teenage years. Causes of tethered cord syndrome can be primary (resulting from defects in neurulation) or can be secondary (acquired). Impaired neural canalization and defects such as meningocele are developmental causes of tethered cord syndrome, whereas scarring from prior infection, or the presence of lipomatous masses can result in tethering [17].

33. Which of the following landmarks is commonly used for the administration of caudal epidural anesthesia?
    a. Intervertebral foramina
    b. Median sacral crest
    c. Superior iliac crest
    d. Cornua of the sacral hiatus
    e. Posterior sacral foramina

Preferred Response: (d) Cornua of the sacral hiatus. Caudal anesthesia is used to anesthetize the sensory nerves from the perineum. It is frequently used in surgical anesthesia for children as well as for chronic pain management in adults. The objective is to deliver local anesthetic to the epidural space via the sacral hiatus. The cornua of the sacral hiatus provides an opening through which a needle may be directed. The superior iliac crest and median sacral crest are both located cranial to the sacral hiatus. The intervertebral foramina and posterior sacral foramina are not palpable external landmarks [18].

34. At which of the following spinal levels does the spinal cord of a newborn end?
    a. L1
    b. L2
    c. L3
    d. L4
    e. L5
    f. S1

Preferred Response: (c) L3. In the newborn, the spinal cord ends at L3. During development, the spinal cord "ascends" to the lower border of L1 as an adult, as the vertebral column lengthens in relation to the neural elements. In some pathologic states, the cord may become "tethered," precluding normal ascent and resulting in a low-lying conus medullaris on subsequent imaging [19].

35. Manual stereognosis is dependent upon the integrity of which of the following pathways?
    a. Dorsal column medial lemniscus tract
    b. Lateral spinothalamic tract
    c. Ventral spinothalamic tract
    d. Vestibulospinal tract
    e. Rubrospinal tract

Preferred Response: (a) Dorsal column medial lemniscus tract. Manual stereognosis is the ability to distinguish the identity of an unseen object placed in one's hand based on 3-dimensional form and texture. This is a function of the dorsal column. The lateral spinothalamic tract mediates itch, pain, and temperature sensation. The ventral spinothalamic tract is concerned with light touch. The vestibulospinal tract is coordinates maintenance of extensor tone. The rubrospinal tract is important in the maintenance of flexor tone.

36. Which of the following changes does not occur at the spinomedullary junction?
    a. Decussation of the pyramids
    b. Synapse between hypothalamic radiations and sympathetic trunk
    c. Replacement of Lissauer's tract by spinal trigeminal tract
    d. Replacement of the spinal gray by the cranial nerve nuclei
    e. Termination of the fasciculi cuneatus and gracilis

Preferred Response: (b) Synapse between hypothalamic radiations and sympathetic trunk. The synapse between the hypothalamic radiations and the sympathetic trunk occurs at the level of C8-T1 at the ciliospinal center. This is the first synapse in the oculosympathetic chain, the second being the synapse at the superior cervical ganglion. The decussation of the pyramids, replacement of Lissauer's tract by spinal trigeminal tract, spinal gray by cranial nerve nuclei, and termination of the fasciculi cuneatus and gracilis all occur at the spinomedullary junction.

37. Which of the following tracts is responsible for conveying unconscious proprioceptive input from the upper extremity?
    a. Dorsal spinocerebellar tract
    b. Cuneocerebellar tract
    c. Vestibulospinal tract
    d. Ventral spinocerebellar tract
    e. Lateral corticospinal tract

Preferred Response: (b) Cuneocerebellar tract. The cuneocerebellar tract transmits proprioception, touch, and pressure from the upper extremity to the cerebellum. The dorsal spinocerebellar tract is analogous to the cuneocerebellar tract for the lower extremities. The vestibulospinal tract is involved in the maintenance of extensor tone. The ventral spinocerebellar tract conveys information regarding lower limb posture and coordination. The lateral corticospinal tract coordinates voluntary skilled movements.

38. An isolated lesion to the cell bodies of which of the following structures would be most likely to cause Horner's syndrome?
    a. Anterior gray horn of the spinal cord
    b. Spinal ganglia
    c. Lateral gray horn of the spinal cord
    d. Posterior gray horn of the spinal cord
    e. Anterior commissure of the spinal cord

Preferred Response: (c) Lateral gray horn of the spinal cord. Horner's syndrome is characterized by dysfunction of the sympathetic pathway. Symptoms include miosis, ptosis, and anhidrosis, among others. The cell bodies of the sympathetic nerves are found within the lateral gray horn of the spinal cord, therefore a lesion in this area would be most likely to generate Horner's syndrome. The anterior gray horn contains cell bodies for somatic efferent fibers, while the posterior gray horn contains sensory fibers from the spinal ganglia cell bodies. The anterior commissure is a white matter tract that does not contain neuronal cell bodies.

39. A 38-year-old male with a several month history of gradually progressive low back/buttock pain, worse on the right side, presents to the office for evaluation. As part of the examination, the patient lies supine, and the physician flexes the right hip and leg, abducts the leg, places the patient's right ankle on the left knee, and allows the patient's right knee to drop parallel to the floor. Which of the following findings would be most suggestive of a sacroiliac source of pain?
    a. Ipsilateral buttock pain
    b. Ipsilateral groin pain
    c. Restriction of movement
    d. Ipsilateral anterior hip pain
    e. Ipsilateral lateral hip tenderness

Preferred Response: (a) Ipsilateral buttock pain. The FABER (Flexion, ABduction, and External Rotation) test is a provocative test that can aid in identifying the hip as a pain generator in an individual with buttock pain. Pain in the groin or anterior/lateral hip is more suggestive of a primary hip disorder, while pain in the low back/buttock region is more suggestive of a sacroiliac source. This test has a sensitivity of 71% and specificity of 75% in the identification of sacroiliac joint inflammation [20].

40. In addition to the capsule of the zygapophyseal joint, which of the following structures forms the posterior border of the lumbar intervertebral foramen?
    a. Posterolateral vertebral body
    b. Intervertebral disc
    c. Ligamentum flavum
    d. Pedicle of the superior vertebrae
    e. Pedicle of the inferior vertebrae

Preferred Response (c) Ligamentum flavum. The ventral border of the intervertebral foramen is formed by the intervertebral disc and posterolateral aspect of the vertebral body, the superior and inferior borders formed by the pedicles, and the posterior border formed by the ventral aspect of the zygapophyseal joint capsule and the ligamentum flavum.

41. A patient with history of brachial plexus avulsion secondary to motor vehicle collision is being evaluated for persistent upper extremity pain. As one of his treatment options, his surgeon discusses spinal cord Dorsal Root Entry Zone (DREZ) lesioning. The spinal DREZ underlies which of the following structures?
    a. Posterolateral sulcus
    b. Posteromedian sulcus
    c. Posterior gray commissure
    d. Anterior median fissure
    e. Dorsal root ganglion

Preferred Response: (a) Posterolateral sulcus. The DREZ is the region of the spinal cord at which the dorsal roots (carrying nociceptive and somatosensory information) of the upper limb terminate. The DREZ is a surgical term thought to encompass both Lissauer's tract and superficial layers of the dorsal horn gray matter. The DREZ is located lateral to the posteromedian sulcus. The anterior median fissure, posterior gray commissure, and dorsal root ganglion are not on the surface of the spinal cord at which the fibers enter [21].

42. The corticospinal tract is responsible for the coordination of voluntary motor movements. The origin of the corticospinal tract originates from the primary motor cortex within the precentral gyrus. Through which of the following structures does the corticospinal tract pass prior to entering the spinal cord?
    a. Anterior limb of the internal capsule
    b. Retrolenticular part of the internal capsule
    c. Sublenticular part of the internal capsule
    d. Posterior limb of the internal capsule

Preferred Response: (d) Posterior part of the posterior limb of the internal capsule. The corticospinal tract occupies the posterior half of the posterior limb of the internal capsule. The anterior limb contains the anterior thalamic peduncle, the retrolenticular part contains the visual projects, and the sublenticular contains auditory projections. Lesions to this area (e.g. lacunar infarctions) can cause neurological deficits consistent with upper motor neuron dysfunction with an otherwise intact spinal cord.

43. A patient is undergoing elective repair of an abdominal aortic aneurysm. Intraoperatively, his aorta is temporarily clamped. Anastomoses from which of the following arteries will likely be responsible for preventing ischemia of the spinal cord in this patient?
    a. Anterior spinal artery
    b. Posterior spinal arteries
    c. Radicular branches of the intercostal arteries and artery of Adamkiewicz
    d. Segmental arteries from the vertebral, intercostal, superficial epigastric, lumbar, and medial sacral arteries
    e. Segmental arteries from the vertebral, intercostal, lumbar, spinal anterior, and posterior and lateral sacral arteries

Preferred Response: (e) Segmental arteries from the vertebral, intercostal, lumbar, spinal anterior, and posterior and lateral sacral arteries. In the presence of abdominal aortic clamping, the anterior and posterior spinal arteries will not provide adequate blood flow to maintain the demand of the spinal cord. At various vertebral levels, the segmental spinal arteries arise predominantly from the vertebral and deep cervical arteries, which will provide the additional supply along the course of the spinal cord. The radicular branches of the intercostal arteries branch from the aorta and will likely not have sufficient blood flow if the aorta is clamped.

44. Which of the following is true regarding first-order neurons of the ventral spinocerebellar tract?
    a. They are responsible for the afferent limb of muscle stretch reflexes
    b. These neurons are located within the dorsal root ganglia of the thoracic spine
    c. They project axons onto the medial root entry zone
    d. Their axons decussate in the anterior white commissure
    e. They enter the fasciculus gracilis

Preferred Response: (a) They are responsible for the afferent limb of muscle stretch reflexes. The first-order neurons of the ventral spinocerebellar tract receive input from muscle spindles, golgi tendon organs, and pressure receptors. They are located within the dorsal root ganglia from L1 to S2, not the thoracic spine. The ventral spinothalamic tract and dorsal spinocerebellar tracts project axons onto the medial root entry zone. The second-order neurons of the ventral spinocerebellar tract decussate within the anterior white commissure of the spinal cord. The fasciculus gracilis and cuneatus are associated with the dorsal column medial lemniscus tract, not the ventral spinocerebellar tract [22].

45. A pregnant woman in labor elects for epidural anesthesia prior to delivery. Which of the following structures is not perforated by the needle to access the epidural space?
    a. Subcutaneous tissue
    b. Ligamentum flavum
    c. Posterior longitudinal ligament
    d. Interspinous ligament
    e. Supraspinous ligament

Preferred Response: (c) Posterior longitudinal ligament. The order of structures pierced in epidural anesthesia administration is skin, subcutaneous tissue, muscle, supraspinous ligament, interspinous ligament, and ligamentum flavum. The posterior longitudinal ligament is located posterior to the vertebral body and anterior to the cord; it cannot be reached by epidural anesthesia [23].

46. A patient is being evaluated in the emergency department for severe low-back pain following a fall from a ladder. Initial radiographs of the lumbar spine reveal bilateral fractures of the pars interarticularis at L5. Which of the following radiographic views would provide the best visualization of these fractures?
    a. Anteroposterior
    b. Oblique
    c. Lateral
    d. Posteroanterior

Preferred Response: (b) Oblique. In the anteroposterior or posteroanterior views, the vertebral bodies obscure the view of the pars interarticularis. In the lateral view, the pedicles may be superimposed on the pars interarticularis and therefore preclude complete visualization. The oblique is the ideal radiographic view for suspected pars interarticularis fracture.

47. A 33-year-old female is being evaluated in the emergency department following a motor vehicle collision in which she was the restrained driver. MRI of the cervical spine revealed a unilateral tear of the alar ligament without injury to any other ligaments. Upon physical

exam, the range of motion of which of the following cervical spine movements is most likely present as a result of this tear?
a. Increased flexion
b. Decreased flexion
c. Increased extension
d. Decreased extension
e. Increased lateral flexion
f. Decreased lateral flexion
g. Increased rotation
h. Decreased rotation

Preferred Response: (g) Increased rotation. The alar ligament attaches the odontoid process to the medial surface of the occipital condyles and functions to limit excessive atlantoaxial rotation. Disruption of this ligament would therefore result in increased range of motion upon cervical spine rotation. Flexion and extension occur at the atlantooccipital joints and zygapophyseal joints. Lateral flexion occurs as a combination of movements at the uncovertebral joints. The alar ligament has no influence on these movements.

48. Which of the following reflexes is the fifth lumbar nerve associated with?
a. Patellar
b. Achilles
c. Cremasteric
d. Anal wink
e. All of the above
f. None of the above

Preferred Response: (e) None of the above. The L5 nerve root is not associated with a known reflex. Primary associations for the other named reflexes are as follows: patellar, L4; Achilles, S1, cremasteric, L1-L2; anal wink, S3-S4 [24].

49. Upon exiting its respective intervertebral foramen, which of the following nerve roots is oriented most obliquely?
a. T4
b. T8
c. T12
d. L3
e. L5
f. S1

Preferred Response: (f) S1. Because the vertebral column is longer than the spinal cord itself, spinal nerve roots become longer and increasingly more obliquely oriented from the cervical to coccygeal region.

50. In the operating room, a patient undergoing elective spinal fusion surgery is positioned prone. Prior to draping, the attending physician draws a horizontal line connecting the inferior aspects of the scapula. What vertebral level does this line traverse?
a. T5
b. T6
c. T7
d. T8
e. T9

Preferred Response: (c) T7. The T7 vertebrae can be readily identified by a line across the inferior tip of the scapula to the other. Because the presence of the scapula can render this level difficult to identify on a lateral radiograph, this tip is useful for identifying T7 in the operating room.

51. Which of the following external landmarks can be utilized to identify the level of C3?
a. Hyoid bone
b. Thyroid cartilage
c. Cricoid cartilage
d. Carotid bifurcation

Preferred Response: (a) Hyoid bone. In most humans, C3 can be identified by the presence of the hyoid bone anteriorly. The thyroid cartilage is typically located at the level of C4-C5. The cricoid is typically located opposite of C6. The carotid bifurcation typically occurs around the level of C4-C5 but is not a reliably identifiable external landmark.

52. On what imaging modality is acute transverse myelitis most readily identified?
a. X-ray
b. CT without contrast
c. CT with contrast
d. T1-weighted MRI
e. T2-weighted MRI

Preferred Response: (e) T2-weighted MRI. Although imaging is frequently normal, transverse myelitis can sometimes be identified on MRI as high T2 signal involving gray and adjacent white matter. Plain radiography and CT scan can be used to rule out several acute neurosurgical indications but are unrevealing in transverse myelitis specifically [25].

53. A patient with a history of progressive neck and left arm pain with numbness presents to the office for evaluation. As part of the physical exam, the physician places downward pressure on the vertex and tilts the patient's

head towards the left. The patient's left arm pain is reproduced. What is the name of this finding?
   a. Positive Lhermitte's sign
   b. Positive Hoffman's sign
   c. Positive Spurling's test
   d. Positive Adson's test
   e. Positive neck distraction test

Preferred Response: (c) Positive Spurling's test. Spurling's test is a provocative maneuver in which the patient's head is flexed laterally towards the symptomatic side, and downward axial force is applied. This narrows the intervertebral foramen and can provoke radicular symptoms, analogous to the straight leg raise for the lumbar spine [26].

54. A 65-year-old man presents to the office with progressive hand clumsiness, difficulty typing quickly, balance difficulties, and neck stiffness. As part of the physical exam, the physician provides passive snapping flexion to the distal phalanx of the patient's middle finger. The patient's ipsilateral thumb and index finger flex and adduct in response. What is the name of this finding?
   a. Positive Lhermitte's sign
   b. Positive Hoffman's sign
   c. Positive Spurling's test
   d. Positive Adson's test
   e. Positive neck distraction test

Preferred Response: (b) Positive Hoffman's sign. Hoffman's sign is a provocative maneuver first described in the early 1900s, in which flicking the middle finger of a patient with cervical myelopathy provokes a flexion/adduction response in the ipsilateral thumb/index finger [26].

55. Which of the following conditions is least likely to present with a positive Lhermitte's sign?
   a. Amyotrophic lateral sclerosis
   b. Multiple sclerosis
   c. Cervical myelopathy
   d. Subacute combined degeneration
   e. Transverse myelitis

Preferred Response: (a) Amyotrophic lateral sclerosis. Lhermitte's sign is most classically associated with multiple sclerosis but can also be seen in other conditions such as cervical myelopathy, subacute combined degeneration, transverse myelitis, and cervical disc herniation. Lhermitte's sign is not reported to occur in amyotrophic lateral sclerosis [27].

56. Autonomic hyperreflexia occurs with spinal cord lesions above which vertebral level?
   a. C3
   b. C7
   c. T1
   d. T6
   e. T10

Preferred Response: (d) T6. Symptoms of autonomic hyperreflexia include cutaneous vasodilation, hyperhidrosis, and headache, among others. Mechanistic understanding of autonomic hyperreflexia following spinal cord injury remains poor, although early recognition of these symptoms is paramount as appropriate management can minimize long-term sequelae 28.

57. Which of the following is not a common characteristic of conus medullaris syndrome?
   a. Preserved patellar reflex
   b. Flaccid bladder with overflow incontinence
   c. Asymmetric motor deficits
   d. Hyperreflexia
   e. Low back pain

Preferred Response: (c) Asymmetric motor deficits. Conus medullaris syndrome typically presents with symmetric neurological deficits, as opposed to cauda equina syndrome, which is typically asymmetric. Preserved patellar reflex, flaccid bladder, hyperreflexia, and low back pain are all common features of conus medullaris syndrome [29].

58. A patient comes to the office for evaluation of gait ataxia. During the physical examination, the patient is asked to place his feet together and stand up straight. He is able to do this with his eyes open, but with closed eyes, he falls over. Dysfunction of which pathway is most likely responsible for this finding?
   a. Dorsal spinocerebellar tract
   b. Dorsal column medial lemniscus
   c. Lateral spinothalamic tract
   d. Lateral corticospinal tract

Preferred Response: (b) Dorsal column medial lemniscus. This patient is able to stand up without falling when their eyes are open, but not with their eyes closed, indicating sensory dystaxia, or Romberg sign. This is a manifestation of dorsal column dysfunction. The dorsal spinocerebellar tract is analogous to the cuneocerebellar tract for the lower extremities in transmitting proprioceptive input. The lateral spinothalamic tract mediates itch, pain, and temperature sensation. The lateral corticospinal tract coordinates voluntary skilled movements.

59. An adolescent male with mid-back pain is evaluated in the office for abnormal findings on recent radiographs.

The radiologist reports a hemivertebra of the thoracic spine. Which of the following findings is also most likely present on imaging?
a. Scoliosis
b. Osteoporosis
c. Thoracolumbar spondylolisthesis
d. Sacralization of L5
e. Hyperlordosis of the lumbar spine

Preferred Response: (a) Scoliosis. A hemivertebra is a condition in which part of one or more vertebrae does not develop. This generates an abnormal lateral bend towards the side of the developmental deficit and is thus a nidus for scoliotic deformity. Rotational deformity may also be present. Osteoporosis is a condition in which the cortical bone loses its normal density and may predispose to fracture. Spondylolisthesis is anterior displacement of a portion of the vertebra upon another, usually secondary to a fracture of the pars interarticularis. Lumbar hyperlordosis is characterized by increased anterior curvature of the lumbar spine. Sacralization of the L5 vertebrae is a congenital fusion of the L5 vertebra to the sacrum.

60. A patient is being evaluated in the emergency department for acute onset of severe back pain. CT of the thoracolumbar spine reveals a fracture of the pars interarticularis of L5 with normal alignment of the vertebral body over the sacrum. Based on this information, which of the following is the most likely diagnosis?
a. Spondylosis
b. Spondylolysis
c. Spondylolisthesis
d. Spondylitis

Preferred Response: (b) Spondylolysis. Spondylolysis is a fracture of the pars interarticularis. Spondylosis is a nonspecific term used to describe degenerative conditions of the spine. Spondylolisthesis is anterior displacement of the vertebral body after fracture of the pars interarticularis. Spondylitis is a nonspecific term used to describe inflammatory conditions of the spine.

61. Which of the following statements is not true regarding the vestibulospinal tract?
a. It arises from the giant cells of Deiters in the ipsilateral vestibular nucleus
b. Plays a role in maintenance of extensor tone
c. It is located ventral to the rubrospinal tract
d. It is located medial to the ventral corticospinal tract

Preferred Response: (d) It is located medial to the ventral corticospinal tract. The vestibulospinal tract arises from the giant cells of Deiters in the ipsilateral vestibular nucleus and is an important tract in the maintenance of extensor tone. It is located in the ventral funiculus, lateral to the ventral corticospinal tract, and ventral to the ventral horn of the spinal gray matter. Decerebrate posturing is a tonic, static reflex that is maintained by the reticular formation and vestibulospinal system.

62. Which of the following spinal tracts is concerned with the control of trunk muscles?
a. Dorsal spinocerebellar
b. Vestibulospinal
c. Ventral corticospinal
d. Lateral corticospinal
e. Lateral spinothalamic

Preferred Response: (c) Ventral corticospinal. The ventral corticospinal tract is involved in the control of the axial muscles, including those of the trunk and head. The dorsal spinocerebellar tract is analogous to the cuneocerebellar tract for the lower extremities in transmitting proprioceptive input. The lateral spinothalamic tract mediates itch, pain, and temperature sensation. The lateral corticospinal tract coordinates voluntary skilled movements.

63. A 44-year-old male presents to the emergency department after the sudden onset of pain while lifting a heavy box. He states that the pain originates in the right buttock, travels down the lateral aspect of the thigh to the front of the leg, and through the dorsum of the foot. His anterior thigh is unaffected. Which of the following nerve roots is most likely affected?
a. L3
b. L4
c. L5
d. S1

Preferred Response: (c) L5. The pain described in the vignette follows an L5 dermatomal distribution. The L3 and L4 distributions involve the anterior thigh. The S1 dermatome involves posterior thigh pain that radiates to the lateral aspect of the leg.

64. An epidural abscess is most commonly encountered in which segment of the spine?
a. Cervical
b. Thoracic
c. Lumbar

Preferred Response (b) Thoracic. Spinal epidural abscesses are infectious processes that most commonly occur in individuals with history of intravenous drug abuse. These should be suspected in patients presenting with focal pain, signs of infection, and elevated inflammatory markers. These infections are distinct from vertebral osteomyelitis, which most commonly occurs in the lumbar spine.

65. In the normal anatomical state, what percentage of the total area of the lumbar intervertebral foramen is occupied by the neurovascular bundle?
    a. 10–20%
    b. 20–50%
    c. 40–70%
    d. 60–90%

Preferred Response: (b) 20–50%. In the lumbar spine, in the absence of significant degenerative processes and/or foraminal stenosis, the neurovascular bundle (nerve root, paired arteries/veins, fat) occupies approximately 20–50% of the total cross sectional foraminal area. Significant narrowing of foraminal area can cause radicular symptoms [30].

66. On which of the following days of development do the anterior and posterior neuropore close, respectively?
    a. 21 and 23
    b. 23 and 25
    c. 25 and 27
    d. 27 and 25
    e. 25 and 23

Preferred Response: (c) 25 and 27. A key concept of spinal development is the closure of the neuropores during week 4. The anterior neuropore closes prior to the posterior neuropore. Disruption or failure of either of these processes can lead to pathologies such as myelomeningocele, meningocele and anencephaly [31].

67. Normal lordotic curvature of the cervical spine is within which of the following ranges?
    a. 10–15°
    b. 15–20°
    c. 20–25°
    d. 25–30°

Preferred Response: (b) 15–20°. Under normal conditions, the cervical and lumbar spine are lordotic, and the thoracic spine is kyphotic. In some pathological states, the cervical spine may develop a kyphotic deformity. Recognition of normal cervical lordosis on lateral spine radiographs is essential in the management of cervical spine disorders.

68. Which of the following is not true regarding the uncovertebral joints of the cervical spine?
    a. They are formed by the articulation between the uncinate process and vertebral body
    b. They define the lateral borders for discectomy
    c. They define the midline for cervical plate placement
    d. They have a distinct synovial membrane with synovial fluid
    e. They have a distinct joint capsule

Preferred Response (e) They have a distinct joint capsule. The uncovertebral joints of the cervical spine are an important intraoperative landmark at the lateral aspects of the upper surfaces of typical vertebrae. They define the lateral borders for corpectomy and discectomy, as well as the midline for implant placement. Although the uncovertebral joints have a synovial membrane with fluid, they do not have their own joint capsule.

69. At which vertebral level is the apex of thoracic kyphosis typically located?
    a. T4
    b. T5
    c. T6
    d. T7
    e. T8
    f. T9

Preferred Response: (d) T7. The normal kyphosis of the thoracic spine ranges from 10 to 40°. The apex of kyphosis occurs at T7 in most individuals. Some surgeons choose to avoid ending spinal constructs at the thoracic kyphotic apex and the thoracolumbar junction in order to prevent instrumentation failures and progressive deformity.

70. A patient with suspected L5 radiculopathy undergoes an electromyography (EMG) approximately 4 weeks after onset of symptoms. What are the most likely findings?
    a. Normal insertion but very long-duration, rapid-firing motor units
    b. Prolonged latencies on both motor and sensory nerve conduction studies
    c. Abnormal insertion with fibrillations and positive waves

   d. Normal insertion, but poor activation of muscles in the L5 myotome

Preferred Response: (c) Abnormal insertion with fibrillations and positive waves. These reflect denervation changes (axonal injury). These changes are evident 3 to 4 weeks following initial insult; until then, it is more common to see normal insertion with poor muscle activation (d).

71. Which of the following ligaments is not responsible for suspending the sacrum between the ilia?
   a. Anterior sacroiliac
   b. Posterior sacroiliac
   c. Sacrotuberous
   d. Interosseous

Preferred Response: (c) Sacrotuberous. The anterior and posterior sacroiliac together with the interosseous ligaments limit motion at the sacroiliac joint. The most important ligaments in this function are the posterior sacroiliac and the interosseous. The sacrotuberous ligament attaches the sacrum to the ischial tuberosity but does not function to suspend the sacrum within the ilia.

72. Which of the following nerves is at greatest risk during dissection of the anterior surface of the psoas major muscle?
   a. Genitofemoral nerve
   b. Ilioinguinal nerve
   c. L5 nerve root
   d. S1 nerve root

Preferred Response (a) Genitofemoral nerve. The genitofemoral nerve is formed within the belly of the psoas muscle by union of the anterior rami of L1 and L2. The nerve courses within the muscle and then emerges on its anterior surface distally. This is of significance in anterior/lateral approaches to the thoracolumbar spine.

73. Which of the following is true regarding the denticulate ligament?
   a. It is a type of pia mater
   b. Is present between all dorsal and ventral roots
   c. Is continuous with the dural sac
   d. Tethers the radicular arteries in place

Preferred Response: (a) It is a type of pia mater. The denticulate ligaments are specialized portions of pia mater extending from the lateral surface of the pia, which aids in suspending the spinal cord within the subarachnoid space. These ligaments are not present between all of the dorsal and ventral rootlets of the spine, are not continuous with the dural sac, and are not related to the radicular arteries.

74. Which of the following veins/venous systems are anatomically predisposed to permit the spread of metastases throughout the vertebral column?
   a. Basilic veins
   b. Cephalic veins
   c. Dorsal scapular veins
   d. Batson's venous plexus
   e. Transverse cervical

Preferred Response: (d) Batson's venous plexus. Batson's venous plexus is valveless and thus is clinically important in the spread of metastatic disease. All other veins listed above have valves.

75. The dural sac and subarachnoid space end at which vertebral level?
   a. L4
   b. L5
   c. S1
   d. S2
   e. S4

Preferred Response: (d) S2. The dural sac and subarachnoid space end at S2. The filum terminale extends from the caudal end of the dural sac to attach to the coccyx inferiorly.

76. At which of the following levels is a patient most likely to develop a cervical disc herniation?
   a. C4-C5
   b. C5-C6
   c. C6-C7
   d. C7-T1

Preferred Response: (c) C6-C7. A cervical disc herniation at C6-C7, which results in compression of the C7 nerve root, accounts for approximately 69% of all cervical disc syndromes. The next most commonly affected level is C5-C6, accounting for approximately 19% of all cervical disc herniations. Of the above options, C4-C5 is the least common.

77. In early development, which of the following structures forms the boundary between the ventral mantle layer and the dorsal mantle layer?

a. Sulcus limitans
b. Basal plate
c. Ventral plate
d. Floor plate

Preferred Response: (a) Sulcus limitans. During the process of neural development, neuroblasts form a mantle layer around the neuroepithelial layer that forms the gray matter of the spinal cord. The ventrally located motor horn, or basal plates, are separated from the dorsally located sensory horn, or alar plates, by the sulcus limitans.

78. In the process of informed consent for patients undergoing lumbar decompression for degenerative disc disease, which of the following factors is expected to improve patient recall of potential surgical risks/complications?
    a. Attainment of informed consent by attending surgeon rather than surgical trainee
    b. Shorter consent-to-surgery time
    c. Longer consent-to-surgery time
    d. Older patient age

Preferred Response: (c) Longer consent-to-surgery time. In a study of 108 patients undergoing elective lumbar decompression, investigators found that younger patient age, as well as a consent-to-surgery time of > 14 days were associated with greater recall of perioperative adverse events compared to those with a consent-to-surgery time of < 2 days. Seniority of the consenting surgeon is not associated with patient recall of the informed consent process.

79. Isolated loss of cutaneous sensation in the webbed space of skin between the hallux and second toe is typically associated with injury to which of the following structures?
    a. L4 nerve root
    b. L5 nerve root
    c. Superficial peroneal nerve
    d. Deep peroneal nerve
    e. Medial calcaneal nerve

Preferred Response: (d) Deep fibular nerve. The medial branch of the deep fibular nerve innervates the skin of the space in question. Although the L4 and L5 nerve roots may contribute to the deep fibular nerve, injury to these structures would be most likely to cause sensory deficit in a dermatomal pattern. The superficial fibular nerve innervates the anterior leg and dorsum of the foot. The medial calcaneal nerve (from the tibial nerve) innervates the region of the heel.

80. In individuals without history of prior spinal surgery, which of the following lumbar discs are most likely to herniate?
    a. L3-L4 and L4-L5
    b. L4-L5 and L5-S1
    c. L3-L4 and L5-S1

Preferred Response: (b) L4-L5 and L5-S1. These two levels account for 95% of all cases of lumbar disc herniation. Disc herniation above this level is more common in people aged over 55 years [32].

81. A 44-year-old female presents to your office with severe axillary hyperhidrosis that has persisted despite conservative measures. Surgical dissection and splitting of which of the following structures is most appropriate to provide relief of these symptoms?
    a. T2 nerve root
    b. Thoracic sympathetic chain
    c. Ventral ramus at T3
    d. Dorsal root ganglion

Preferred Response: (b) Thoracic sympathetic chain. The candidate procedure described is known as a sympathectomy, which is ablation of the postganglionic sympathetic fibers of the sympathetic chain at a given level. This procedure can be considered in patients with severe axillary hyperhidrosis that has not responded to medications. Destruction of the dorsal root ganglion, ventral rami, and nerve roots would not specifically provide relief of the patient's bothersome symptoms.

Reference: Cheng AV, Tadi P. Neuroanatomy, White Rami Communicans. 2021 Jul 31. In: StatPearls [Internet]. Treasure Island (FL): StatPearls Publishing; 2022 Jan–. PMID: 31,751,100.

82. Prolonged maintenance of which of the following biomechanical positions results in the greatest amount of intradiscal pressure in the normal human lumbar discs?
    a. Sitting upright
    b. Sitting upright with a forward bend (flexion)
    c. Standing upright
    d. Standing upright with a forward bend (flexion)
    e. Supine recumbent position
    f. Left/Right lateral decubitus position

Preferred Response: (b) Sitting upright with a forward bend (flexion). This position, commonly referred to as "slouching" in a chair, results in the highest intradiscal pressure of any of the noted positions. Conversely, the supine recumbent position results in the lowest amount of intradiscal pressure. This may in part explain the subjective worsening of herniated disc symptoms in patients based on posture [33].

83. A 60-year-old male with symptomatic degenerative spondylolisthesis at L4-L5 without response to conservative management undergoes L4-L5 posterior interbody fusion with posterolateral pedicular screw fixation. At which of the following levels is the patient most likely to develop adjacent segment degeneration?
    a. L3-L4
    b. L5-S1
    c. Both L3-L4 and L5-S1 simultaneously

Preferred Response: (a) L3-L4. Adjacent segment disease, as defined by clinical and radiographic evidence of degenerative spinal disease (disc degeneration, stenosis, or spondylolisthesis) requiring reoperation at a level adjacent to a prior intervention, is a known cause of reoperation following lumbar fusion procedures. Retrospective cohort studies have demonstrated that rostral adjacent segment disease is more common than caudal adjacent segment disease (in one series, an incidence of 18% versus 2%, respectively). Clinically insignificant rates of adjacent segment disease at the L5-S1 segment following L4-L5 fusion suggest that preemptive extension of fusion to the sacrum to avoid reoperation for this complication is perhaps not necessary [34].

84. Via which of the following structures do the sympathetic fibers exit the spinal cord to travel to the sympathetic trunk?
    a. White rami communicantes
    b. Gray rami communicantes
    c. Dorsal root
    d. Spinal ganglion

Preferred Response: (a) White rami communicantes. The white ramus communicans is a structure that lies anterior to the spinal cord and connects the spinal nerve to the sympathetic trunk. Sympathetic neurons pass through the white ramus as preganglionic neurons, synapse onto a ganglion, and then innervate their respective organs as postganglionic neurons.

85. Upon evaluation, a 34-year-old man is found to have an isolated injury of the rami communicans at the level of T3-T4. Which of the following physiologic consequences is most likely to result from this injury?
    a. Elimination of tremor due to lower motoneuron destruction
    b. Relief of upper trunk spasticity
    c. Atrophy of the thenar eminence
    d. Palmar anhidrosis

Preferred Response: (d) Palmar anhidrosis. The rami communicans provides an interface between the sympathetic chain and the spinal cord. Ramicotomy is a procedure that is sometimes performed for the treatment of refractory palmar and axillary hyperhidrosis; other surgical options may include sympathycotomy. The other options would not be expected findings following an isolated lesion to the rami communicans [35].

86. A 72-year-old man is being evaluated in the surgical intensive care unit following thoracic aortic aneurysm repair. Since the procedure, the patient states that he has lost sensation in the bilateral upper extremities and has difficulty using his hands to grab objects. Intraoperative embolization resulting in spinal cord ischemia is suspected. Occlusion of which of the following would most likely explain this patient's symptoms?
    a. Anterior spinal artery
    b. Posterior spinal artery
    c. Segmental artery
    d. Intercostal artery

Preferred response: (c) Segmental artery. Arterial blood supply to the thoracic spinal cord via the anterior spinal artery is substantially less prominent than its role in the cervical and lumbar regions of the spine. In much of the thoracic spine, especially in the mid thoracic region, blood flow to the spinal cord is provided by the segmental arteries branching from the aorta at these levels.

87. Which of the following is the major finding on plain radiographs of patients with a lumbar disc herniation?
    a. Disc space narrowing
    b. Loss of segmental lordosis
    c. Lumbar hyperlordosis
    d. Anterior displacement of the vertebral body compared to the caudal level
    e. Ventral vertebral body osteophytosis

Preferred Response: (a) Disc space narrowing. Although the x-ray examination is one of the fundamental diagnostic tools for patients with low back pain, its utility in suspected lumbar disc herniation is low. While data support the use of magnetic resonance imaging for the establishment of a diagnosis of disc herniation, plain radiographs represent an inexpensive, less time-consuming diagnostic aid to exclude other potential pathologies, such as spondylolisthesis [36].

88. An 18-year-old man presents to his primary care provider for a clinical examination. At the visit, the examiner taps the brachioradialis tendon with a reflex hammer to elicit a reflex arc. Which of the following options most accurately describes the afferent and efferent nerve/nerve roots involved in eliciting this finding?
    a. Musculocutaneous nerve; C5-C6
    b. Radial nerve; C5-C6
    c. Musculocutaneous nerve; C6-C8
    d. Posterior interosseous nerves; C6-C7
    e. Radial nerve; C6-C7

Preferred Response (b) Radial nerve; C5-C6. The above vignette describes the brachioradialis reflex, which is elicited by induction of a rapid stretch in the brachioradialis tendon, which sends an afferent action potential to the spinal cord via the radial nerve. A post-synaptic potential returns to the same muscle group via nerve roots C5-C6, provoking reflexive contraction of the brachioradialis muscle. This is an example of a myotatic spinal reflex.

89. An 18-year-old man presents to his primary care provider for a clinical examination. At the visit, the examiner taps the brachioradialis tendon with a reflex hammer to elicit a reflex arc. In this example, which of the following ventral nerve roots is inhibited to permit relaxation of the antagonist muscle group?
    a. C5-C6
    b. C6-C7
    c. C7-C8
    d. C8-T1
    e. C6-C8

Preferred Response: (e) C6-C8. An aspect of the myotatic spinal reflex is simultaneous relaxation of the antagonist muscle group. In the brachioradialis reflex, the antagonist muscle group is the triceps muscle, which is primarily innervated by nerve roots C6-C8. Therefore, inhibition of the C6-C8 nerve roots permits reflexive contraction of the brachioradialis muscle. Inhibition of C5-C6 would result in relaxation of the biceps. Inhibition of C8-T1 would result in relaxation of the flexor digitorum profundus.

90. Approximately what percentage of patients without back pain will demonstrate a disc herniation on magnetic resonance imaging?
    a. 5%
    b. 10%
    c. 15%
    d. 25%
    e. 40%

Preferred Response: (d) 25%. Some studies have demonstrated that approximately 27% of patients without back pain have been found to have a disc herniation on imaging, which highlights the importance of clinical correlation in establishing the diagnosis of one's primary complaint. Additionally, identification of incidental disc herniation on imaging does not predict future development of back pain/radiculopathy.

91. A clinical researcher uses a reflex hammer to briskly tap on the Achilles tendon of a healthy volunteer. Which of the following is the correct pair of stimulated and inhibited nerve roots in this maneuver?
    a. S1-S2 stimulated; L2-L4 inhibited
    b. S1-S2 stimulated; L5-S1 inhibited
    c. L5-S1 stimulated; L3-L4 inhibited
    d. S1-S2 stimulated; L4-L5 inhibited
    e. L5-S1 stimulated; L2-L3 inhibited

Preferred Response: (a) L5-S1 stimulated; L2-L4 inhibited. The exam maneuver described is the Achilles reflex. In this reflex, an afferent action potential is carried via the S1-S2 nerve roots to the spinal cord, which returns via S1-S2 to the same nerve roots, resulting in contraction of the triceps surae. L2-L4 is simultaneously inhibited, resulting in relaxation of the tibialis anterior.

92. A 55-year-old man undergoing anterior cervical fusion is intubated and sedated. On the operating table, the surgeon palpates the thyroid cartilage and draws a horizontal mark just off midline on the patient's left side. At approximately what vertebral level is the thyroid cartilage encountered in most individuals?
    a. C3
    b. C4
    c. C5
    d. C6

Preferred Response: (b) C4-C5. In most individuals, the level of the C4 vertebral body can be approximated at the level of the thyroid cartilage. Note that the exact relations of these traditional landmarks to the true vertebral levels is dependent upon the position of the patient's neck; in one series, slight extension of the neck to achieve cervical lordosis resulted in the C4 vertebral body being located at the thyroid cartilage in approximately 42% [37].

93. Approximately what percentage of cervical spine rotation is conferred by the atlantoaxial joint?
    a. 0–10%
    b. 25%
    c. 50%
    d. 75%

Preferred Response: (c) 50%. The primary movement of the atlantoaxial joint is rotation, with 50% of rotation occurring at this segment.

94. Which of the following statements is false regarding the C7 vertebra?
    a. It has the largest vertebral body of any of the cervical vertebrae
    b. It has the largest vertebral foramen of any of the cervical vertebrae
    c. It does not transmit the vertebral arteries
    d. The C7 nerve roots exit superior to the C7 vertebra
    e. It has inferior facets and spinous processes

Preferred Response: (b) It has the largest vertebral foramen of any of the cervical vertebrae. C7 is a unique vertebra in many ways; it has the largest vertebral body in the cervical spine, it does not transmit the vertebral arteries in most individuals, and is regarded as a "transitional level" as it resembles the thoracic vertebrae, given its inferior zygapophyseal (facet) joints. The C7 vertebra has a smaller vertebral foramen than the other cervical vertebrae.

95. A 24-year-old female is evaluated in the trauma bay following a motor vehicle collision in which she was the restrained passenger. During the accident, her neck rapidly extended backwards. She did not lose consciousness and self-extricated from the vehicle. She was diagnosed with a whiplash injury. Cervical spine imaging suggests damage to the suboccipital triangle. Injury to the suboccipital nerve would result in weakness of which of the following muscles?
    a. Obliquus capitis superior
    b. Serratus posterior superior
    c. Trapezius
    d. Occipitofrontalis
    e. Digastric

Preferred Response: (a) Obliquus capitis superior. The suboccipital triangle is outlined by the rectus capitis posterior major, obliquus capitis superior, and obliquus capitis inferior. These suboccipital muscles share common innervation by the suboccipital nerve, which arises from the dorsal rami of C1. Serratus posterior superior is located at the upper back and is innervated by the intercostal nerves. The trapezius is innervated by cranial nerve XI. The occipitofrontalis muscle is the long and wide muscle of the scalp, innervated by cranial nerve VII. The anterior belly of the digastric muscle is innervated by the mylohyoid nerve and is located anterior to the cervical spine.

96. Which of the following is the most common presenting symptom/examination findings in acute lumbosacral radiculopathy?
    a. Pain radiating into the foot
    b. Paresthesias
    c. Midline low back pain
    d. Muscular weakness
    e. Claudication

Preferred Response: (b) Paresthesias. Approximately 63–72% of patients with lumbar radiculopathy will experience paresthesia, 35% will experience pain, and weakness is present in up to 37%. Weakness is less common as a presenting symptom as most of the muscles of the lower extremities are innervated by several nerve roots.

97. Which of the following descriptions of radiographic spinopelvic parameters accurately describes pelvic incidence?
    a. Horizontal distance from the posterior edge of the S1 endplate to a plumb line dropped from the mid-C7 vertebral body
    b. Angle between the top of S1 and the top of L1
    c. Angle between a line drawn from center of T1 to the center of the femoral head, and the line from the femoral head to the center of the S1 endplate
    d. Angle between the horizontal reference line and the S1 endplate
    e. Angle between a point perpendicular to the S1 endplate and a line drawn from the midpoint of the femoral head to the midpoint of the S1 endplate

Preferred Response: (e) Angle between a point perpendicular to the S1 endplate and a line drawn from the midpoint of the femoral head to the midpoint of the S1 endplate. Normal pelvic incidence is approximately 50° and becomes fixed upon attainment of skeletal maturity.

98. Which of the following descriptions of radiographic spinopelvic parameters accurately describes T1 pelvic angle (TPA)?

a. Horizontal distance from the posterior edge of the S1 endplate to a plumb line dropped from the mid-C7 vertebral body
b. Angle between the top of S1 and the top of L1
c. Angle between a line drawn from center of T1 to the center of the femoral head, and the line from the femoral head to the center of the S1 endplate
d. Angle between the horizontal reference line and the S1 endplate
e. Angle between a point perpendicular to the S1 endplate and a line drawn from the midpoint of the femoral head to the midpoint of the S1 endplate

Preferred Response: (c) Angle between a line drawn from center of T1 to the center of the femoral head, and the line from the femoral head to the center of the S1 endplate. Normal TPA is approximately 20°.

99. Which of the following descriptions of radiographic spinopelvic parameters accurately describes sagittal vertical alignment (SVA)?
  a. Horizontal distance from the posterior edge of the S1 endplate to a plumb line dropped from the mid-C7 vertebral body
  b. Angle between the top of S1 and the top of L1
  c. Angle between a line drawn from center of T1 to the center of the femoral head, and the line from the femoral head to the center of the S1 endplate
  d. Angle between the horizontal reference line and the S1 endplate
  e. Angle between a point perpendicular to the S1 endplate and a line drawn from the midpoint of the femoral head to the midpoint of the S1 endplate

Preferred Response: (a) Horizontal distance from the posterior edge of the S1 endplate to a plumb line dropped from the mid-C7 vertebral body, which is typically within 5 cm. Numbers are considered positive if the plumb line is anterior.

100. In a patient with acute radiculopathy, after how many weeks of symptoms do electromyography (EMG) or nerve conduction studies demonstrate diagnostic value?
  a. 1
  b. 2
  c. 3
  d. 4
  e. 6
  f. 12

Preferred Response: (c) 3. EMG/nerve conduction studies are accurate only after three weeks of persistent radiculopathy, as they depend on fibrillation potentials after an acute injury, which typically do not develop until 2 to 3 weeks following injury [38].

101. Which of the following cervical vertebrae has the smallest lateral mass, on average, in terms of width and depth?
  a. C3
  b. C4
  c. C5
  d. C6
  e. C7

Preferred Response: (e) C7. In the subaxial cervical spine, the size and volume of the lateral masses tend to decrease in most individuals from the upper to the lower cervical spine [39].

102. Which of the following segments of the cervical spine are the least mobile?
  a. C2-C3
  b. C3-C4
  c. C6-C7
  d. C7-T1

Preferred Response: (d) C7-T1. The transitional segment, or cervicothoracic junction, has been shown in biomechanical studies to confer the least mobility to neck flexion/extension/lateral bending compared to other segments of the cervical spine.

103. In a patient with central cord syndrome, which of the following is the most common presenting neurological symptom?
  a. Upper extremity motor deficit > lower extremity motor deficit
  b. Lower extremity motor deficit > upper extremity motor deficit
  c. Loss of pain and temperature sensation at the level of the lesion
  d. Loss of stereognosis in the upper extremities

Preferred Response: (a) Upper extremity motor deficit > lower extremity motor deficit. Central cord syndrome is an incomplete cord syndrome that most commonly results following hyperextension injury of the cervical spine. Due to the somatotopic organization of the lateral cortical spinal tract, with arm function lying more medial within the tract, most patients tend to experience upper extremity weakness to a greater degree than lower extremity weakness.

104. A 30-year-old man is being evaluated in the trauma bay following a motor vehicle collision. On initial

examination, he is unable to move his upper and lower extremities. To aid with prognostication, the examiner tests the bulbocavernosus reflex. Which of the following nerve roots does this reflex assess?
   a. L5-S1
   b. S1-S2
   c. S1-S3
   d. S2-S3
   e. S3-S4
   f. S2-S4

Preferred Response: (f) S2-S4. Several structures such as the pelvic splanchnic nerves, the pudendal nerve, and others are comprised of nerve rootlets from S2-S4. The presence of reflexes in this region is important in the grading of spinal cord injury and thus potential for functional recovery [40].

105. A patient is being evaluated in the office with complaints of low back pain. With the patient supine, the examiner raises the patient's right leg, keeping the knee extended. Which of the following findings is considered a positive straight-leg-raise, or Laségue's sign?
   a. Low back pain upon elevation of the foot < 60°
   b. Pain and paresthesia of a nerve root distribution upon elevation of foot < 60°
   c. Low back pain upon elevation of the foot < 35°
   d. Pain and paresthesia of a nerve root distribution upon elevation of foot < 35°

Preferred Response: (b) Pain and paresthesia of a nerve root distribution upon elevation of foot < 60°. Note that some authors use a cutoff of < 45°. At the 60° level, the straight-leg-raise is positive in 83% of cases of nerve root compression. Sensitivity is highest for suspected involvement of L5 or S1 nerve roots rather than upper lumbar nerve roots.

106. Which of the following is true regarding the posterior longitudinal ligament (PLL)?
   a. It extends from the occiput to S1
   b. It is adherent to the posterior surface of the vertebral bodies
   c. It functions to limit extension of the spine
   d. The tectorial membrane is a rostral extension of the PLL

Preferred Response: (d) The tectorial membrane is a rostral extension of the PLL. The PLL, which extends from C1/C2 to the sacrum, is one of the major ligaments of the spine and limits flexion. It also reinforces the anulus posteriorly. Although the PLL spans the length of the spine, it is adherent only to the annulus (not the vertebral bodies).

107. A 50-year-old man undergoes an uneventful anterior lumbar interbody fusion at L5-S1 for degenerative disc disease with loss of lumbar lordosis. After the procedure, he is diagnosed with retrograde ejaculation, but has no other symptoms. Which of the following structures was most likely injured during the procedure?
   a. Lumbar plexus within the psoas major muscle
   b. Superior hypogastric plexus
   c. L5 nerve root
   d. Inferior mesenteric plexus

Preferred Response: (b) Superior hypogastric plexus. The superior hypogastric plexus is a complex collection of nervous tissue in the lumbosacral region below the level of the aortic bifurcation. It is a part of the autonomic nervous system that is at risk during approaches to the lumbosacral spine. One of such consequences of injury is retrograde ejaculation in males, which has reported rates ranging from 0.42% to 5.9%. Although the L5 nerve root runs just anterior to the sacroiliac joint and is susceptible to injury, it would not be expected to cause retrograde ejaculation without other deficits [41].

108. A patient with longstanding low back pain and leg pain presents to the office for evaluation. During the physical examination, the patient lays prone on the table, the examiner applies pressure to the sacrum while simultaneously applying a traction force caudally on the leg. Reproduction of the patient's symptoms indicates which of the following?
   a. The patient's symptoms are likely due to primary spinal pathology
   b. The patient's symptoms are likely due to primary sacral pathology
   c. The patient's symptoms are suggestive of trochanteric bursitis
   d. The patient's symptoms are likely representative of a factitious disorder

Preferred Response: (b) The patient's symptoms are likely due to primary sacral pathology. This maneuver is known as the shear test. A positive finding is reproduction of the patient's symptoms and is useful for differentiating sacroiliac joint pain from lumbar nerve root compression.

109. A 35-year-old female with a history of prior spine fusion for adolescent idiopathic scoliosis is being worked up for lumbar radiculopathy. Which of the following is not considered an absolute contraindication to magnetic resonance imaging?
   a. Presence of Harrington rods

b. Metallic intraocular foreign bodies
c. Swan-Ganz catheter
d. Implantable cardioverter defibrillators
e. Ferrous aneurysm clip

Preferred Response: (a) Presence of Harrington rods. Patients with Harrington rods can be safely scanned on a 1.5 T magnetic resonance scanner. Each of the other listed choices are considered absolute contraindications to MRI. If it is unclear whether the patient has ever had any facial injury with metal or ever welded without eye protection, an orbit x-ray must be taken and reviewed prior to magnetic resonance imaging.

110. A 41-year-old female presents to clinic with a 3-week history of weakness in arm abduction and diminished sensation over the shoulder. The patient has no other focal neurological deficits. Plain radiographs of the cervical spine are unrevealing. Which of the following is most likely to be identified on magnetic resonance imaging?
a. Acute cervical disc herniation at C4-C5
b. Acute cervical disc herniation at C5-C6
c. Acute cervical disc herniation at C6-C7

Preferred Response: (a) Acute cervical disc herniation at C4-C5. Disc herniation at C4-C5 is rare, comprising only 2% of all cervical disc herniations. Herniation at this level typically results in compression of C5, which results in weakness of the deltoid and paresthesia over the shoulder. Cervical disc herniation at the other levels, although more common, are unlikely to cause this clinical presentation.

111. According to Modic's classification of MRI characteristics of vertebral body marrow changes, which of the following constellations of findings is most suggestive of bone marrow edema associated with acute or subacute inflammation?
a. T1WI intensity ↑; T2WI intensity ↓
b. T1WI intensity ↓; T2WI intensity ↓
c. T1WI intensity ↑; T2WI intensity ↑
d. T1WI intensity ↓; T2WI intensity ↑
e. T1WI intensity iso or ↑; T2WI intensity ↓
f. T1WI intensity ↓; T2WI intensity iso or ↓
g. T1WI intensity ↑; T2WI intensity iso or ↑

Preferred Response: (d) T1WI intensity ↓; T2WI intensity ↑. This pattern of MRI findings is known as Type 1 Modic changes. Notably, these changes disappear on STIR images. Back pain in individuals with these findings may respond to treatment with spinal fusion. Answer choice (g) represents Type 2 Modic changes, i.e. replacement of bone marrow by fat. Answer choice (b) represents Type 3 Modic changes, i.e. reactive subchondral osteosclerosis [42].

112. Spinal implants (e.g. pedicle screws, interbody devices) composed of which of the following materials results in the least amount of metal artifact on magnetic resonance imaging?
a. Polymer
b. Titanium
c. Cobalt chrome
d. Stainless steel

Preferred Response: (a) Polymer. Magnetic resonance imaging is considered the gold-standard imaging modality to establish the diagnosis of a wide variety of spinal pathologies. However, the presence of metallic implants from prior spinal intervention may preclude visualization of the spine due to imaging artifact. Different implant composition may affect the amount of artifact present. Of the answer choices presented above, the amount of artifact, from least to greatest, is approximately the following: polymer < titanium < stainless steel < cobalt chrome [43].

113. Approximately what percentage of patients with acute lumbar disc herniation on imaging with corresponding clinical symptoms will improve without surgical intervention within 6 weeks?
a. 30%
b. 50%
c. 75%
d. 85%
e. 95%

Preferred Response: (d) 85%. For this reason, most clinicians advocate for a clinical observation period of 5 to 8 weeks after the onset of radiculopathy prior to offering surgical intervention to the patient.

114. Which of the following imaging modalities is recommended for the assessment of dynamic instability in the setting of possible vertebral body displacement?
a. Magnetic resonance imaging
b. Plain lateral radiographs
c. Flexion–extension lateral radiographs
d. Computed tomography

Preferred Response: (c) Flexion–extension lateral radiographs. The assessment of dynamic instability requires a dynamic imaging modality, namely, flexion–extension lateral radiographs. The spinal architecture is assessed with the patient in each of these positions and compared for displacement. Each of the other provided choices represent static images that would have less utility in diagnosing instability.

115. Which of the following is true regarding the crossed straight-leg-raise test for herniated lumbar disc?
   a. It is elicited by performing a straight-leg-raise on the painful leg, and observing for symptoms in the painless leg
   b. It is more sensitive than the conventional straight-leg-raise for a herniated lumbar disc
   c. It is more specific than the conventional straight-leg-raise for a herniated lumbar disc
   d. It may correlate with a more lateral disc herniation, rather than central
   e. Less leg elevation is usually required to produce a positive finding compared to the conventional straight leg raise

Preferred Response: (c) It is more specific than the conventional straight-leg-raise for a herniated lumbar disc. The crossed straight-leg-raise (AKA Fajersztajn's sign) is elicited by performing a straight-leg-raise on the painless leg. It is considered positive when the contralateral leg experiences pain. It is less sensitive, but more specific for herniated lumbar disc (up to 97% of patients undergoing surgery with this sign have confirmed herniated lumbar disc). It may suggest a more central disc herniation.

116. Which of the following clinical history/physical examination findings is most suggestive of a herniated lumbar disc at the level of L3-L4?
   a. Pain radiating down anterior thigh
   b. Decreased sensation over the lateral malleolus and lateral foot
   c. Pain radiating down posterior lower extremity
   d. Extensor hallucis longus weakness with foot drop
   e. Diminished Achilles reflex
   f. (a) and (d)
   g. (c) and (d)
   h. (b) and (e)

Preferred Response: (a) Pain radiating down anterior thigh. In most cases, a herniated lumbar disc at the level of L3-L4 will cause compression of the L4 nerve root. Corresponding symptoms that would support this diagnosis include diminished knee jerk reflex, weakness of knee extension, pain distribution in the anterior thigh, and decreased sensation over the medial malleolus and medial foot [44].

117. Which of the following clinical history/physical examination findings is most suggestive of a herniated lumbar disc at the level of L4-L5?
   a. Pain radiating down anterior thigh
   b. Decreased sensation over the lateral malleolus and lateral foot
   c. Pain radiating down posterior lower extremity
   d. Extensor hallucis longus weakness with foot drop
   e. Diminished Achilles reflex
   f. (a) and (d)
   g. (c) and (d)
   h. (b) and (e)

Preferred Response: (g) Pain radiating down anterior thigh. In most cases, a herniated lumbar disc at the level of L4-L5 will cause compression of the L5 nerve root. Although posterior lower extremity pain and weakness of the extensor hallucis longus are both features that could be seen in compression of the S1 nerve root (e.g. by herniation at L5-S1), the presence of foot drop makes this constellation of findings more suggestive of L4-L5 disc herniation with compression of L5 [44].

118. Approximately what percentage of patients with symptomatic acute cervical disc herniation will improve without surgery?
   a. 50%
   b. 70%
   c. 80%
   d. 90%
   e. 98%

Preferred Response: (d) 90%. Most cervical disc herniations can be managed successfully without surgical treatment. Progression of neurologic loss is uncommon [45].

119. Which of the following external landmarks can be utilized to identify the level of C6-C7?
   a. Hyoid bone
   b. Thyroid cartilage
   c. Cricoid cartilage
   d. Cricothyroid membrane

Preferred Response: (c) Cricoid cartilage. In most humans, the cricoid cartilage can be identified at the level of C6-C7 and is identified caudal to the thyroid cartilage. This can serve as an intraoperative landmark to identify cervical layers while the patient is under general anesthesia [46].

120. Which of the following is true regarding the anterior longitudinal ligament (ALL)?
   a. It extends from the basiocciput to L5 vertebral body
   b. In the upper cervical region, it is known as the tectorial membrane
   c. Functions to limit hyperflexion of the spine

d. The segment rostral to C1 is known as the anterior atlanto-occipital membrane
e. (a) and (b)
f. (a) and (d)
g. (a) and (c)

Preferred Response: (d) The segment rostral to C1 is known as the anterior atlanto-occipital membrane. The anterior longitudinal ligament is a structure that spans the anterior surface of the vertebral bodies from the basiocciput to S1, and functions to limit extension of the spine. From C1 to the anterior basion, it is also known as the atlanto-occipital membrane. The tectorial membrane represents the rostral extension of the posterior longitudinal ligament.

121. Which of the following clinical history/physical examination findings is most suggestive of a herniated cervical disc at C5-C6?
   a. Diminished biceps reflex
   b. Diminished brachioradialis reflex
   c. Weakness in forearm extension with wrist drop
   d. Paresthesia over the second and third digits, all fingertips
   e. (a) and (b)
   f. (a) and (d)
   g. (b) and (c)
   h. (c) and (d)

Preferred Response: (e) Diminished biceps and brachioradialis reflexes. Herniation of the intervertebral disc at C5-C6 typically results in compression of the C6 nerve root. This clinical syndrome is typically marked by biceps and brachioradialis hyporeflexia, weakness in forearm flexion, and paresthesia in the upper arm, thumb, and radial forearm [44].

122. Which of the following clinical history/physical examination findings is most suggestive of a herniated cervical disc at C6-C7?
   a. Diminished biceps reflex
   b. Diminished brachioradialis reflex
   c. Weakness in forearm extension with wrist drop
   d. Paresthesia over the second and third digits, all fingertips
   e. (a) and (b)
   f. (a) and (d)
   g. (b) and (c)
   h. (c) and (d)

Preferred Response: (h) Weakness in forearm extension with wrist drop and paresthesia over the second and third digits, all fingertips. Herniation of the intervertebral disc at C6-C7 typically results in compression of the C7 nerve root. This clinical syndrome is typically marked by diminished triceps reflex, weakness in forearm extension (wrist drop), and paresthesia in the noted distribution [44].

123. With the neck in a slightly extended position, which of the following external anatomical landmark-cervical level pairs is the most reliable, in terms of percentage of patients having the landmark at that level?
   a. Angle of the mandible—C2 vertebral body
   b. Hyoid bone—C2-C3 intervertebral disc
   c. Thyroid cartilage—C4 vertebral body
   d. Cricoid cartilage—C5-C6 intervertebral disc

Preferred Response: (a) Angle of the mandible—C2 vertebral body. In a series of 96 healthy volunteers, the angle of the mandible was located at the C2 vertebral body in 95.5%. The hyoid bone was located at the C2-C3 intervertebral disc in 51.7%, the thyroid cartilage was located at the C4 vertebral body in 42%, and the cricoid cartilage was located at the C5-C6 intervertebral disc in 43.4% [47].

124. Which of the following clinical signs is suggestive of a lower motor neuron rather than upper motor neuron disorder?
   a. Spasticity
   b. Hyperreflexia
   c. Positive Babinski sign
   d. Sustained clonus
   e. Fasciculations

Preferred Response: (e) Fasciculations. An upper motor neuron lesion is a lesion anywhere from the cortex to the corticospinal tract. This, among other things, may cause findings such as hyperreflexia, spasticity, Babinski sign, and sustained clonus. Conversely, lower motor neuron lesions are localized to anywhere between the anterior horn of the spinal cord, the peripheral nerve, neuromuscular junction, or the muscle. Findings may include flaccid paralysis, hyporeflexia, and fasciculations. Clinical differentiation of these two subgroups of findings may aid in clinical localization and correlation with imaging findings.

125. Which of the following statements is false regarding the tectospinal tract?
   a. Fibers of the superior colliculi interface with the medial longitudinal fasciculus before reaching the cervical spinal cord
   b. Synapses of the tectospinal tract reach to the level of T1 of the spinal cord

c. The primary purpose of the tectospinal tract is to coordinate reflex posture movements in response to visual stimuli
d. None of the above

Preferred Response: (b) Synapses of the tectospinal tract extend to the level of T1 of the spinal cord. The tectospinal tract is a component of the extrapyramidal system of the descending motor pathway. Its primary function is to coordinate reflex posture movements, such as to move the head towards visual stimuli. It appears to play a lesser role in humans than some other animals and is not completely understood. The tectospinal tract consists of projections from the superior colliculi to the medial longitudinal fasciculus at the medulla that travel in the anterior funiculus to the cervical levels C1-C4.

126. Which of the following is true regarding the innervation of the lumbar zygapophyseal joints?
    a. Each joint is typically innervated solely by branches of lumbar nerves exiting at that level
    b. The articular branches arise from the lateral branch of the posterior primary rami
    c. The same branches that innervate the zygapophyseal joints also innervate neighboring structures such as the multifidus muscle and the interspinous ligament
    d. None of the above

Preferred Response: (c) The same branches that innervate the zygapophyseal joints also innervate neighboring structures such as the multifidus muscle and the interspinous ligament. Zygapophyseal joint pain is a potential cause of low back pain. The lumbar zygapophyseal joints are innervated by the medial branches of the posterior primary rami. Each zygapophyseal joint receives dual innervation, from the primary rami exiting at that level, as well as adjacent levels. As an example, the L4-L5 zygapophyseal joints are innervated by the L4 branch as well as the L3 branch [48].

127. Which of the following structures is not involved in the transmission of proprioceptive input?
    a. Pacinian corpuscles
    b. Ruffini's end organs
    c. Extremity Golgi tendon organs
    d. Superficial free nerve endings

Preferred Response: (d) Superficial free nerve endings. The Pacinian corpuscles, Ruffini's end organs, and Golgi tendon organs all generate impulses that are conveyed via various ascending tracts to eventually synapse at the cerebellum.

128. On plain radiographs of the cervical spine, which of the following represents average spinal canal diameter (spinolaminar line to posterior vertebral body) from C3-T1?
    a. 10 mm
    b. 12 mm
    c. 15 mm
    d. 17 mm

Preferred Response: (c) 15 mm. Various cutoffs for the normal minimum AP diameter have been suggested, although this measurement is mostly used as an inference, as direct compression of the spinal cord can be demonstrated directly with MRI. Most authors agree that stenosis is present with AP diameter < 12 mm in an adult [49].

129. Which of the following statements is accurate regarding radiculopathy due to compression?
    a. Only the dorsal roots are typically involved
    b. Only the ventral roots are typically involved
    c. The most common cause is vascular in origin
    d. The most common cause is intervertebral disc herniation
    e. They occur only within the intervertebral foramen

Preferred Response: (d) The most common cause is intervertebral disc herniation. Compressive radiculopathy is the result of nerve irritation as it exits the spine. Paresthesia, pain, and weakness are common clinical features, although not all of these may be present at original presentation. A common cause of compressive radiculopathy is intervertebral disc herniation: vascular or neoplastic causes are relatively less common. While many cases of compressive radiculopathy are the result of nerve compression as it exits the intervertebral foramen, radiculopathy can be caused by compression distal or proximal to this site [50].

130. Which of the following spinal tracts is most involved in conveying cutaneous and group 1b receptor impulses from the dorsal root ganglia?
    a. Dorsal spinocerebellar
    b. Vestibulospinal
    c. Ventral corticospinal
    d. Spino-olivary
    e. Lateral spinothalamic

Preferred Response: (c) Spino-olivary. The spino-olivary tract conveys cutaneous and group 1b receptor impulses from the DRG to the posterior columns, which are carried via the nuclei cuneatus and gracilis to the accessory olivary nucleus and eventually the cerebellum. The dorsal spinocerebellar tract is analogous to the cuneocerebellar tract for the lower extremities in transmitting proprioceptive input. The lateral spinothalamic tract mediates itch, pain, and temperature sensation.

131. In a patient with radiculopathy due to lumbar disc herniation, which of the following prognostic factors are most likely to positively affect functional outcomes after lumbar discectomy?
   a. Younger patient age
   b. Longer duration of symptoms (>3 months)
   c. Prior treatment with epidural steroid injections with good response
   d. Level of lumbar spine affected
   e. Shorter duration of symptoms (<3 months)
   f. (a) and (b)
   g. (c) and (e)
   h. (a) and (e)

Preferred Response: (h) Younger patient age and shorter duration of symptoms (<3 months). Although there is insufficient evidence to make recommendations regarding the influence of many potential prognostic factors on outcomes following medical/surgical treatment of lumbar disc herniation with radiculopathy, there is level II evidence to suggest that patient age (under 40 years of age) and shorter duration of symptoms (<3 months) are associated with better outcomes in patients undergoing percutaneous lumbar discectomy [51].

132. Hypertrophy of which of the following structures can contribute to spinal canal stenosis in the cervical region?
   a. Dura
   b. Articular facets
   c. Ligamentum flavum
   d. Posterior longitudinal ligament
   e. Lamina
   f. (b), (c), and (d)
   g. (b), (d), and (e)
   h. All of the above

Preferred Response: (h) All of the above. Cervical spinal canal stenosis can be caused by a wide variety of pathologies, including age-related degenerative conditions. Any of the above-named structures can hypertrophy and abut the cervical spinal cord, thus resulting in canal stenosis. Note that in the lumbar spine, facet joint hypertrophy can result in lateral recess stenosis, compressing the nerve root just before it exits the foramen.

133. Which of the following statements is true regarding cervical spinal canal stenosis?
   a. Exacerbation of stenosis is more common in flexion than with extension
   b. Segmental or diffuse ossification of the anterior longitudinal ligament can cause cervical stenosis, most common in Japanese populations
   c. Cervical spondylosis is the most common cause of myelopathy in patients > 55 years of age
   d. Histologically, the central gray matter is usually preserved at the level of compression, even in symptomatic patients
   e. None of the above

Preferred Response: (c) Cervical spondylosis is the most common cause of myelopathy in patients > 55 years of age. Age-related degenerative conditions of the spine are an important cause of myelopathy in older individuals. Cervical stenosis is generally exacerbated in extension due to buckling of the posterior longitudinal ligament in this position. Ossification of the posterior, not anterior, longitudinal ligament is another potential cause of cervical spinal stenosis. Histopathological studies show degeneration of the central gray matter at the level of compression, in the posterior columns above the lesion, and demyelination in the lateral columns [52].

134. In the three-column model of the spine, which of the following represents the anterior column?
   a. Anterior 1/2 of the disc and vertebral body
   b. Anterior 1/2 of the disc and vertebral body and anterior longitudinal ligament
   c. Anterior 2/3 of the disc and vertebral body
   d. Anterior 2/3 of the disc and vertebral body and anterior longitudinal ligament
   e. Disc, vertebral body, and anterior longitudinal ligament

Preferred Response: (b) Anterior 1/2 of the disc and vertebral body and anterior longitudinal ligament. The three-column model of the spine was developed to assist in the prognostication of the stability of thoracolumbar fractures. In this model, the anterior column contains the anterior longitudinal ligament as well as the anterior half of the vertebral body/disc space [53]

135. A 70-year-old patient with a history of coronary artery disease presents to clinic with a several month history of leg pain while walking more than three city blocks. Which of the following features, when present on history/examination, is most suggestive of a vascular, rather than neurogenic cause of this patient's symptoms?

a. Triggering of pain with standing, alleviation with sitting
b. Triggering of pain with standing, alleviation with sitting, and pain located above the knees
c. Triggering of pain with standing, alleviation with sitting, and pain located below the knees/in the calves
d. Triggering of pain with standing, alleviation with sitting, and positive shopping cart sign

Preferred Response: (c) Triggering of pain with standing, alleviation with sitting, and pain located below the knees/in the calves. Intermittent claudication is a symptom characterized by pain in the legs while walking, more common in elderly patients. The two most common causes of intermittent claudication are lumbar spinal stenosis ("neurogenic claudication") and peripheral vascular disease ("vascular claudication"). While differentiation of these two entities can sometimes be challenging based on clinical history alone, there are several features that may suggest one diagnosis over the other. Cohort studies indicate that the most specific indicator of vascular claudication, rather than neurogenic claudication, is pain located in the calves [54].

136. At what antero-posterior spinal canal diameter on plain radiographs would one be considered to have significant stenosis in the lumbar region?
   a. 10 mm
   b. 12 mm
   c. 14 mm
   d. 16 mm

Preferred Response: (a) 10 mm. Normal diameter of the lumbar spinal canal is > 12 mm. Although the diagnosis of lumbar spinal stenosis can be accomplished with clinical findings and magnetic resonance imaging, it can be inferred based on plain radiographs. Absolute stenosis is defined as less than 10 mm in diameter.

137. Which of the following Rexed's laminae, also known as the substantia gelatinosa, receives input from the posterior columns, dorsolateral, and lateral funiculi with C fibers and functions to modulate sensation?
   a. Layer I
   b. Layer II
   c. Layer V
   d. Layer VII
   e. Layer VIII
   f. Layer IX

Preferred Response: (b) Layer II. The Rexed laminae are a proposed model for the organization of the spinal cord. Layer II, or the substantia gelatinosa, is a gray matter structure primarily involved in transmission and modulation of pain, temperature, and touch. It spans the entire spinal cord rostrally into the medulla oblongata, receiving input from peripheral sensory fibers of the dorsal root ganglia.

138. Which of the following Rexed's laminae, also known as the zona intermedia, is located between the anterior and posterior horns, and contains the dorsal nucleus of Clarke from C8-L2?
   a. Layer I
   b. Layer II
   c. Layer V
   d. Layer VII
   e. Layer VIII
   f. Layer IX

Preferred Response: (b) Layer VII. The Rexed laminae are a proposed model for the organization of the spinal cord. Layer VII, or the zona intermedia, transmits the Dorsal nucleus of Clarke, the central nucleus of Clarke, and the intermediolateral cell column.

139. Which of the following is true regarding the use of electromyography (EMG) in the diagnosis of radiculopathy?
   a. A normal motor exam is usually associated with a normal EMG
   b. EMG is highly sensitive for radiculopathy
   c. Abnormal EMG findings are associated with low specificity
   d. Cervical EMG is particularly useful to test nerve roots C3-C4

Preferred Response: (a) A normal motor exam is usually associated with a normal EMG. In the workup of radiculopathy, if a reliable motor examination can be obtained, EMG is unlikely to add any substantial new information. In a patient with questionable radiculopathy, EMG has low sensitivity, but when findings are abnormal, high specificity. Therefore, EMG perhaps has best value in cases where the patient cannot be reliably assessed. In the cervical spine, it is most useful for nerve roots C5-T1, as there are no muscles that can reliably test C3-C4.

140. A 45-year-old man with grade 1 spondylolisthesis undergoes uneventful left-sided lateral lumbar interbody fusion. After the procedure, the patient notes weakness in flexing his left hip. The right hip is unaffected. Which of the following is the most likely explanation of this patient's new symptoms?
   a. Local trauma to the psoas major muscle

b. Injury to the anterior femoral cutaneous nerve
c. Injury to the femoral nerve
d. Genitofemoral neuralgia

Preferred Response: (a) Local trauma to the psoas major muscle. Hip flexor weakness is a common, self-limiting finding following lateral, transpsoas approaches to the lumbar spine [55].

141. In the three-column model of the spine, which of the following represents the middle column?
   a. Posterior 2/3 of the vertebral body and disc
   b. Posterior 2/3 of the vertebral body and disc, and posterior longitudinal ligament
   c. Posterior 1/2 of the vertebral body and disc, and posterior longitudinal ligament
   d. Posterior 1/2 of the vertebral body and disc, posterior longitudinal ligament, and ligamentum flavum
   e. Posterior 1/2 of the vertebral body and disc

Preferred Response: (c) Posterior 1/2 of the vertebral body and disc, and posterior longitudinal ligament. The three-column model of the spine was developed to assist in the prognostication of the stability of thoracolumbar fractures. In this model, the middle column contains the posterior half of the vertebral body and the posterior longitudinal ligament [53].

142. Which of the following sources is the most common cause of spontaneous vertebral osteomyelitis?
   a. Soft tissue infection
   b. Odontogenic infection
   c. Respiratory tract infection
   d. Urinary tract infection

Preferred Response: (d) Urinary tract infection. Vertebral osteomyelitis comprises a minority of all osteomyelitis cases and is usually the result of hematogenous spread. Of these, urinary tract infection is the most commonly identified source. Direct extension (e.g. following surgery) is also possible. In about one-third of cases, no source is ever identified [56].

143. A 25-year-old male is evaluated in the trauma bay following a motor vehicle collision. After a detailed examination, he is deemed to have an American Spinal Injury Association (ASIA) B injury at the C7 level, such that C7 is the last level with intact sensation and antigravity strength, and everything below this level has intact sensation and no motor function. Which of the following findings on physical exam would NOT be consistent with this injury classification?
   a. 0/5 strength in the intrinsic hand muscles
   b. Intact sensation on the lateral forearm
   c. Intact sensation on the medial forearm
   d. 0/5 strength in elbow flexion
   e. 5/5 strength in shoulder abduction

Preferred Response: (d) 0/5 strength in elbow flexion. The ASIA scale provides an organization structure for the classification of spinal cord injuries and determines whether injuries are incomplete or complete. As explained in the vignette, the ASIA B injury is characterized by intact sensation but motor deficit below the level of injury. The intrinsic hand muscles (interossei and finger flexion) are provided by C8 and T1, which is consistent with ASIA B C7 injury. Similarly, sensation over the lateral and medial forearm are conserved as sensation is expected to be intact. Shoulder abduction is expected to be preserved, as function of the C5 level is expected to be unaffected. Elbow flexion, conferred by C6, should also be expected to be preserved in an injury at C7. Therefore, 0/5 strength in elbow flexion is inconsistent with the reported injury [57].

144. A 40-year-old female presents to the clinic for evaluation of low back pain. Which of the following findings, when present on physical examination, are most suggestive of a non-psychogenic basis of the patient's symptoms?
   a. Positive straight-leg-raise while supine and while distracted sitting upright
   b. Non-dermatomal sensory deficit pattern in the lower extremities
   c. Low back pain elicited with axial loading of the head
   d. Tenderness on light palpation of a wide area of lumbar paraspinal skin

Preferred Response: (a) Positive straight-leg-raise while supine and while distracted sitting upright. Orthopedic surgeon Gordon Waddell described a group of clinical signs known as Waddell signs. The purpose of these signs was to identify patients who are unlikely to experience a good functional outcome following lumbar spine surgery. Distracted straight-leg-raise discrepancy is identified by performing a straight-leg-raise with the patient supine, usually with a positive finding, and then testing the straight-leg-raise again while upright without informing the patient by elevating the leg for some other reason, e.g. to test knee/ankle strength. Patients more likely to have a psychogenic cause of back pain will sometimes complain of pain when being tested in the supine position, but not while upright. Findings (b)-(d) are also considered Waddell signs.

145. In a healthy adult patient, which of the following vertebral levels has the smallest transverse pedicle diameter?
  a. T1
  b. T3
  c. T6
  d. T12
  e. L3

Preferred Response: (c) T6. A general understanding of pedicle dimensions is important for thoracic pedicle screw placement. Anatomical studies of pedicle diameter have found that the average pedicle diameter is smallest at T6 and largest at L5. Thoracic pedicle diameter is generally maximal at T1 and T12, with a "dip" at T6 [58].

146. Which of the following statements regarding the cervical spine is accurate?
  a. In most patients, all subaxial cervical vertebrae have foramina transversaria
  b. The vertebral artery traverses the foramen transversarium at all levels of the subaxial spine in most patients
  c. The orientation of the superior articular facets transitions from posterolateral facing to posteromedial facing going caudally down the subaxial cervical spine,
  d. On axial imaging, the inferior articular process is anterior to the superior articular process
  e. (a) and (b)
  f. (a), (c), (d)
  g. All of the above

Preferred Response: (a) In most patients, all subaxial cervical vertebrae have foramina transversaria. Although all subaxial cervical vertebrae have these foramina, the vertebral artery does not traverse these foramina at the level of C7 in most individuals. When traveling rostrally to caudally, the orientation of the facets moves from posteromedial facing to posterolateral facing, which permits increased rotation at the rostral levels. On axial imaging, the superior articular process is generally anterior to the inferior articular process [59].

147. Which of the following physical exam findings is NOT characteristic of cervical myelopathy?
  a. Posturing of the hand in flexion of the metacarpophalangeal joints and extension of the interphalangeal joints ("intrinsic plus hand")
  b. Difficulty with rapid alternating movements of the hand
  c. Involuntary flexion of the thumb/index finger upon flicking of the fingernail of the 3rd digit
  d. Intrinsic muscular atrophy of the hand

Preferred Response: (a) Posturing of the hand in flexion of the metacarpophalangeal joints and extension of the interphalangeal joints ("intrinsic plus hand"). Intrinsic plus hand is typically the result of spasticity of the intrinsic hand muscles or weakness of the extrinsic hand muscles; it is not typically associated with cervical myelopathy. Rapid alternating movements can be assessed by asking the patient to open/close a fist as fast as possible for 15 s and is typically decreased in cervical myelopathy. Flexion of the thumb/index finger upon flicking of the 3rd fingernail describes Hoffman sign [60].

148. A 67-year-old man undergoes cervical decompression for myelopathy via a posterior approach. Afterwards, he develops new symptoms suggestive of postoperative C5 palsy. Which of the following options best describes the likely new clinical history/examination findings in this patient?
  a. Lateral shoulder pain/paresthesia
  b. Wrist extensor weakness
  c. Triceps muscle weakness
  d. Pain/paresthesia of the medial upper forearm
  e. Shoulder abduction weakness

Preferred Response: (e) Shoulder abduction weakness. Postoperative C5 palsy is a known potential complication following posterior cervical spine surgery and is posited to result from tethering of the nerve root as the cord migrates dorsally. Retrospective studies of patients with postoperative radiculopathy following posterior cervical decompression found that the most common presenting pattern of this complication is a motor-dominant radiculopathy, manifesting with weakness of the deltoid. Although lateral shoulder pain/paresthesia can be encountered in C5 palsy, the motor-dominant shoulder abduction weakness is more common [61].

149. Which of the following statements regarding age-related intervertebral disc changes is true?
  a. Proteoglycan concentration increases with age
  b. Water content increases with age
  c. Acidity decreases with age
  d. There is conversion to fibrocartilage along the endplate
  e. Disc height increases
  f. (a) and (b)
  g. (c) and (d)
  h. All of the above

Preferred Response: (d) There is conversion to fibrocartilage along the endplate. Age-related intervertebral disc changes have been studied in previous laboratory experiments. Boos et al. in 2002 found that as age increases, proteoglycan and water concentration decline, pH decreases, degradative enzyme activity increases, and the fibrocartilage composition increases. Knowledge of these concepts and advancements in basic science may guide future therapeutic options for individuals with age-related degenerative pathologies [62].

150. Which of the following structures is NOT considered a component of the posterior ligamentous complex (PLC)?
    a. Supraspinous ligament
    b. Interspinous ligament
    c. Ligamentum flavum
    d. Posterior dura
    e. Facet capsule ligament

Preferred Response: (d) Posterior dura. The PLC is thought to contribute significantly to the stability and alignment of the thoracolumbar spine. The PLC resists bending, compressive loads, and limits excessive motion. Obvious dislocation of a vertebral interspace is often clearly suggestive of disruption of the PLC. The PLC is comprised of four primary structures: the supraspinous ligament, interspinous ligament, facet capsule ligament, and the ligamentum flavum. The dura is not considered a component of the PLC[63].

References

1. Drake RL, Vogl AW, Mitchell AWM. Back. In: Gray's Anatomy for Students. Philadelphia, PA: Elsevier; 2013:82
2. Whitney E, Alastra AJ. Neuroanatomy, Decerebrate Rigidity. 2020 Aug 10. In: StatPearls [Internet]. Treasure Island (FL): StatPearls Publishing; 2021 Jan–. PMID: 31613467
3. Lang IM, Hughes DG, Jenkins JP, St Clair Forbes W, McKenna F. MR imaging appearances of cervical epidural abscess. Clin Radiol. 1995 Jul;50(7):466–71. https://doi.org/10.1016/s0009-9260(05)83162-9. PMID: 7614792. (2) Sun B, Wang C, Wang J, Liu A. MRI features of intramedullary spinal cord ependymomas. J Neuroimaging. 2003 Oct;13(4):346–51. PMID: 14569827
4. Viswanathan A, Burton AW, Rekito A, McCutcheon IE. Commissural myelotomy in the treatment of intractable visceral pain: technique and outcomes. Stereotact Funct Neurosurg. 2010;88(6):374–82. https://doi.org/10.1159/000319041. Epub 2010 Oct 15 PMID: 20948242.
5. Ku J, Morrison EH. Neuroanatomy, Anterior White Commissure. 2020 Jul 31. In: StatPearls [Internet]. Treasure Island (FL): StatPearls Publishing; 2021 Jan–. PMID: 31536221.
6. Konrad P. Dorsal root entry zone lesion, midline myelotomy and anterolateral cordotomy. Neurosurg Clin N Am. 2014;25(4):699–722. https://doi.org/10.1016/j.nec.2014.07.010. PMID: 25240658.
7. Green R. Vitamin B12 deficiency from the perspective of a practicing hematologist. Blood. 2017;129(19):2603–11. https://doi.org/10.1182/blood-2016-10-569186. Epub 2017 Mar 30 PMID: 28360040.
8. Texakalidis P, Tora MS, Boulis NM. Neurosurgeons' Armamentarium for the Management of Refractory Postherpetic Neuralgia: A Systematic Literature Review. Stereotact Funct Neurosurg. 2019;97(1):55–65. https://doi.org/10.1159/000499476. Epub 2019 Apr 17 PMID: 30995653.
9. Ishak B, G Dupont, S Lachkar, E Yilmaz, AV Glinski, J Altafulla, S Kikuta, J Iwanaga, Chapman JR, Oskouian R, Tubbs RS. Update on the Biomechanics of the Craniocervical Junction-Part I: Transverse Atlantal Ligament in the Elderly. Global Spine J. 2021 Mar;11(2):180–6. https://doi.org/10.1177/2192568219896544. Epub 2020 Jan 7. PMID: 32875854; PMCID: PMC7882814.
10. Liao S, Jung MK, Hörnig L, Grützner PA, Kreinest M. Injuries of the upper cervical spine-how can instability be identified? Int Orthop. 2020;44(7):1239–53. https://doi.org/10.1007/s00264-020-04593-y. Epub 2020 May 25 PMID: 32451654.
11. Drake RL, Vogl AW, Mitchell AWM. Back. In: Gray's Anatomy for Students. Philadelphia, PA: Elsevier; 2013:78
12. Baaj AA, Mummaneni PV, Uribe JS, Vaccaro AR, Greenberg MS. Embryology of the Spine. In: Handbook of Spine Surgery. New York, NY. Thieme Medical Publishers 2016:15
13. Stiell IG, Clement CM, McKnight RD, Brison R, Schull MJ, Rowe BH, Worthington JR, Eisenhauer MA, Cass D, Greenberg G, MacPhail I, Dreyer J, Lee JS, Bandiera G, Reardon M, Holroyd B, Lesiuk H, Wells GA. The Canadian C-spine rule versus the NEXUS low-risk criteria in patients with trauma. N Engl J Med. 2003;349(26):2510–8. https://doi.org/10.1056/NEJMoa031375. PMID: 14695411.
14. Johal J, Loukas M, Fisahn C, Oskouian RJ, Tubbs RS. Bergmann's ossicle (ossiculum terminale persistens): a brief review and differentiation from other findings of the odontoid process. Childs Nerv Syst. 2016;32(9):1603–6. https://doi.org/10.1007/s00381-016-3199-7. Epub 2016 Jul 27 PMID: 27465675.
15. Kumar Y, Hayashi D. Role of magnetic resonance imaging in acute spinal trauma: a pictorial review. BMC Musculoskelet Disord. 2016;22(17):310. https://doi.org/10.1186/s12891-016-1169-6.
16. Elton S, Oakes WJ. Dermal sinus tracts of the spine. Neurosurg Focus. 2001;10(1): e4. https://doi.org/10.3171/foc.2001.10.1.5. PMID:16749756.\.
17. Agarwalla PK, Dunn IF, Scott RM, Smith ER. Tethered cord syndrome. Neurosurg Clin N Am. 2007;18(3):531–47. https://doi.org/10.1016/j.nec.2007.04.001. PMID: 17678753.
18. Kao SC, Lin CS. Caudal Epidural Block: An Updated Review of Anatomy and Techniques. Biomed Res Int. 2017;2017:9217145. https://doi.org/10.1155/2017/9217145. Epub 2017 Feb 26. PMID: 28337460; PMCID: PMC5346404.
19. Sahin F, Selçuki M, Ecin N, Zenciroğlu A, Unlü A, Yilmaz F, Maviş N, Saribaş S. Level of conus medullaris in term and preterm neonates. Arch Dis Child Fetal Neonatal Ed. 1997;77(1):F67–9. https://doi.org/10.1136/fn.77.1.f67.PMID:9279188;PMCID: PMC1720669.
20. Castro MP, Stebbings SM, Milosavljevic S, Pedersen SJ, Bussey MD. Assessing the construct validity of clinical tests to identify sacroiliac joint inflammation in patients with non-radiographic axial spondyloarthritis. Int J Rheum Dis. 2019;22(8):1521–8. https://doi.org/10.1111/1756-185X.13606. Epub 2019 May 27 PMID: 31131990.
21. Gebreyohanes AMH, Ahmed AI, Choi D. Dorsal Root Entry Zone Lesioning for Brachial Plexus Avulsion: A Comprehensive Literature Review. Oper Neurosurg (Hagerstown). 2021;20(4):324–33. https://doi.org/10.1093/ons/opaa447. PMID: 33469654.
22. Koh M, Markovich B. Neuroanatomy, Spinocerebellar Dorsal Tract. 2020 Sep 29. In: StatPearls [Internet]. Treasure Island (FL): StatPearls Publishing; 2021 Jan–. PMID: 32310473.

23. Iwanaga J, Ishak B, Saga T, Singla A, Impastato D, Chapman JR, Oskouian RJ, David G, Porzionato A, Reina MA, Macchi V, de Caro R, Tubbs RS. The Lumbar Ligamentum Flavum Does Not Have Two Layers and Is Confluent with the Interspinous Ligament: Anatomical Study with Application to Surgical and Interventional Pain Procedures. Clin Anat. 2020;33(1):34–40. https://doi.org/10.1002/ca.23437. Epub 2019 Aug 9 PMID: 31325341.
24. Russell SM. The lumbosacral anatomy of the lumbosacral plexus. In: Examination of Peripheral Nerve Injuries: An Anatomical Approach. New York, NY: Thieme Medical Publishers; 2006: 150–63
25. Absoud M, Greenberg BM, Lim M, Lotze T, Thomas T, Deiva K. Pediatric transverse myelitis. Neurology. 2016;87(9 Suppl 2): S46-52. https://doi.org/10.1212/WNL.0000000000002820. PMID: 27572861.
26. Malanga GA, Landes P, Nadler SF. Provocative tests in cervical spine examination: historical basis and scientific analyses. Pain Physician. 2003;6(2):199–205 PMID: 16883381.
27. Gutrecht JA. Lhermitte's sign. From observation to eponym Arch Neurol. 1989;46(5):557–8.
28. Rabinstein AA. Autonomic Hyperactivity. Continuum (Minneap Minn). 2020;26(1):138–53. https://doi.org/10.1212/CON.0000000000000811. PMID: 31996626.
29. Harrop JS, Hunt GE Jr, Vaccaro AR. Conus medullaris and cauda equina syndrome as a result of traumatic injuries: management principles. Neurosurg Focus. 2004;16(6): e4. https://doi.org/10.3171/foc.2004.16.6.4. PMID: 15202874.
30. Garfin, Steven R., et al. Rothman-Simeone and Herkowitz's the Spine. Seventh edition. ed. Philadelphia: Elsevier, Inc., 2018. Print
31. Baaj AA, Mummaneni PV, Uribe JS, Vaccaro AR, Greenberg MS. Embryology of the Spine. In: Handbook of Spine Surgery. New York, NY. Thieme Medical Publishers 2016:3
32. Jordan J, Konstantinou K, O'Dowd J. Herniated lumbar disc. BMJ Clin Evid. 2009 Mar 26;2009:1118. PMID: 19445754; PMCID: PMC2907819
33. Humphreys SC, Eck JC. Clinical evaluation and treatment options for herniated lumbar disc. Am Fam Physician. 1999 Feb 1;59 (3):575–82, 587–8. PMID: 10029785.
34. Maragkos GA, Atesok K, Papavassiliou E. Prognostic Factors for Adjacent Segment Disease After L4–L5 Lumbar Fusion. Neurosurgery. 2020;86(6):835–42. https://doi.org/10.1093/neuros/nyz241. PMID: 31245812.
35. Vanaclocha V, Guijarro-Jorge R, Saiz-Sapena N, Granell-Gil M, Ortiz-Criado JM, Mascarós JM, Vanaclocha L. Selective T3–T4 sympathicotomy versus gray ramicotomy on outcome and quality of life in hyperhidrosis patients: a randomized clinical trial. Sci Rep. 2021;11(1):17628. https://doi.org/10.1038/s41598-021-96972-7.PMID:34475473;PMCID:PMC8413289.
36. Bell GR, Ross JS. Diagnosis of nerve root compression. Myelography, computed tomography, and MRI. Orthop Clin North Am. 1992 Jul;23(3):405–19. PMID: 1620535.
37. Siribumrungwong K, Sinchai C, Tangtrakulwanich B, Chaiyamongkol W. Reliability and Accuracy of Palpable Anterior Neck Landmarks for the Identification of Cervical Spinal Levels. Asian Spine J. 2018 Feb;12(1):80–84. https://doi.org/10.4184/asj.2018.12.1.80. Epub 2018 Feb 7. PMID: 29503686; PMCID: PMC5821937.
38. Albeck MJ, Taher G, Lauritzen M, Trojaborg W. Diagnostic value of electrophysiological tests in patients with sciatica. Acta Neurol Scand. 2000;101(4):249–54. https://doi.org/10.1034/j.1600-0404.2000.101004249.x. PMID: 10770521.
39. Mohamed E, Ihab Z, Moaz A, Ayman N, Haitham AE. Lateral mass fixation in subaxial cervical spine: anatomic review. Global Spine J. 2012;2(1):39–46. https://doi.org/10.1055/s-0032-1307261. PMID:24353945;PMCID:PMC3864406.
40. Previnaire JG. The importance of the bulbocavernosus reflex. Spinal Cord Ser Cases. 2018;10(4):2. https://doi.org/10.1038/s41394-017-0012-0.PMID:29423307;PMCID:PMC5798690.
41. Eid S, Iwanaga J, Chapman JR, Oskouian RJ, Loukas M, Tubbs RS. Superior Hypogastric Plexus and Its Surgical Implications During Spine Surgery: A Review. World Neurosurg. 2018;120:163–7. https://doi.org/10.1016/j.wneu.2018.08.170. Epub 2018 Aug 30 PMID: 30172971.
42. Jones A, Clarke A, Freeman BJ, Lam KS, Grevitt MP. The Modic classification: inter- and intraobserver error in clinical practice. Spine (Phila Pa 1976). 2005 Aug 15;30(16):1867–9. https://doi.org/10.1097/01.brs.0000173898.47585.7d. PMID: 16103857
43. Ernstberger T, Buchhorn G, Heidrich G. Artifacts in spine magnetic resonance imaging due to different intervertebral test spacers: an in vitro evaluation of magnesium versus titanium and carbon-fiber-reinforced polymers as biomaterials. Neuroradiology. 2009 Aug;51(8):525–9. https://doi.org/10.1007/s00234-009-0537-4. Epub 2009 May 26. PMID: 19468722; PMCID: PMC3085728.
44. Patel EA, Perloff MD. Radicular Pain Syndromes: Cervical, Lumbar, and Spinal Stenosis. Semin Neurol. 2018;38(6):634–9. https://doi.org/10.1055/s-0038-1673680. Epub 2018 Dec 6 PMID: 30522138.
45. Saal JS, Saal JA, Yurth EF. Nonoperative management of herniated cervical intervertebral disc with radiculopathy. Spine (Phila Pa 1976). 1996 Aug 15;21(16):1877–83. https://doi.org/10.1097/00007632-199608150-00008. PMID: 8875719.
46. Rosen RD, Winters R. Physiology, Lower Esophageal Sphincter. 2021 Apr 20. In: StatPearls [Internet]. Treasure Island (FL): StatPearls Publishing; 2022 Jan–. PMID: 32491384.
47. Siribumrungwong K, Sinchai C, Tangtrakulwanich B, Chaiyamongkol W. Reliability and Accuracy of Palpable Anterior Neck Landmarks for the Identification of Cervical Spinal Levels. Asian Spine J. 2018 12(1):80–4. https://doi.org/10.4184/asj.2018.12.1.80 . Epub 2018 Feb 7. PMID: 29503686; PMCID: PMC5821937.
48. Saravanakumar K, Harvey A. Lumbar Zygapophyseal (Facet) Joint Pain. Rev Pain. 2008;2(1):8–13. https://doi.org/10.1177/204946370800200103.PMID:26525677;PMCID:PMC4589934.
49. Zhang L, Chen HB, Wang Y, Zhang LY, Liu JC, Wang ZG. Cervical spinal canal narrowing and cervical neurological injuries. Chin J Traumatol. 2012;15(1):36–41 PMID: 22300918.
50. Corey DL, Comeau D. Cervical radiculopathy. Med Clin North Am. 2014;98(4):791–9, xii. https://doi.org/10.1016/j.mcna.2014.04.001. PMID: 24994052
51. Kreiner DS, Hwang SW, JE Easa, DK Resnick, JL Baisden, S Bess, CH Cho, MJ DePalma, P Dougherty, R Fernand, G Ghiselli, AS Hanna, T Lamer, AJ Lisi, DJ Mazanec, RJ Meagher, RC Nucci, RD Patel, JN Sembrano, AK Sharma, JT Summers, CK Taleghani, WL Jr Tontz, JF Toton. North American Spine Society. An evidence-based clinical guideline for the diagnosis and treatment of lumbar disc herniation with radiculopathy. Spine J. 2014;14(1):180–91. https://doi.org/10.1016/j.spinee.2013.08.003. Epub 2013 Nov 14. PMID: 24239490
52. Lee Y, Kim SY, Kim K. A Dynamic Magnetic Resonance Imaging Study of Changes in Severity of Cervical Spinal Stenosis in Flexion and Extension. Ann Rehabil Med. 2018;42(4):584–90. https://doi.org/10.5535/arm.2018.42.4.584. Epub 2018 Aug 31. PMID: 30180528; PMCID: PMC6129716.
53. Panjabi MM, Oxland TR, Kifune M, Arand M, Wen L, Chen A. Validity of the three-column theory of thoracolumbar fractures. A biomechanic investigation. Spine (Phila Pa 1976). 1995;20 (10):1122–7. https://doi.org/10.1097/00007632-199505150-00003 . PMID: 7638654.
54. Nadeau M, Rosas-Arellano MP, Gurr KR, Bailey SI, Taylor DC, Grewal R, Lawlor DK, Bailey CS. The reliability of differentiating neurogenic claudication from vascular claudication based on

symptomatic presentation. Can J Surg. 2013;56(6):372–7. https://doi.org/10.1503/cjs.016512.PMID:24284143;PMCID:PMC3859778.
55. Von Glinski, Alexander, et al. "Complications from Lateral Transpsoas Approaches to the Lumbar Spine." Surgical Anatomy of the Lateral Transpsoas Approach to the Lumbar Spine, Elsevier, Edinburgh, 2020, pp. 219–31.
56. Sapico FL, Montgomerie JZ. Pyogenic vertebral osteomyelitis: report of nine cases and review of the literature. Rev Infect Dis. 1979 Sep-Oct;1(5):754–76. https://doi.org/10.1093/clinids/1.5.754 . PMID: 542761.
57. Roberts TT, Leonard GR, Cepela DJ. Classifications In Brief: American Spinal Injury Association (ASIA) Impairment Scale. Clin Orthop Relat Res. 2017;475(5):1499–504. https://doi.org/10.1007/s11999-016-5133-4. Epub 2016 Nov 4. PMID: 27815685; PMCID: PMC5384910.
58. Scoles PV, Linton AE, Latimer B, Levy ME, Digiovanni BF. Vertebral body and posterior element morphology: the normal spine in middle life. Spine (Phila Pa 1976). 1988;13(10):1082–6. https://doi.org/10.1097/00007632-198810000-00002. PMID: 3206263.
59. Pal GP, Routal RV, Saggu SK. The orientation of the articular facets of the zygapophyseal joints at the cervical and upper thoracic region. J Anat. 2001;198(Pt 4):431–41. https://doi.org/10.1046/j.1469-7580.2001.19840431.x.PMID:11327205;PMCID: PMC1468229.
60. Lebl DR, Hughes A, Cammisa FP Jr, O'Leary PF. Cervical spondylotic myelopathy: pathophysiology, clinical presentation, and treatment. HSS J. 2011;7(2):170–8. https://doi.org/10.1007/s11420-011-9208-1. Epub 2011 Jun 22. PMID: 22754419; PMCID: PMC3145857.
61. Dai L, Ni B, Yuan W, Jia L. Radiculopathy after laminectomy for cervical compression myelopathy. J Bone Joint Surg Br. 1998;80(5):846–9. https://doi.org/10.1302/0301-620x.80b5.8580. PMID: 9768896.
62. Boos N, Weissbach S, Rohrbach H, Weiler C, Spratt KF, Nerlich AG. Classification of age-related changes in lumbar intervertebral discs: 2002 Volvo Award in basic science. Spine (Phila Pa 1976). 2002 Dec 1;27(23):2631–44. https://doi.org/10.1097/00007632-200212010-00002. PMID: 12461389.
63. Li Y, Shen Z, Huang M, Wang X. Stepwise resection of the posterior ligamentous complex for stability of a thoracolumbar compression fracture: An in vitro biomechanical investigation. Medicine (Baltimore). 2017;96(35): e7873. https://doi.org/10.1097/MD.0000000000007873.PMID:28858098;PMCID: PMC5585492.

Surgical Anatomy and Techniques to the Spine

2

Asham Khan, Moleca M. Ghannam, Ryan M. Hess, Slah Khan, Alexander O. Aguirre, Cathleen C. Kuo, Ali Y. Elkady, Ahmed H. Omar, Mohammad Elbaroody, and Mohamed A. R. Soliman

Question 1

What structures are connected by the iliolumbar ligaments?

A. The L5 transverse process and posterior iliac crest.
B. The lateral surface of the sacrum to the posterior iliac crest
C. The L5 transverse process with the sacral ala.
D. None of the above.

Response (**A**) The iliolumbar ligaments connect the L5 transverse process and posterior iliac crest (see Fig. 2.1); The lumbosacral ligaments connect the L5 transverse process with the sacral ala; The posterior sacral ligaments originate from lateral sacral surfaces and connect the sacrum to the posterior ilium [1].

Question 2

A 55-year-old male presents with severe neck pain after a whiplash injury, sustained when his car was struck from behind. Radiologic studies reveal trauma to the ligament lying on the anterior surface of the cervical vertebral bodies. Which ligament is most likely disrupted?

A. Posterior longitudinal ligament.
B. Ligamentum flavum
C. Nuchal ligament
D. Anterior longitudinal ligament
E. Transverse ligament

Response (**D**) The anterior longitudinal ligament lies anterior to the vertebral bodies along the vertebral column. The ligamentum flavum connects the laminae of two adjacent vertebrae. The nuchal ligament is a continuation of the supraspinous ligament above C7, which connects spinous processes. The posterior longitudinal ligament lies on the posterior margin of the vertebral bodies. The transverse ligament, a component of the cruciate ligament, lies behind the dens [2].

Question 3

A 19-year-old man is diagnosed with a cervical herniated disc, but he has no symptoms of spinal cord injury. In the event of intervertebral disc herniation in the cervical region, which of the following ligaments is in an anatomic position to protect the spinal cord from direct compression?

A. Supraspinous ligament
B. Posterior longitudinal ligament
C. Anterior longitudinal ligament
D. Ligamentum flavum

A. Khan · M. M. Ghannam · R. M. Hess · S. Khan · A. O. Aguirre · C. C. Kuo · M. A. R. Soliman (✉)
Department of Neurosurgery, University at Buffalo, Buffalo, NY, USA
e-mail: msolim8@uwo.ca

A. Khan
e-mail: akhan@ubns.com

M. M. Ghannam
e-mail: mghannam@ubns.com

R. M. Hess
e-mail: rhess@ubns.com

S. Khan
e-mail: slahkhan@buffalo.edu

A. O. Aguirre
e-mail: aa284@buffalo.edu

C. C. Kuo
e-mail: ckuo9@buffalo.edu

A. Y. Elkady · A. H. Omar · M. Elbaroody · M. A. R. Soliman
Department of Neurosurgery, Cairo University, Cairo, Egypt
e-mail: ayousri54@gmail.com

A. H. Omar
e-mail: a.hussein.omar1990@gmail.com

M. Elbaroody
e-mail: mohammad.elbaroody@kasralainy.edu.eg

C. Gragnaniello et al. (eds.), *MCQs in Spine Surgery*,
https://doi.org/10.1007/978-3-031-69332-8_2

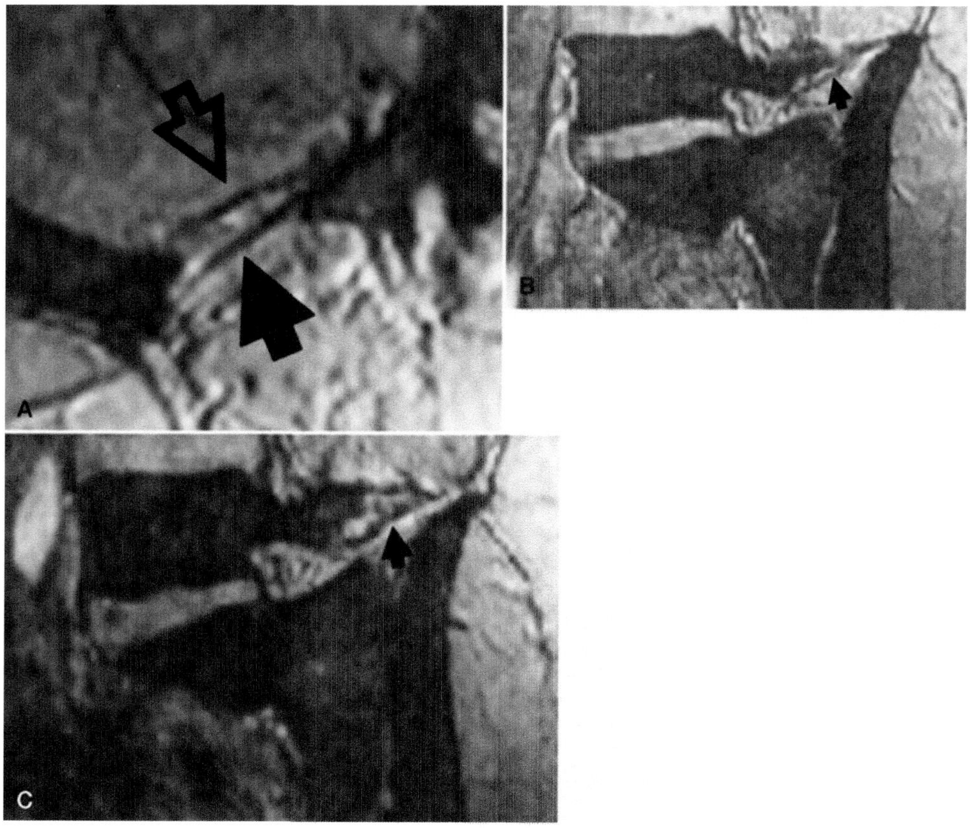

Fig. 2.1 Magnetic resonance 3D computer reformatted volume image of the iliolumbar ligament representing the size and breadth of the iliolumbar ligament. **A**, Reformatted coronal section of the anterior and posterior bands. **B**, Reformatted sagittal section of the anterior band. **C**, Reformatted sagittal section of the posterior band

Response (**B**) The posterior longitudinal ligament extends along the posterior surface of the vertebral bodies and intervertebral discs. With intervertebral disc herniation, the nucleus pulposus of the intervertebral disc protrudes posterolaterally. The anterior longitudinal ligament traverses the anterior side of the vertebral bodies and thus would not protect the spinal cord from direct compression. The supraspinous and ligamentum flavum ligaments are posterior to the cord [3].

Question 4

A 40-year-old woman is diagnosed with stenosis of the cervical vertebral canal. A laminectomy of two vertebrae is performed. Which of the following ligaments will most likely also be removed?

A. Anterior longitudinal ligament
B. Denticulate ligament
C. Ligamentum flavum
D. Cruciate ligament

Response (C) The anterior longitudinal ligament runs along the anterior-most aspect of the vertebral column from C1 to the sacrum and would therefore be unaffected by a laminectomy. The denticulate ligaments extend intradurally laterally from the pia mater to the arachnoid mater along the length of the spinal cord and should not be encountered in this approach. The ligamentum flavum is one of the two ligaments found in the vertebral canal and it arises from the lower half of the anterior surface of the lamina above and inserted in the posterior surface and upper margin of the lamina below and often greatly thickened in spinal pathology. It is thus simultaneously removed upon excision of the lamina. The cruciate ligament is an incorrect answer because it is located anterior to the spinal cord, posterior to the dens and therefore would not be involved in the laminectomy4.

Question 5

A 28-year-old pregnant woman is admitted to the obstetrics department for delivery. In the final stages of labor, a caudal anesthetic is administered via the sacral hiatus. Which of the following spaces in the sacral canal is the anesthetic drug placed?

A. Vertebral canal
B. Epidural space
C. Subarachnoid space
D. Subdural space

Response (**B**) The spinal epidural space is superficial to the dura. It is a fat-filled space extending from foramen magnum to the sacrum. It is the site of epidural anesthesia. The subarachnoid space is found within the CNS, and the subdural space is a potential space between the dura and arachnoid, and usually, these two layers are fused due to the presence of CSF in the subarachnoid space [4].

Question 6

A 53-year-old man was in a head-on vehicle collision that resulted in compression of his spinal cord by the dens (odontoid process) of the axis, with resulting quadriplegia. Which of the following ligaments was most probably torn?

A. Anterior longitudinal ligament
B. Transverse ligament of the atlas
C. Ligamentum flavum.
D. Supraspinous ligament
E. Nuchal ligament

Response (**B**) The anterior longitudinal ligament runs on the anterior aspect of the vertebrae and disruption would not result in atlantoaxial instability. The transverse ligament of the atlas anchors the dens laterally to prevent posterior displacement of the dens. It embraces the neck of the odontoid process posteriorly. Injury to this ligament will cause posterior dislocation of the dens and compression on the spinal cord leading to quadriplegia. The ligamentum flavum is found on the posterior aspect of the vertebral canal. The supraspinous ligament is located along the spinous processes of the vertebrae. The nuchal ligament is a longitudinal extension of the supraspinous ligament above the level of C7 [5].

Question 7

A forty-four-year-old patient presenting after a fall from height with odontoid fracture and disturbed transverse atlantal ligament. The decision was to fuse C1-C2 levels. A preoperative CT angiography was done to delineate the course of the vertebral artery. The groove for the vertebral artery is located on which aspect of the atlas?

A. Superior surface of the posterior arch.
B. Superior surface of the anterior arch.
C. Inferior surface of the posterior arch.
D. Inferior surface of the anterior arch.

Response (**A**) The groove for vertebral artery is located on the superior aspect of the posterior arch of C1 after exiting the foramen transversarium of the atlas on its way to enter the intradural space through the foramen magnum [6].

Question 8

Which of the following muscles is NOT attached to the atlas?

A. Levator scapulae muscle
B. Rectus capitis posterior minor muscle
C. Rectus capitis posterior major muscle
D. Oblique capitis inferior muscle

Response (**C**) The rectus capitis posterior major arises by a pointed tendon from the spinous process of the axis and is inserted into the lateral part of the inferior nuchal line of the occipital bone and the surface of the bone immediately below the line (see Fig. 2.2) [7].

Question 9

The atlanto-occipital articulation is classified as a _______ articulation.

A. Ball and socket
B. Condyloid
C. Syndesmosis
D. Cartilaginous

Response (**B**) Condylar joint (condyloid joint) is formed of an ovoid head of one bone moves in an elliptical cavity of another, the atlas bone and the occipital bone. It consists of a pair of condyloid joints. It is a synovial joint.

Question 10

Which spinal nerve emerges from the vertebral canal above its respective vertebra?

A. L1
B. T1
C. T12
D. C7

Response (**D**) The cervical spinal nerves are named according to the vertebra above which they emerge with the exception of C8. In contrast, thoracic, lumbar, sacral, and coccygeal spinal nerves are numbered according to the vertebra below.

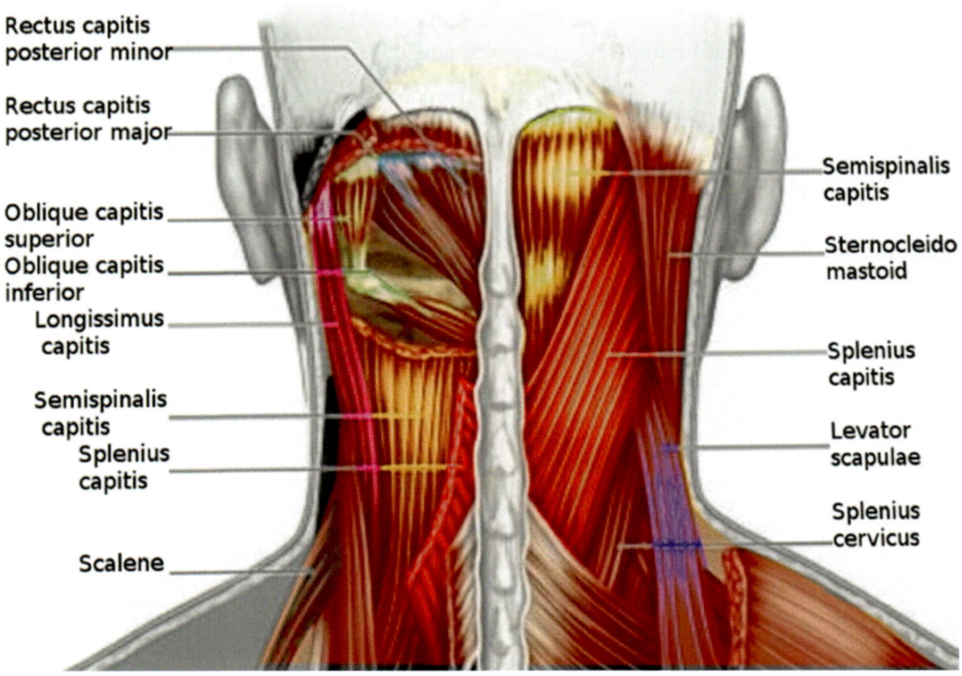

Fig. 2.2 Artist's rendering demonstrating the different layers of the posterior cervical musculature

Question 11

The blood supply of the cervical cord arises from which arterial supply?

A. Vertebral artery
B. Deep cervical artery
C. Ascending cervical artery
D. All of the above

Response (**D**) All the vessels listed supply the spinal cord in the cervical region.

Question 12

What range of angulation in degrees is considered normal for thoracic kyphosis?

A. 15° to 30°
B. 25° to 55°
C. 20° to 40°
D. 30° to 60°

Response (**C**) The typical range for thoracic kyphosis is 20° to 40°. The other choices are incorrect.

Question 13

Which of the following includes all thoracic vertebral bodies with costotransverse facets on their transverse process?

A. T1 to T12
B. T2 to T11
C. T1 to T10
D. T2 to T9

Response (**C**) All the thoracic vertebrae have a costotransverse facet on their transverse process except T11 and 12.

Question 14

What artery runs through the anterior median fissure of the spinal cord and originates from the vertebral and radicular arteries?

A. Anterior intercostal artery
B. Anterior spinal artery
C. Posterior spinal artery
D. Ascending cervical artery

Response (**B**) The anterior spinal artery is the only artery that runs through the median fissure [8].

Question 15

At what vertebral level and anatomical side does the artery of Adamkiewicz most commonly arise from?

A. Left T7
B. Left T9
C. Right T7
D. Right T10

Response (**B**) In 80% of people, this artery originates on the left side of the body. Of those people, a large majority of them have the artery extend from T9 to L2 vertebral bodies [9].

Question 16

Which of the following is considered the posterior border of the intervertebral foramen?

A. Posterior borders of the adjacent vertebral bodies and discs
B. Inferior border of the pedicle for the superior vertebrae
C. Pars interarticularis and facet joints
D. Superior border of the pedicle of the inferior vertebrae

Response (**C**) The pars interarticularis is located posteriorly along with the facet joints, and they serve as the posterior border of the intervertebral foramen [10].

Question 17

The cauda equina receives blood from all of the following **EXCEPT**:

A. Lumbar arteries
B. Lateral sacral arteries
C. Anterior sacral arteries
D. Median sacral arteries

Response (**C**) The cauda equina receives blood from the lumbar arteries, the lateral sacral arteries, and the median sacral arteries [11].

Question 18

Which of the following is an indication for a posterior cervical foraminotomy?

A. Cervical instability
B. Cervical myelopathy
C. Severe kyphosis
D. Recurrent surgery, with cervical root compression

Response (**D**) Recurrent surgery with cervical root compression is an indication for posterior cervical foraminotomy. It provides the greatest improvements for patients who have repeated cervical spine problems [12].

Question 19

Of the following surgical complications after an Anterior Lumbar Interbody Interbody Fusion (ALIF), which can cause retrograde ejaculation?

A. Deep vein thrombosis
B. Injury to the superior hypogastric plexus
C. Injury to the testicular artery
D. Abdominal hernia

Response (**B**) The superior hypogastric plexus controls the process of ejaculation, and damage to it leads to the retrograde flow of sperm. The remaining options could be surgical complications of the ALIF approach but do not change the pattern of ejaculation [13].

Question 20

What anatomical landmark should serve as the lateral marker during a lumbar laminectomy?

A. Bilateral transverse process
B. Bilateral pedicle
C. Bilateral pars
D. Bilateral lamina

Response (**C**) The correct lateral anatomical landmark for a lumbar laminectomy is the pars located on both sides of the lamina to minimize the potential for instability [14].

Question 21

The most common complication following transoral odontoidectomy:

A. Injury of the vertebral artery
B. Injury of the hypoglossal nerve
C. CSF leakage
D. Infection

Response (**D**) Infections from the oral flora due to the poor pharynx and soft palate closure is the most common complication following the transoral approach [15].

Question 22

Regarding Spinal Cord Stimulation (SCS), all of the following are true **EXCEPT**:

A. In cases of extensive scarring, laminectomy is recommended to pass the lead without resistance
B. Cervical and upper extremity stimulation is attainable at the level of C1-C2
C. SCS lead is usually placed at T8-9 epidural space
D. Active infection is a contraindication for the technique

Response (**A**) While multiple laminotomies may be needed with extensive epidural scarring, a total laminectomy is avoided, as there will be no remaining bone to keep the lead apposed snuggly against the dura.

Question 23

Regarding Closed Cervical Traction (CCT), all of the following are true **EXCEPT**:

A. Coexistence of skull fracture may contraindicate the technique.
B. Posterior pin placement will apply an extension to the cervical spine.
C. Correct pin placement is ½ an inch above ear pinna in line with the external auditory meatus.
D. Too superior pins are at high risk of pullout.
E. If over distraction or neurologic deterioration occurs, the weights should be immediately removed.

Response (**B**) Posterior pin placement will apply a flexion (not extension) to the cervical spine [16].

Question 25

Regarding retroperitoneal approach to the lumbar spine, which one of the following is true:

A. It can easily provide exposure above L2
B. Muscle sparing is more painful than muscle incising approach
C. Placement of graft cannot be done utilizing this approach
D. This approach is indicated for patients with moderate spine deformity in the form of scoliosis < 40° or kyphosis < 25°

Response (**D**) This approach can expose from L2-S1. Muscle sparing is less painful than muscle incising approach. The direct anterior exposure facilitates graft placement and anterior decompression [17].

Question 26

Regarding vascular injury in anterior lumbar approach, all of the following are true, **EXCEPT**:

A. The middle sacral artery and vein usually lie directly over the L5-S1 disc
B. The great vessels bifurcate at the level of L4 vertebral body
C. The incidence of vascular injury during anterior lumbar spine surgery is 1–15%
D. Exposure for pathology at the L5-S1 level needs extensive vascular exposure.

Response (**D**) If exposure of only the L5–S1 disc is needed, this can be easily achieved typically without mobilizing any great vessels (see Fig. 2.3). However, extensive vascular mobilization is required if exposure is needed to the L4–L5 level or to multiple anterior disc levels, and the exposure will be more complex [18].

Question 27

Regarding cervical degenerative disease, which one of the following is true:

A. The rate of pseudoarthrosis is higher when an anterior plate is not used in single-level fusion.
B. Dislodgment of graft is the most common complication following Anterior Cervical Discectomy and Fusion (ACDF).
C. The posterior approach is associated with a longer hospital stay after surgery.
D. Four-level involvement is a contraindication for the anterior approach.

Response (**C**) The rate of pseudoarthrosis for single-level fusion is the same 0–5% with or without plate. Dysphagia is the most common complication following ACDF. Four-levels involvement is not a contraindication of anterior approach [19].

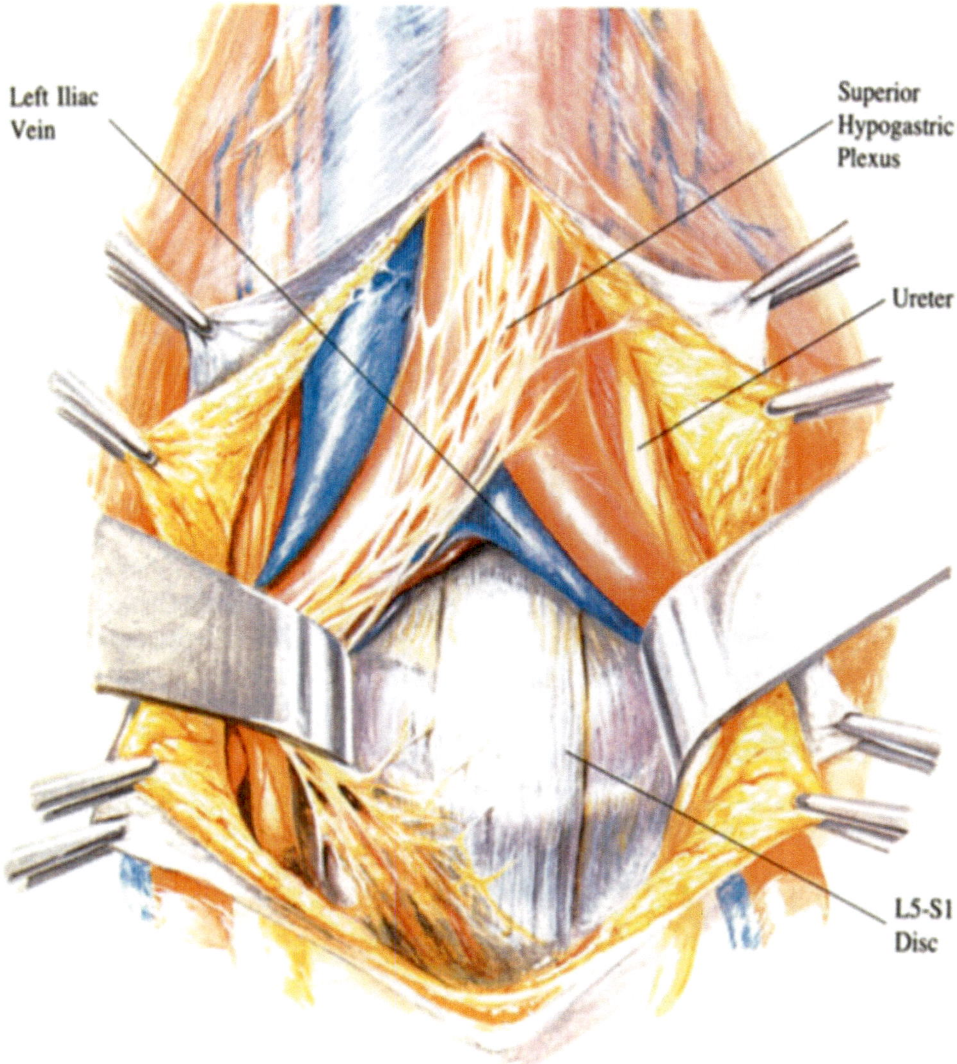

Fig. 2.3 Artist's rendering of the bifurcation of the aorta below which the anterior surface of LS-S1 is visualized (adapted with permission, Watkins) [18]

Question 28

Regarding spinal cord tracts, which one of the following is true:

A. Sensory fibers directed to the dorsal columns entering the spinal cord below T6 enter the gracilis and travel medially.
B. The posterior column transmits pain and temperature sensations.
C. The tectospinal tract, arising from the superior colliculus, controls the muscle tone of flexor muscle groups.
D. The rubrospinal tract, arising from the red nucleus, mediates reflex postural movements in response to visual stimuli.

Response (A) The anterolateral system transmits pain and temperature sensations; the tectospinal tract mediates reflex postural movements in response to visual stimuli; the rubrospinal tract colliculus controls muscle tone of flexor muscle groups.

Question 29

All of the following ligaments connect C1 to the occipital bone, **EXCEPT**:

A. Anterior atlanto-occipital membrane
B. Posterior atlanto-occipital membrane
C. Cruciate ligament
D. Tectorial membrane

Response (D)The tectorial membrane runs from the posterior aspect of the body of C3, C2, and the dorsal aspect of the odontoid process to the anterior aspect of the foramen magnum [20].

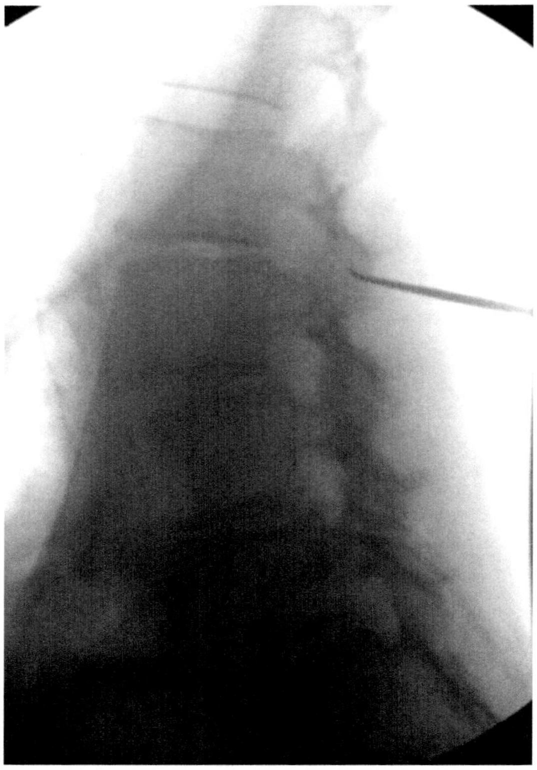

Fig. 2.4 Lateral intraoperative XR demonstrating the placement of a curette to localize the level of interest

Question 30

Regarding nerve roots, all of the following are true, **EXCEPT**:

A. C3, C4, C5 form the phrenic nerve
B. L3 root exits through the L3/4 foramen
C. C4 root exits through the C4/5 foramen
D. T7 root exits through the T7/8 foramen

Response (**C**) C5 root exits through the C4/5 foramen. Unique to the cervical spine, the nerve roots exit above their respective vertebral level except C8. There are eight nerve roots, with the first one exiting between the occiput and the atlas. From T1 downwards, the nerve root exit below its corresponding vertebral body pedicle [21].

Question 31

In the following image, the instrument's tip is located under which structure (see Fig. 2.4)?

A. Pedicle
B. Spinous Process
C. Superior Articulating Facet
D. Lamina
E. Inferior Articulating Facet

Response (**D**) The tip of the angled curette is resting just under the lamina of L2. This is a method of intraoperative level localization commonly utilized.

Question 32

Which of the following is not considered a risk or disadvantage unique to anterior lumbar interbody fusion (ALIF) compared to posterior interbody fusion techniques?

A. Risk of injury to the iliac vein
B. Venous thromboembolism secondary to venous retraction
C. Postoperative ileus due to manipulation of abdominal viscera
D. Retrograde ejaculation
E. Postoperative neuropraxia

Response (**E**) Answers A-D are all complications, risks, or disadvantages considered unique to the approach of the ALIF. Though postoperative neuropraxia is possible after ALIF, the risk is far less than posterior interbody techniques as retraction of neural elements is not required to insert the interbody graft or expose the disk space.

Question 33

Damage to which structure during anterior lumbar interbody fusion (ALIF) can lead to retrograde ejaculation?

A. Superior hypogastric nerve plexus
B. Genitofemoral nerve
C. Obturator nerve
D. Pudendal nerve
E. Common peroneal nerve

Response (**A**) The superior hypogastric plexus is seated just inferior to or along the bifurcation of the aorta. Damage to these nerves results in regulatory issues with the internal vesicular sphincter resulting in semen entering the bladder during ejaculation leading to retrograde ejaculation in males. It is often due to thermal injury from the monopolar electrocautery during exposure and dissection.

Question 34

The anterior longitudinal ligament extends from the anterior sacrum to C1 then continues rostrally as which named ligamentous structure?

A. Cruciate ligament
B. Anterior atlanto-occipital membrane
C. Ligamentum flavum
D. Accessory tectorial membrane
E. Transverse ligament

Response (**B**) The anterior atlanto-occipital membrane extends from the anterior ring of C1 to the ventral skull base. It serves as a continuation of the anterior longitudinal ligament of the spine.

Question 35

A 40 years old male presents to your clinic for surgical consultation for severe radicular pain refractory to medical management. He describes to you pain originating in his low back radiating down his right leg into the dorsal aspect of his right foot and great toe. Based on this description, what is the location of the disc herniation if the patient were to have a single disc herniation that resulted in all of his symptoms?

A. Far lateral disc herniation at L5-S1
B. Paracentral disc herniation at L5-S1
C. Far lateral disc herniation at L4-5
D. Paracentral disc herniation at L3-4
E. Far lateral disc herniation at L3-4

Response (**A**) It is important to distinguish which nerve root is affected by the different types of disc herniations. Far lateral disc herniations affect the exiting nerve root, while paracentral disc herniations affect the traversing nerve root. The patient, in this case, is describing a classic L5 radiculopathy. Therefore, a far lateral disc herniation at L5-S1 would explain this as the disc would impinge upon the exiting L5 nerve root at this level.

Question 36

In a patient undergoing minimally invasive microdiscectomy for a far lateral disc herniation at L4-5, what anatomical structures are used as docking points for the retractor?

A. L5 pars interarticularis and transverse process
B. L4 lamina and superior articulating process
C. L4 pars interarticularis and transverse process
D. L4 lamina and inferior articulating process
E. L4 lamina and pars interarticularis

Response (**C**)When performing a minimally invasive far lateral microdiscectomy, the retractor is docked on the pars and transverse process at the level of the impinged exiting nerve root. This offers a lateral working corridor to visualize and protect the exiting nerve root and offer room for disc removal [22].

Question 37

Which cranial nerve controls the most superficial muscle encountered during an anterior cervical discectomy and fusion (ACDF)?

A. Cranial nerve XI
B. Cranial nerve VII
C. Cranial nerve XII
D. Cranial nerve VIII
E. Cranial Nerve IX

Response (**B**) The platysma is the most superficial neck muscle seen during an ACDF dissection. This muscle is innervated by the cervical branch of the facial nerve (cranial nerve VII) [23].

Question 38

In what percentage of people does the vertebral artery enters the transverse foramen at C6?

A. 75%
B. 25%
C. 90%
D. 5%
E. 50%

Response (**C**) In 90% of people, the vertebral artery enters the transverse foramen at C6. However, there are anatomic anomalies, with 1% entering at C3, 2% entering at C4, 5% entering at C5, and 2% entering at C7.

Question 39

How many degrees of kyphotic correction does a Smith-Peterson Osteotomy typically achieve?

A. 5–10 degrees
B. 10–15 degrees

C. 15–20 degrees
D. 15–30 degrees
E. 20–25 degrees

Response (**A**) A Smith-Peterson Osteotomy typically achieves 5–10 degrees of correction of kyphotic deformity in the sagittal plane [24].

Question 40

How many degrees of kyphotic correction does a Pedicle Subtraction Osteotomy typically achieve?

A. 5–10 degrees
B. 10–12 degrees
C. 12–20 degrees
D. 15–30 degrees
E. 20–25 degrees

Response (**D**)A Pedicle Subtraction Osteotomy typically achieves 15–30 degrees of correction of kyphotic deformity in the sagittal plane (see Fig. 2.5) [25].

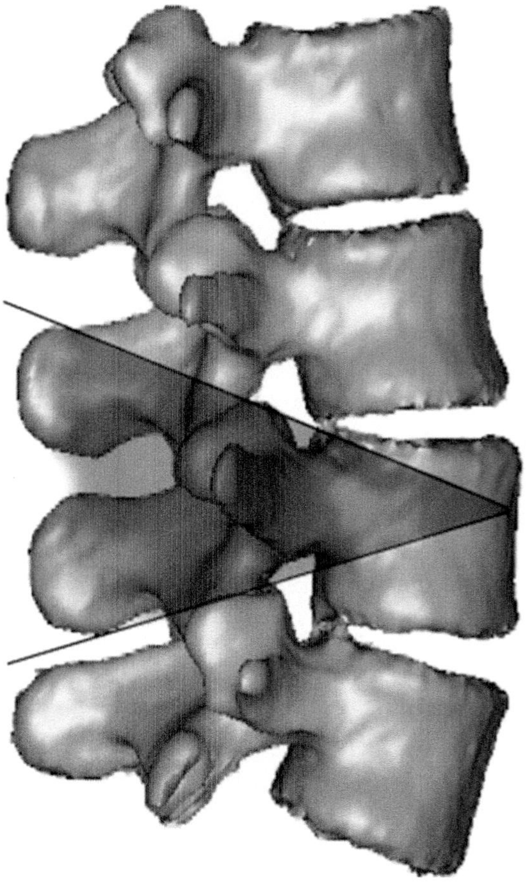

Fig. 2.5 Lateral drawing of PSO angulation and shape of the osteotomy

Question 41

When performing a Smith Peterson or Ponte Osteotomy (SPO) at L2, which of the following structures is preserved?

A. Inferior articulating process of L2
B. L2 pedicle
C. Superior articulating process of L3
D. L2 spinous process
E. L2 lamina

Response (**B**) During an SPO or Ponte osteotomy, the following bony structures are removed to complete the osteotomy: At the osteotomy level, the spinous process, lamina, and inferior articulating process and at the level below, the superior articulating process. The pedicles are removed in pedicle subtraction osteotomy [26].

Question 42

During a transoral odontoidectomy, the exposure of which ligamentous structure indicates the maximal depth of dissection has been reached?

A. Apical ligament
B. Anterior atlantooccipital membrane
C. Posterior atlantooccipital membrane
D. Tectorial membrane

Response (**D**) When performing a transoral odontoidectomy the tectorial membrane lies deep to the odontoid and is the ligamentous structure that is just ventral to the thecal sac. It marks the deep extent of exposure for this procedure as visualization of this structure typically signifies adequate spinal cord decompression has been achieved.

Question 43

Which diagnosis requires a sympathectomy procedure involving resection of the sympathetic chain only at the second and third rib?

A. Palmar hyperhidrosis
B. Craniofacial hyperhidrosis
C. Axillary hyperhidrosis
D. Clavicular hyperhidrosis

Response (**A**) Palmar hyperhidrosis is the only approach that is limited to the second and third rib. Craniofacial hyperhidrosis involves the 2nd, 3rd, and 4th ribs resection. Axillary hyperhidrosis involves the 3rd, 4th, and 5th ribs resection. Clavicular hyperhidrosis is not associated with the second or third ribs [27].

Question 44

What is the external anatomic landmark used to help identify the location of the C4-5 disc space?

A. Hyoid bone
B. Thyroid cartilage
C. Cricoid cartilage
D. Chassaignac's tubercle
E. Midpoint of the sternocleidomastoid

Response (**B**) The thyroid cartilage approximates the location of the C4-C5 disc space [28].

Question 45

When performing lateral trans-psoas approach to the lumbar spine, which of the following is considered a safe working zone?

A. Middle of the L1/2 disc space
B. Middle of the L2/3 disc space
C. Middle of the L3/4 disc space
D. Middle of the L4/5 disc space
E. Posterior third of the L4/5 disc space

Response (**D**) The safe working areas during lateral trans-psoas approach to the lumbar spine are the posterior third of the disc space from L1-L4 and the middle for the disc space at L4-5. The operation here decreases rates of retraction-related morbidity of the lumbar plexus such as thigh numbness and hip flexor weakness [29].

Question 46

What is the most common complication following lateral trans-psoas lumbar fusion?

A. Retrograde ejaculation
B. Transient thigh numbness or hip flexor weakness
C. Ileus
D. Retroperitoneal hematoma
E. Bowel perforation

Response (**B**) Following lateral transpsoas approaches, patients commonly experience transient anterior thigh numbness or hip flexor weakness secondary to traction on the psoas muscle as well as branches of the lumbar plexus. The rate of weakness has been reported at 0.7–33.6%, and the rate of sensory changes was reported at 0–75%. There have been few organ- or vascular-related complications in the published literature on this approach.

Question 47

When Smith-Peterson osteotomies (SPO) performed in conjunction with transforaminal lateral interbody fusion (TLIF), how many degrees of lordosis per level can be achieved?

A. 0–5 degrees
B. 5–10 degrees
C. 10–15 degrees
D. 15–20 degrees
E. 20–25 degrees

Response (**D**) According to data from Shaffrey and collegues, performing an SPO at the level undergoing TLIF can increase lordosis approximately 5–10 degrees at each level. This gain in lordosis is additive, meaning that this 5–10 degree is in addition to the lordosis achieved by the TLIF itself. Shaffrey reports a total increase in lordosis at 15–20 degrees per level when using this technique [30].

Question 48

For which of the following spinal levels is lateral lumbar interbody fusion (LLIF) not recommended?

A. L1-2
B. L3-2
C. L3-4
D. L4-5
E. L5-S1

Response (**E**) It is suggested to refrain from using the LLIF approach for fusion at the L5-S1 level due to the risk of damage to the iliac vessels as well as unfavorable access to the disk space due to the iliac crest.

Question 49

Which of the following is not considered an advantage of cervical laminoplasty over anterior cervical discectomy and fusion (ACDF)?

A. Lower incidence of complications compared to ACDF
B. Lower incidence of adjacent segment disease compared to ACDF
C. Preserved cervical range of motion
D. Allows foraminotomy to be performed simultaneously if needed
E. Allows for correction of alignment

Response (E) Cervical laminoplasty does not allow for the correction of alignment as opposed to ACDF, which can help restore cervical lordosis.

Question 50

Which of the following are types of laminoplasty?

A. Open door laminoplasty
B. Double open-door laminoplasty
C. Closed-door laminoplasty
D. A and B
E. B and C

Response (D) The two types of laminoplasty include the open door and double open-door approaches. The open-door approach involves drilling a trough on one side of the vertebra to create a hinge and then drilling out an open area of the lamina on the contralateral side. The spinous process is also removed at the base and is used as a graft on the open side to expand the canal. In the double open-door laminoplasty, bilateral laminar troughs are drilled. Additionally, a trough is drilled in the spinous process until dura is exposed. Finally, either iliac or artificial graft is placed within the spinous process window [31].

Question 51

Which of the following is not true regarding postoperative C5 palsy post cervical decompression?

A. Patients whose muscle power is antigravity often have a low likelihood of recovering function.
B. Patients with poor motor exams as a result of the palsy have a low likelihood of recovering function.
C. It is thought to be due to dorsal migration of the spinal cord resulting in traction of the C5 nerve root.
D. It is most likely to occur after laminectomy and fusion.
E. The mean recovery time is 21 weeks.

Response (A) All of the above are true regarding postoperative C5 palsy except answer A. Patients with preserved antigravity function often recover to full strength, unlike patients with significant postoperative deficits.

Question 52

Which of the following is the most suitable surgical approach for a patient with central and calcified thoracic disc herniation but has bronchiectasis?

A. Traditional open thoracotomy
B. Retro-pleural approach using a tubular retractor
C. Transforaminal endoscopic approach
D. Mini-thoracotomy approach
E. Oblique paraspinal approach using tubular micro-endoscopic discectomy

Response (B)The traditional open thoracoscopy and mini-thoracotomy approaches are considered the gold standard for central disc herniations. However, both procedures require entry into the chest cavity, increasing the risk of postoperative pulmonary complications such as atelectasis, pneumonitis, pleuritis, and intercostal neuralgia. An oblique retropleural approach using a tubular retractor is developed to overcome this difficulty. It uses a smaller incision site and provides equally good access to the disc as the transthoracic approaches [32].

Question 53

Which of the following condition is not a contraindication for lateral lumbar interbody fusion (LLIF)?

A. History of diverticulitis
B. L5/S1 disc space access
C. Lumbar spinal stenosis of Schizas grade D
D. Rising psoas sign at L4-L5 level
E. Nerve root anomaly

Response (E)LLIF is suitable for degenerative diseases that require the restoration of the disc height and has a particular advantage in revision cases. Contraindications are mainly secondary to conditions that prevent safe lateral approaches. These can include prior retroperitoneal surgery, L5–S1 disease, high-grade spondylolisthesis, and extreme spinal canal stenosis. However, nerve root anomaly is a relative contraindication for the transforaminal approach, as it can increase the risk of iatrogenic nerve injury in the nerve roots [33].

Question 54

Which of the following is not a benefit of performing image-guided punctate midline myelotomy (PMM) in comparison to the traditional approach?

A. Less disturbance to the posterior structures of the spine
B. Decreased the possibility of subarachnoid hemorrhage
C. Decreased the risk of respiratory dysfunction after the surgery
D. Decreased the length of hospital stay
E. Decreased neurological complications because patients are capable of reporting abnormal sensation or motor function intraoperatively

Response (B) PMM is a surgical procedure that damages the ascending fibers of the postsynaptic dorsal column pathway to interrupt visceral pain transmission. It has the potential to be performed using a minimally invasive approach. However, the feasibility of this technique is still questionable. The percutaneous needle may pierce the meandering dorsal spinal vein, leading to subarachnoid haemorrhage [34].

Question 55

A selective dorsal rhizotomy is one of the oldest standard surgical techniques in treating spasticity. What is the most common perioperative complication after selective dorsal rhizotomy?

A. Bladder dysfunction
B. Paraplegia
C. Lower extremity hyperesthesia
D. Incidental durotomy
E. Deep wound infection

Response (C) Selective dorsal rhizotomy is a procure that divides the posterior nerve rootlets in the lumbosacral region to reduce the level of spasticity, in particular muscle groups of the lower extremity. Despite uncommon, complications of selective dorsal rhizotomy still occur, including paraplegia, sensory loss, hyperesthesia, bowel or bladder incontinence, cerebrospinal leak, and infection. Among these complications, hyperesthesia in the legs is the most common that can last for several months.

Question 56

How many primary ossification centers do C1, C2, and C3 vertebrae contain, respectively?

A. 3, 5, 3
B. 3, 3, 3
C. 5, 3, 1
D. 2, 4, 2
E. 4, 2, 2

Response (A) C1 (atlas) and C2 (axis) vertebrae show unique patterns of ossification. The atlas develops from three primary ossification centers: one anterior arch and two neural arches. The axis develops from five primary ossification centers: two vertically oriented odontoid centers, two neural arches, and one centrum. C3 through L5 vertebrae have a similar pattern of development. Each of these vertebrae has three primary ossification centers: one centrum and two neural arches; however, the shapes of the ossification centers vary between the cervical, thoracic, and lumbar spine.

Question 57

Punctate midline myelotomy (PMM) can be valuable for patients with chronic, intractable visceral pain associated with malignancy of the abdominal or pelvic regions. In managing the pelvic visceral pain that originates from genitalia, rectum, and colon cancer, the incision is commonly made at which spinal cord level?

A. T2
B. T5
C. T9
D. T12
E. L2

Response (C) It is well known that the level of the thoracic spinal cord is usually several segments higher than the corresponding vertebral level. The lesion level is better placed several segments above the innervating segment of the spinal cord. Genitalia, rectum, and colon are innervated by spinal cord segments S2 to S4. An incision at the T9 spinal cord is remote from the spinal segments innervated by afferents of the pelvic organs and thus is generally successful in managing intractable pain associated with these malignancies.

Question 58

Which of the following is not a contraindication for performing an anterior lumbar interbody fusion?

A. Severe loss of disc space height
B. High-grade spondylolisthesis
C. Spinal infection
D. Isthmic spondylolisthesis at L5/S1
E. Solitary kidney on the side of exposure

Response (**A**)Severe loss of disc space height is not a contraindication for ALIF Procedure. In grade 3 and 4 spondylolisthesis, the nerve roots are stretched, which places patients at high risk for nerve root injury without first decompressing the nerve roots. Spinal infection is a contraindication to interbody fusion, given that a foreign body is being placed into infected tissue. For isthmic spondylolisthesis, addition of posterior fusion should strongly be considered because of the inherent instability. Solitary kidney on the side of the exposure would also be considered a contraindication because the anterior approach poses a risk of injury to the ureter [35].

Question 59

A 19-year-old female is brought to the emergency room after a motor vehicle collision. She complains of persistent neck pain without any radiation. On examination, she is neurologically intact. A CT scan of the spine shows bilateral fracture of the C2 pars interarticular is with a displacement of 5.5 mm, severe anterior angulation, and C2-3 facet subluxation. Which of the following is the most rational management strategy for this patient?

A. Soft cervical collar
B. Hard cervical collar
C. Reduction with traction followed by halo immobilization
D. Open reduction and internal fixation
E. Halo-vest orthosis

Response (**D**)Traumatic spondylolisthesis of the axis, also known as a Hangman's Fracture, is a fracture of the pedicles or pars interarticularis of the C2 vertebra. This patient has a type III Hangman's fracture that is greater than 5mm displacement with significant angulation and facet capsule disruption, making reduction with surgical stabilization the most ideal treatment strategy. Cervical collar, halo-vest orthosis, and closed reduction with halo immobilization are only indicated when the patient has either a type I Hangman's fracture (< 3mm horizontal displacement) or type II with 3 to 5 mm displacement [36].

Question 60

Which of the following is not an advisable indication for posterior and transforaminal lumbar interbody fusion approach?

A. Degenerative scoliosis
B. Infection
C. Spondylolisthesis
D. Pseudarthrosis
E. Severe spinal instability

Response (**B**)Acceptable indications for PLIF and TLIF include spondylolisthesis, failure of posterolateral fusion (pseudarthrosis), and degenerative scoliosis. Relative indications for these approaches include degenerative disc disease, high-grade spinal instability, and recurrent disc herniation. Active infection, on the contrary, is a contraindication to PLIF and TLIF due to the high risk of dural tear and possible meningitis. Additionally placement of foreign body in the setting of infection is avoided when able.

Question 61

A 30-year-old woman sustained a complete spinal cord injury after a gunshot to her back. Following the acute phase of injury, she regainedher patellar reflex. Which of the following component must have been intact?

A. Cell bodies in the lower thoracic spinal cord
B. Cell bodies in the lumbar prominence of the spinal cord
C. Corticospinal tract between the brain and lumbar spinal cord
D. Dorsal column–medial lemniscus pathway between the brain and lumbar spinal cord

Response (**B**) A "reflex arc" is made up of five components: a receptor (muscle spindle), an afferent fiber, an integration center (lamina IX of the spinal cord), an efferent fiber (alpha motor neuron), and an effector (muscle). It primarily occurs without the involvement of the central nervous system; the brain only works to suppress the reflex when all spinal circuitry is intact (see Fig. 2.6). This patient had a patellar reflex

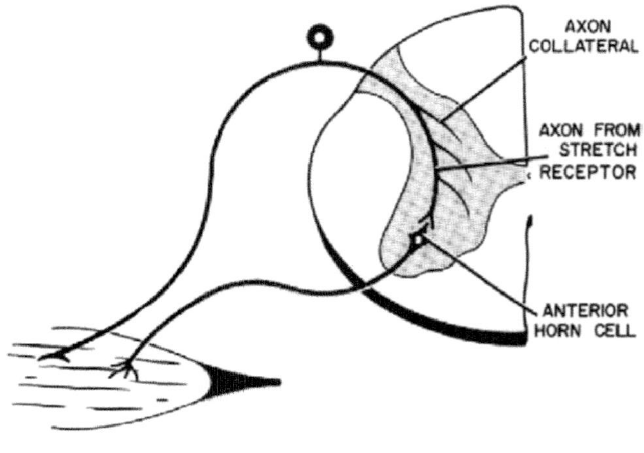

Fig. 2.6 Schematic representation of the monosynaptic stretch reflex

after the injury because her sensory nerves from the patellar tendon, the cell bodies within the lumbar spinal cord, and the motor neurons at the same level were all intact [37].

Question 62

A 41-year-old male was emergently transported to the emergency room after a motor vehicle collision. He was restrained in the front seat with a three-point belt. The patient complained of severe lower back pain but was able to ambulate at the scene. On physical examination, he was fully conscious and vital signs were stable. He has normal motor power in all extremities and no sensory deficit. An antero-posterior radiograph revealed an empty vertebral body sign at T12 level and widening of interspinous processes from T11 to L1. Which of the following is an indication for spine surgery in this patient?

A. Normal neurological exam
B. Additional intrabdominal injury
C. Kyphosis less than 15 degree
D. Ligamentous injury
E. Purely osseous injury

Response (**D**) Chance fracture is a transverse vertebral splitting that extends from the posterior spinal complex to the anterior vertebral body, with no rotation or lateral displacement of the fracture fragments. Treatment options include conservative management through immobilization and surgical stabilization. Unstable posterior elements and ligamentous chance fracture with neurological deficits are indicative for emergent open reduction surgery followed by rehabilitation. In a patient with a bony type of Chance fractures, no neurological deficit, and less than 15-degree kyphosis, conservative management is appropriate.

Question 63

A 61-year-old male with a history of intravenous drug use and diabetes mellitus presents to the clinic with fevers, chills, neck pain, and worsening gait instability. His symptoms have been persistent for more than two weeks. On exam, he has bilateral upper and lower extremity weakness. An MRI of the spine shows anterior cervical epidural access with spinal stenosis. What is the most appropriate next step for this patient?

A. Broad-spectrum intravenous antibiotics
B. CT-guided biopsy and culture
C. Cervical collar with intravenous methylprednisolone
D. Posterior decompressive laminectomy
E. Anterior debridement and interbody fusion with strut grafting

Response (**E**) This patient presents with risk factors (IV drug use, diabetes) and exam findings (fever, motor weakness) concerning spinal epidural abscess. Access draining, necrotic bone debridement, and instrumentation and fusion are necessary for this patient, as he has multiple risk factors. Prophylactic antibiotics should not be given until intraoperative cultures are obtained. Surgical delay for IV steroids is also not supported because this patient has neurological symptoms. The posterior approach is not the best option, given that the cervical abscess is anterior in this patient [38].

Question 64

At which of the following spinal cord levels can the ciliospinal center of Budge be found?

A. C5
B. T1
C. T6
D. L4
E. S1

Response (**B**) The ciliospinal center is located in the intermediolateral horn between C8 and T2. It is a sympathetic nucleus that receives input from the pretectum and sends output to the superior cervical ganglion. It innervates the iris dilator muscle.

Question 65

A 20-year-old student was sent to the emergency room after hitting a sandbank as he dived into the waves. A CT scan of the spine was ordered and found a complete spinal cord injury at the C7 level. Which of the following sets of motions is most likely to still be working in this student?

A. Wrist extension, shoulder abduction, finger flexion, tricep reflex
B. Wrist flexion, elbow extension, thumb extension, bicep reflex,
C. Wrist extension, elbow flexion, forearm supination, brachioradialis reflex
D. Wrist flexion, elbow flexion, thumb extension, bicep reflex

Response (**C**) Patients with a complete injury at C7 level cannot move their legs or trunk. They have weakness in breathing and coughing and have limited use of their hands and fingers. Motions, including finger flexion (C8), wrist flexion (C7), elbow extension (C7), thumb extension (C8), and finger abduction (T1), may be affected by such injury.

Question 66

Which of the following is not an indication for surgical management of rheumatoid arthritis in the cervical spine?

A. A cervico-medullary angle between 135 and 175 degrees
B. Atlantoaxial impaction represented by odontoid migration $\geq$ 5 mm rostral to McGregor's line
C. Progressive neurological deficit
D. Sagittal canal diameter $\leq$ 14 mm in patients with sub axial subluxation
E. Posterior atlantodental interval $\leq$ 14 mm in the setting of atlantoaxial subluxation

Response (A) The cervico-medullary angle can be measured on MRI by drawing a line along the anterior aspect of the cervical spinal cord and the medulla. This angle is an effective indicator of cord distortion from superior migration of the odontoid. It is normally between 135 and 175 degrees. With progressive craniocervical disease, the brainstem angulates ventrally over the displaced odontoid process, leading to increased obliquity of the cervicomedullary angle. Therefore, when the cervicomedullary angle is less than 135 degrees, surgery is indicated in patients with rheumatoid disease of the cervical spine [39].

Question 67

A 43-year-old male with a history of alcoholism presents to the emergency room after collapsing while having a seizure. He is conscious and reports severe low back pain coupled with leg weakness that makes him unable to walk. On examination, he is ASIA grade B. Initial CT scan reveals a burst fracture at L1 vertebra with 65% retropulsion into the spinal canal and translation of L1 on L2. MRI spine with and without contrast further shows significant edema disrupting interspinous ligaments and ligamentum flavum. Which of the following options is most likely recommended to this patient?

A. Pain control and early mobilization in a turtle shell type brace
B. Reassessment upon return of Osinski reflex
C. Posterior lumbar laminectomy
D. Corpectomy with interbody cage placement
E. Corpectomy with interbody cage placement and instrumented fusion

Response (E) According to the Thoracolumbar Injury Classification and Severity Score (TLICS), this patient has a highly unstable burst fracture with a TLICS of 9 (translation, injured posterior ligamentous complex, and incomplete cord injury) (see Fig. 2.7). Conservative treatment is only indicated in stable burst fracture without neurological deficit. We can also assume from the ASIA impairment scale that the patient's Osinski reflex is intact. The best surgical option to maximize structural stability is decompression through vertebral corpectomy with the placement of an interbody cage, followed by posterior instrumentation [40].

Question 68

With regard to ossification of the posterior longitudinal ligament (OPLL) and degenerative cervical myelopathy, a posterior approach is preferred in which of the following indications?

A. K-line (+) OPLL with canal-occupying ratio < 50 to 60%
B. K-line (−) OPLL regardless of the canal-occupying ratio
C. K-line (+) OPLL with canal-occupying ratio > 60%
D. Preexisting cervical kyphosis
E. None of the above

Response (A) Posterior approach is preferred for K-line (+) OPLL with canal-occupying ratio < 50–60% and for multi-level degenerative cervical myelopathy. The anterior approach is preferred for K-line (−) OPLL, K-line (+) with canal occupying ratio > 60% and degenerative cervical myelopathy with preexisting cervical kyphosis. However, the anterior approach is associated with increased rates of complications and thereby needs to be weighed carefully during the decision-making process [41].

Question 69

After lifting a heavy load, a 46-year-old construction worker presents with an immediate onset of right leg burning pain. The pain exacerbates by coughing, sneezing, and sitting. Physical examination shows severe weakness in hip abduction, knee flexion, and foot dorsiflexion on the right. Which direction is the structure implicated in this patient's presentation most likely displaced?

Fig. 2.7 Table demonstrating the Thoracolumbar injury classification and severity score [40]

TLICS Independent Predictors		Score	Method
Morphology Immediate stability	- Compression	1	Radiographs, CT scan
	- Burst	2	
	- Translation/rotation	3	
	- Distraction	4	
Integrity of PLC Long-term stability	- Intact	0	MRI scan
	- Suspected	2	
	- Injured	3	
Neurological status	- Intact	0	Physical examination
	- Nerve root	2	
	- Complete cord injury	2	
	- Incomplete cord injury	3	
	- Cauda equina	3	
Total Score		0 to 3	Conservative treatment
		4	Surgeon's choice
		>4	Surgery

A. Central posterior
B. Lateral
C. Posterolateral
D. Anterior
E. Inferio-medial

Response (**C**) Protrusions of nucleus pulpous through annulus fibrosis are most likely to occur posterolaterally at the level of L4-L5 or L5-S1. The presence of a thicker posterior longitudinal ligament in the center prevents the disc from herniating directly posteriorly, and the annulus fibrosis is thinner on the posterolateral aspect, making it vulnerable for herniation. Pain from lumbar disc herniation arises from the protruding material exerting pressure on the nerve root(s).

Question 70

A 39-year-old woman presents to the emergency department with postural abnormality. She was admitted to the hospital three weeks ago for a non-traumatic pontine and midbrain intracranial hemorrhage. On examination, the patient had significant head nodding, bilateral flexion of the upper extremities, and bilateral extension of the lower extremities. Which extrapyramidal tract is most likely to facilitate this patient's postural abnormality?

A. Reticulospinal tracts
B. Rubrospinal tract
C. Corticobulbar tract
D. Olivospinal tract
E. Tectospinal tract

Response (**B**)This patient's presentation is consistent with decorticate rigidity. The rubrospinal tract, which originates from the red nucleus, travels adjacent to the lateral corticospinal tract and ends in the upper cervical segments of the spinal cord. When there is an injury distal to the red nucleus, the rubrospinal tract becomes overactivated, leading to an unimpeded flexion reflex of the upper limbs. The vestibulospinal tract is also left disinhibited, thereby induce biased extension of the lower limbs [42].

Question 71

A 13-year-old boy presents to the clinic complaining of progressive low back pain for the last month. He plays ice hockey in school and trains at least four times a week. The pain is located at the lumbar region, non-radiating, and exacerbates by extension or twisting of the spine. What is the most likely diagnosis?

A. Pars interarticularis fracture
B. Lumbar disc herniation
C. Sprain/strain injuries
D. Vertebra fracture

Response (**A**)Spondylolysis is a common identifiable cause of low back pain in young athletes participating in sports, particularly those involving repetitive hyperextension and axial loading of the spine. Gymnastics, weight-lifters, divers, rowers, and tennis players have higher rates of this injury. There is no sciatica or leg pain for a disc herniation diagnosis. Spinal sprain/strain injures may be a possibility, but the symptoms should subside with pain medications and rest within a few weeks. The patient also did not experience acute trauma, making vertebra fracture less likely.

Question 72

A 63-year-old male underwent decompressive laminectomy for lumbar stenosis and neurogenic claudication. The patient complains of persistent pain at the surgical site postoperatively, especially when walking. He has no fever and no wound drainage. His C-reactive protein level and erythrocyte sedimentation rate are within normal limits. What is the next step in management?

A. MRI scan
B. Increase opioid dosage
C. Digital Motion X-ray
D. Antibiotics

Response (**C**) Joint instability is a common complication for laminectomy of the spine because off disruption of many of the bony stabilizing structures during the procedure. Patients experiencing postoperative spinal instability often present with characteristic localized pain, especially during ambulation. Digital motion X-ray (DMX) can provide clear images being able to see the bones in motion. The probability of discitis in this patient is also very low, as his erythrocyte sedimentation rate and C-reactive protein levels are normal as well as there is no constitutional symptoms [43].

Question 73

Generally, the indications for anterior lumbar interbody fusion (ALIF) and lateral lumbar interbody fusion (LLIF) at the L4-5 level are similar. However, which of the following complications seen in ALIF is normally avoided in LLIF when performing the surgery at the L4-L5 level?

A. Vascular injury
B. Interbody subsidence
C. Neurologic injury
D. Retrograde ejaculation
E. Incisional hernia

Response (**D**) Complication rates appear similar to ALIF (26.6%) and LLIF (25%). However, their complication profiles differ slightly. LLIF gains access to the lumbar spine via a lateral approach that passes through the retroperitoneal fat and psoas major. It thus avoids the peritoneal contents, sympathetic chain, and great vessels, which are all potential injury sites in ALIF. The risk of injury to the superior hypogastric plexus, which leads to retrograde ejaculation in men, is reported to be less than 3% in ALIF and has not been reported yet in LLIF.

Question 74

Which of the following ligaments attach to a spinous process?

A. Anterior longitudinal ligament
B. Posterior longitudinal ligament
C. Nuchal ligament
D. Ligamentum flavum

Response (**C**) The inferior part of the nuchal ligament attaches to the C7 spinous process. None of the remaining answers A, B, D attach to any spinous processes.

Question 75

Which of the following correctly lists the embryological progression of somatogenesis?

A. Paraxial mesoderm → Somite → Ventromedial Sclerotomes → Dorsolateral dermomyotomes
B. Somite → Ventromedial Sclerotomes →Paraxial mesoderm → Dorsolateral dermomyotomes
C. Dorsolateral dermomyotomes → Ventromedial Sclerotomes →Paraxial mesoderm → Somite
D. Somite → Paraxial mesoderm → Dorsolateral dermomyotomes → Ventromedial Sclerotomes

Response (**A**) This is the proper progression of somatogenesis for the bony development of the vertebral body.

Question 76

Which gene is specifically responsible for the shape of the vertebral body?

A. ATM
B. FXN
C. HOX
D. ATP7B

Response (**C**) the Hox and SHH gene controls the shape of the vertebral body. ATM gene is associated with ataxia-telangiectasia. FXN is associated with Friedreich ataxia. ATP7B is associated with Wilson disease [44].

Question 77

There are ______ primary ossification centers and ______ secondary ossifications for the bony development of the vertebrae.

A. Two, Four
B. Four, Two
C. Three, Four
D. Three, Five

Response (**D**) C3 through L5 have one primary ossification center for the vertebral body and two primary ossification centers that each contribute to one-half of each vertebral arch. There is one secondary ossification center for superior and inferior endplates, one at each end of the transverse processes, and one for the spinous process [45].

Question 78

Which pair of spinal curves is not present during the fetal period?

A. Thoracic, Lumbar
B. Lumbar, Sacral
C. Thoracic, Cervical
D. Cervical, Lumbar

Response (**D**) The cervical lordosis curve forms after time as the infant works on learning to hold their head up. The lumbar lordosis curve forms later as the infant learn how to walk. The thoracic and sacral curves are present in the fetus.

Question 79

Lateral masses are composed of which of the following?

A. Superior and inferior articulating processes
B. Bilateral lamina
C. Superior and inferior transverse processes
D. Ipsilateral and contralateral lamina

Response (**A**) The lateral mass does not begin until the lateral junction of the lamina and the pedicle. The transverse processes have no contributions to the lateral mass. The lateral masses are made from the superior and inferior articulating surfaces that form the facet joint [46].

Question 80

What is the theoretical benefit of approaching the anterior cervical spine from the left side?

A. Lower risk of bradycardia
B. Lower risk of recurrent laryngeal nerve injury (RLN)
C. Lower risk of postoperative facial droop
D. Elevated risk of thoracic duct injury during a right-sided approach
E. Lower risk of phrenic nerve injury

Response (**B**) Based on a purely anatomical basis, there is thought to be a lower risk of damage to the recurrent laryngeal nerve when using a left-sided approach to the anterior cervical spine. This is due to a more anterolateral course of the nerve outside the tracheoesophageal groove. However, studies have not demonstrated a significant difference in RLN injury in the left-sided approach compared to the right-sided approach.

References

1. Rucco V, Basadonna PT, Gasparini D. Anatomy of the iliolumbar ligament: a review of its anatomy and a magnetic resonance study. Am J Phys Med Rehabil. 1996;75(6):451–5. https://doi.org/10.1097/00002060-199611000-00010. PMID: 8985109
2. Malek E, Faddoul DG, Baydoun H, Omeis I, Makki A. Reversible acute anterior longitudinal ligament calcification with retropharyngeal inflammation. J ClinRheumatol. 2021;27(4):e123–5. https://doi.org/10.1097/RHU.0000000000000878. PMID: 30142115.
3. Ohara Y. Ossification of the ligaments in the cervical spine, including ossification of the anterior longitudinal ligament, ossification of the posterior longitudinal ligament, and ossification of the ligamentum flavum. NeurosurgClin N Am. 2018;29(1):63–8. https://doi.org/10.1016/j.nec.2017.09.018. PMID: 29173437.
4. Gala FB, Aswani Y. Imaging in spinal posterior epidural space lesions: a pictorial essay. Indian J Radiol Imaging. 2016;26(3):299–315. https://doi.org/10.4103/0971-3026.190406.
5. Wu ZH, Zheng Y, Yin QS, Ma XY, Yin YH. Anterior pedicle screw fixation of C2: an anatomic analysis of axis morphology and simulated surgical fixation. Eur Spine J. 2014;23(2):356–61. https://doi.org/10.1007/s00586-013-3042-8.
6. Scali F, Marsili ES, Pontell ME. Anatomical connection between the rectus capitis posterior major and the dura mater, Spine. 2011;36(25):E1612–4

7. Mysorekar VR, Nandedkar AN. Surface area of the atlanto-occipital articulations. Acta Anat (Basel). 1986;126 (4):223–5. https://doi.org/10.1159/000146221. PMID: 3766103.
8. Er U, Fraser F, Lanzino G. The anterior spinal artery origin: a microanatomical study; Spinal Cord. 2008;46(1):45–9. https://doi.org/10.1038/sj.sc.3102060
9. Dominik T, Bendik S, Przemysław AP, Wan CH, Roberto C, Jerzy AW, Shane Tubbs R, Krzysztof AT, Brandon MH. Artery of Adamkiewicz: a meta-analysis of anatomical characteristics. Neuroradiology. 2019;61(8): 869–80. Published online 2019 Apr 27. https://doi.org/10.1007/s00234-019-02207-y. PMCID: PMC6620248
10. Shuaifeng Y, Yunfan Z, Kai W, Yingchao H, Kai Z, Fan H, Jun T. Three-dimensional morphological characteristics of lower lumbar intervertebral foramen with age. Biomed Res Int. 2018;2018:8157061. Published online 2018 Nov 11. https://doi.org/10.1155/2018/8157061. PMCID: PMC6252236
11. Katsunari A. Vascular anatomy of the cauda equina and its implication on the vascular lesions in the caudal spinal structure. Neurol Med Chir (Tokyo) 2016;56(6):310–6. Published online 2016 Mar 28. https://doi.org/10.2176/nmc.ra.2016-0006
12. Jae-Chil C, Hyung-Ki P, Soon-Kwan C. Posterior cervical inclinatory foraminotomy for spondylotic radiculopathy preliminary. J Korean Neurosurg Soc. 2011;49(5):308–13. Published online 2011 May 31. https://doi.org/10.3340/jkns.2011.49.5.308. PMCID: PMC3115157
13. Christensen FB, Bünger CE. Retrograde ejaculation after retroperitoneal lower lumbar interbody fusion. Int Orthop. 1997;21(3):176–80. https://doi.org/10.1007/s002640050145.
14. Enyo Y, Yamada H, Kim JH, Yoshida M, Hutton WC. Microendoscopic lateral decompression for lumbar foraminal stenosis. J Spinal Disord Tech. 2014;27:257–62. https://doi.org/10.1097/BSD.0b013e31828cff6e.
15. Tubbs RS, Demerdash A, Rizk E, Chapman JR, Oskouian RJ. Complications of transoral and transnasal odontoidectomy: a comprehensive review. Childs NervSyst. 2016;32:55–9.
16. Sabiston CP, Wing PC, Schweigel JF, Van Peteghem PK, Yu WI. Closed reduction of dislocations of the lower cervical spine. J Trauma. 1988;28(6):832–5.
17. Ozgur BM, Aryan HE, Pimenta L, Taylor WR. Extreme Lateral Interbody Fusion (XLIF): a novel surgical technique for anterior lumbar interbody fusion. Spine J. 2006;6(4):435–43.
18. Davis TT, Hynes RA, Fung DA, Spann SW, MacMillan M, Kwon B, Liu J, Acosta F, Drochner TE. Retroperitoneal oblique corridor to the L2–S1 intervertebral discs in the lateral position: an anatomic study. J Neurosurg: Spine. 2014;21(5):785–93.
19. Fountas KN, Kapsalaki EZ, Nikolakakos LG, Smisson HF, Johnston KW, Grigorian AA, Lee GP, Robinson JS Jr. Anterior cervical discectomy and fusion associated complications. Spine. 2007;32(21):2310–7.
20. Yüksel KZ, Yüksel M, Gonzalez LF, Baek S, Heiserman JE, Sonntag VK, Crawford NR. Occipitocervical vertical distraction injuries: anatomical biomechanical, and 3-tesla magnetic resonance imaging investigation. Spine. 2008;33(19):2066–73.
21. Leijnse JN, D'Herde K. Revisiting the segmental organization of the human spinal cord. J Anat. 2016;229(3):384–93.
22. Siu TLT, Lin K. Direct tubular lumbar microdiscectomy for far lateral disc herniation: a modified approach. Orthop Surg. 2016;8 (3):301–8. https://doi.org/10.1111/os.12263. PMID: 27627712.
23. Hwang K, Kim JY, Lim JH. Anatomy of the platysma muscle. J Craniofac Surg. 2017;28(2):539–42. https://doi.org/10.1097/SCS.0000000000003318.
24. Yang BP, Ondra SL, Chen LA, Jung HS, Koski TR, Salehi SA. Clinical and radiographic outcomes of thoracic and lumbar pedicle subtraction osteotomy for fixed sagittal imbalance. J Neurosurg Spine. 2006;5(1):9–17. https://doi.org/10.3171/spi.2006.5.1.
25. Yang BP, Ondra SL, Chen LA, Jung HS, Koski TR, Salehi SA. Clinical and radiographic outcomes of thoracic and lumbar pedicle subtraction osteotomy for fixed sagittal imbalance. J Neurosurg Spine. 2006;5(1):9–17. https://doi.org/10.3171/spi.2006.5.1.9.
26. Bunmaprasert T, Chaibhuddanugul N, Keeratiruangrong J, Raphitphan R, Sugandhavesa N, Liawrungrueang W. Corrective osteotomy of global sagittal imbalance in the neglected fracture-dislocation thoracic spine. Trauma Case Rep. 2021;32:100409. https://doi.org/10.1016/j.tcr.2021.100409. eCollection 2021 Apr
27. Vannucci F, Araújo JA. Thoracic sympathectomy for hyperhidrosis: from surgical indications to clinical results. J Thorac Dis. 2017;9(Suppl 3):S178–92. https://doi.org/10.21037/jtd.2017.04.04
28. Siribumrungwong K, Sinchai C, Tangtrakulwanich B, Chaiyamongkol W. Reliability and accuracy of palpable anterior neck landmarks for the identification of cervical spinal levels. Asian Spine J. 2018;12(1):80–4. https://doi.org/10.4184/asj.2018.12.1.80.
29. Uribe JS, Arredondo N, Dakwar E, et al. Defining the safe working zones using the minimally invasive lateral retroperitoneal transpsoas approach: an anatomical study. J Neurosurg Spine. 2010;13:260–6
30. Jagannathan J, Sansur CA, Oslouian RJ, et al. Radiographic restoration of lumbar alignment after transforaminal lumbar interbody fusion. Neurosurgery. 2009;64:955–64
31. Kurokawa R, Kim P. Cervical Laminoplasty: The History and the Future. Neurol Med Chir (Tokyo). 2015;55(7):529-39. https://doi.org/10.2176/nmc.ra.2014-0387
32. Sharma SB, Kim JS. A review of minimally invasive surgical techniques for the management of thoracic disc herniations. Neurospine. 2019;16(1):24–33. https://doi.org/10.14245/ns.1938014.007.
33. Ishii K, Isogai N, Shiono Y, et al. Contraindication of minimally invasive lateral interbody fusion for percutaneous reduction of degenerative spondylolisthesis: a new radiographic indicator of bony lateral recess stenosis using i line. Asian Spine J. 8 2021;15 (4):455–63.https://doi.org/10.31616/asj.2020.0083
34. Hong D, Andrén-Sandberg A. Punctate midline myelotomy: a minimally invasive procedure for the treatment of pain in inextirpable abdominal and pelvic cancer. J Pain Symptom Manage. 2007;33(1):99–109. https://doi.org/10.1016/j.jpainsymman.2006.06.012. PMID: 17196911.
35. Mobbs RJ, Phan K, Malham G, Seex K, Rao PJ. Lumbar interbody fusion: techniques, indications and comparison of interbody fusion options including PLIF, TLIF, MI-TLIF, OLIF/ATP. LLIF and ALIF J Spine Surg. 2015;1(1):2–18. https://doi.org/10.3978/j.issn.2414-469X.2015.10.05.
36. Murphy H, Schroeder GD, Shi WJ, Kepler CK, Kurd MF, Fleischman AN, Kandziora F, Chapman JR, Benneker LM, Vaccaro AR. Management of Hangman's Fractures: A Systematic Review. J Orthop Trauma. 2017;31 Suppl 4:S90-S95. https://doi.org/10.1097/BOT.0000000000000952uns
37. Trontelj MA, Trontelj JV. Reflex arc of the first component of the human blink reflex: a single motoneurone study. J NeurolNeurosurg Psychiatry. 1978;41(6):538–47. https://doi.org/10.1136/jnnp.41.6.538.
38. Al-Hourani K, Al-Aref R, Mesfin A. Upper cervical epidural abscess in clinical practice: diagnosis and management. Global Spine J. 2016;6(4):383–93. https://doi.org/10.1055/s-0035-1565260.
39. Mallory GW, Halasz SR, Clarke MJ. Advances in the treatment of cervical rheumatoid: Less surgery and less morbidity. World J Orthop. 2014;5(3):292–303. Published 2014 Jul 18. https://doi.org/10.5312/wjo.v5.i3.292
40. Lee JY, Vaccaro AR, Lim MR, et al. Thoracolumbar injury classification and severity score: a new paradigm for the treatment

of thoracolumbar spine trauma. J Orthop Sci. 2005;10(6):671–5. https://doi.org/10.1007/s00776-005-0956-y.
41. Kwok SSS, Cheung JPY. Surgical decision-making for ossification of the posterior longitudinal ligament versus other types of degenerative cervical myelopathy: anterior versus posterior approaches. BMC MusculoskeletDisord. 2020;21:823. https://doi.org/10.1186/s12891-020-03830-0.
42. Riddle CN, Edgley SA, Baker SN. Direct and indirect connections with upper limb motoneurons from the primate reticulospinal tract. J Neurosci. 2009;29(15):4993–9. https://doi.org/10.1523/JNEUROSCI.3720-08.2009.
43. Bisschop A, van Royen BJ, Mullender MG, et al. Which factors prognosticate spinal instability following lumbar laminectomy? Eur Spine J. 2012;21(12):2640–8. https://doi.org/10.1007/s00586-012-2250-y.
44. Mallo M, Wellik DM, Deschamps J. Hox genes and regional patterning of the vertebrate body plan. Dev Biol. 2010;344(1):7–15.
45. Baumgart M, Wiśniewski M, Grzonkowska M, et al. Digital image analysis of ossification centers in the axial dens and body in the human fetus. Surg Radiol Anat. 2016;38(10):1195–203.
46. Pait TG, McAllister PV, Kaufman HH. Quadrant anatomy of the articular pillars (lateral cervical mass) of the cervical spine. J Neurosurg. 1995;82(6):1011–4. https://doi.org/10.3171/jns.1995.82.6.1011.

Instrumentation

3

Asham Khan, Moleca M. Ghannam, Ryan M. Hess, Slah Khan, Alexander O. Aguirre, Cathleen C. Kuo, Ali Y. Elkady, Ahmed H. Omar, Mohammad Elbaroody, and Mohamed A. R. Soliman

Question 1

What complication is seen with lateral breach of a lateral mass screw in the fixation of C2?

A. Spinal cord durotomy
B. Vertebral artery injury
C. Disruption of the atlantoaxial joint
D. Screw loosening

Response (**B**) The vertebral artery is located just laterally to the lateral mass of the C2 vertebral body. The other options are associated with a superior or medial breach of the lateral mass screw [1].

A. Khan · M. M. Ghannam · R. M. Hess · S. Khan · A. O. Aguirre · C. C. Kuo · M. A. R. Soliman (✉)
Department of Neurosurgery, University at Buffalo, Buffalo, NY, USA
e-mail: msolim8@uwo.ca

A. Khan
e-mail: akhan@ubns.com

M. M. Ghannam
e-mail: mghannam@ubns.com

R. M. Hess
e-mail: rhess@ubns.com

S. Khan
e-mail: slahkhan@buffalo.edu

A. O. Aguirre
e-mail: aa284@buffalo.edu

C. C. Kuo
e-mail: ckuo9@buffalo.edu

A. Y. Elkady · A. H. Omar · M. Elbaroody · M. A. R. Soliman
Department of Neurosurgery, Cairo University, Cairo, Egypt
e-mail: ayousri54@gmail.com

A. H. Omar
e-mail: a.hussein.omar1990@gmail.com

M. Elbaroody
e-mail: mohammad.elbaroody@kasralainy.edu.eg

Question 2

Which of the following is the benefit of using cross-links in spinal instrumentation?

A. Increase in torsional (rotation) stiffness.
B. Increase resistance to lateral bend.
C. Increase in axial stiffness.
D. Increase resistance to flexion/extension.
E. Increase fusion rate.

Response (**A**) Adding cross-links to spinal instrumentations can increase torsional (rotational) stiffness, which is especially crucial for long constructs. There are no significant changes in implants' axial, flexural/extensional, and lateral stiffness with the addition of either the cross-links or segmental medical screws [2].

Question 3

Which of the following is <u>**not**</u> a known risk factor for proximal junctional kyphosis after a spinal fusion?

A. Large preoperative sagittal parameters.
B. Greater curvature correction.
C. Anterior–posterior spinal fusion.
D. Male sex.

Response (**D**) Large preoperative sagittal parameters, greater curvature correction, and anterior–posterior spinal fusion are all known risk factors that increase the risk of a proximal junctional kyphosis occurring after a spinal fusion [3].

Question 4

In those with SI joint injury undergoing either open or percutaneous placement of sacroiliac screws as part of a

C. Gragnaniello et al. (eds.), *MCQs in Spine Surgery*,
https://doi.org/10.1007/978-3-031-69332-8_3

longer lumbosacral construct, what is required to ensure the safety of the patient and good clinical outcome?

A. Fracture reduction.
B. Dissection of surrounding soft tissue.
C. Removal of any invasive vasculature.
D. Retraction of the pudendal nerve.

Response (**A**) A fracture reduction is mandatory when placing an iliosacral screw as this is key in the final alignment for long term fusion. Complications related to SI screw placement are usually caused by inadequate appreciation of the pelvic anatomy due to osseous injury, anatomical variability, and displacement. Several neurovascular structures are in the vicinity of the posterior ilium and sacrum and can be damaged during this procedure but it is not necessary for these to be exposed, removed, or retracted. The L5, S1, or S2 nerve roots and the common iliac vessels are in close relationship to the sacrum. If a guide wire or drill is aberrantly placed into the greater sciatic notch, damage to the sciatic nerve, superior and inferior gluteal neurovascular bundles, pudendal nerve, and internal pudendal artery/vein could occur. In addition, branches of the superior gluteal neurovascular bundle are at risk during the procedure while passing through the abductor musculature [4].

Question 5

Which of the following is true regarding CT myelography?

A. It is an indirect spinal imaging method.
B. It carries extremely high specificity.
C. Can diagnose the pathology of compressive lesions.
D. It is a non-invasive procedure.

Response (**A**) This procedure carries low specificity, cannot diagnose the pathology of compressive lesions and is an invasive procedure. Therefore, A is the only correct answer. It is an indirect, rather than direct, assessment of extradural compression as diagnosis can be inferred based on changes in the contour of the contrast-filled thecal sac and nerve root sleeves [5].

Question 6

Management of adult spinal deformities often involves long thoracolumbar fusions. What is the major advantage of selecting sacrum over L5 as the caudal extent of fusion?

A. Improved correction and maintenance of sagittal balance.
B. Decreased risk of pseudarthrosis.
C. Improvement in pain and disability.
D. Decreased major medical complication rates.
E. Improved curve correction in the coronal plane.

Response (**A**) Fusion to the sacrum achieves a better correction of sagittal imbalance than fusion to L5. Proponents of ending fusions at L5, on the other hand, often cite three main reasons: decreased complication rate (pseudoarthrosis and implant-related complications), maintenance of lumbosacral motion, and avoiding possible anterior surgery at L5-S1. There is no difference in medical complication rate, coronal plane curve correction, and postoperative pain and disability between these two approaches, as assessed by VAS (visual analogue score) score and ODI (Oswestry disability index), respectively [6].

Question 7

Which of the following is not a risk from ionizing radiation exposure?

A. Temporary or permeant sterility.
B. Glaucoma.
C. Depression of hematopoiesis.
D. Heart disease.

Response (**B**) All the risks are impacted by ionizing radiation, although in the eyes, this manifests as cataracts, not glaucoma. The remaining options are all true.

Question 8

If an autologous bone stem cell harvest were to occur during a spine surgery, what nerve would be at risk by the instrumentation trajectory?

A. Lateral femoral cutaneous nerve.
B. Ilio-hypogastric nerve.
C. Ilioinguinal nerve.
D. All of the above.

Response (**D**) All of the following nerves would be at risk from the instrumentation during this stem cell harvest [7].

Question 9

If a lateral lumbar interbody fusion was completed while the patient was in the right lateral decubitus position and the distal tip was placed too anteriorly, which vessel would be at the greatest risk of injury or rupture?

A. Inferior vena cava.
B. Segmental artery.
C. Abdominal aorta.
D. Iliolumbar vein.

Response (**A**) The patient would be placed with the right side of their body down, with the surgical approach occurring from the left. An anterior cage placement would have the greatest probability of injuring the vessel on the contralateral side, which would be the inferior vena cava. The iliolumbar vein and segmental arteries are more lateral and would not have a risk of damage from the distal tip of the interbody.

Question 10

When doing a posterior lumbar interbody fusion (PLIF) for treating disc pathology, which of the following parts of the vertebral bone must be removed to place the interbody cage safely?

A. Lamina.
B. Facet joint.
C. Both A and B.
D. Neither A nor B.

Response (**A**) At least a part of the lamina MUST be removed to place an interbody through the PLIF approach. The interbody cage can safely be placed while keeping the facet joint intact [8].

Question 11

Regarding dynamic stabilization of the spine, all of the following are true, **EXCEPT**:

A. It is a concept of placing anchors into the spine connected with a flexible longitudinal member (e.g. rod).
B. The goal of this type of implant is to eliminate the motion.
C. This type of implant will produce less stress on the adjacent spinal segments and may prevent adjacent-level degenerative changes.
D. Without concurrent spinal arthrodesis, these implants may loosen or fail prematurely and require revision surgery.

Response (**B**) The goal of this type of implant is to constrain but not eliminate motion. The other answers are correct [9].

Question 12

Regarding anterior spinal instrumentation, which one of the following is true?

A. Restoration of spinal alignment is not required before plate application.
B. Even with significant coronal or sagittal plane deformity, the plating system can be placed.
C. In short-segment spinal problems, anterior plating systems permit corrective forces to be applied directly to spinal segments, thereby restoring spinal alignment.
D. The anterior plating system can be used alone for tumors, burst fractures, and degenerative spinal disorders requiring anterior fusion over one or two levels.

Response (**C**) Restoration of spinal alignment is mandatory before plate application. Technical difficulties for the anterior plating system arise because restoration of spinal alignment is required before plate application, especially in the presence of significant spinal deformity. Tumors, burst fractures, and degenerative spinal disorders requiring anterior fusion over one or two levels are indications for using an anterior plating system however this is in conjunction with decompression of cord or nerves as well as it is recommended to posteriorly supplement it [10].

Question 13

Regarding spinal implants, all of the following are true, **EXCEPT:**

A. Short-term stabilization of the spine is provided by spinal implants, while long-term stabilization of the spine is traditionally provided by fusion.
B. Autograft bone (e.g. fibula) can be used as an intercolumn implant to promote fusion.
C. Polymethylmethacrylate [PMMA] cannot be used as a spacer to reconstruct an anterior spinal column defect.
D. Disc spacer can be used to maintain segmental mobility, stability, and disc space height without fusion.

Response (**C**) Certain intracolumn implants (e.g. polymethylmethacrylate [PMMA]) are intended to function as an anterior column spacer despite lack of potential for biologic incorporation; PMMA is used as a spacer to reconstruct an anterior spinal column defect; anterior spinal reconstruction of metastatic vertebral body lesions in patients with a finite lifespan; or reconstruction of osteoporotic compression fractures. Vertebroplasty and kyphoplasty procedures involve the injection of PMMA into the vertebral bodies to alleviate pain secondary to acute and subacute fractures.

Question 14

Regarding C2 screws, which one of the following is **false**?

A. C2 pedicle screw trajectory is more medial and superior than the pars screw.
B. C2 pedicle screw has greater risk of injury to a high riding vertebral artery.
C. A longer screw may be achieved using a C2 pedicle screw than C2 pars screw.
D. C2 pars screw can be safely placed with bi-cortical screw purchase.

Response (**D**) A C2 pars screw is typically a unicortical screw that stops short of the transverse foramen to prevent potential injury to the vertebral artery. The C2 pedicle is located medial to the pars and is more superiorly oriented. High riding vertebral artery and narrow C2 pedicle are two anatomical variations that increase risk of vertebral artery injury in placement of cervical pedicle screws [11, 12].

Question 15

Regarding C1–C2 screws, which one of the following is true?

A. In case of vertebral artery anomalies, transarticular screw is less preferred.
B. Transarticular screws are more versatile than C1–C2 screw-rod systems.
C. Preoperative reduction of the C1–C2 joints is mandatory before the placement of the C1–C2 screw-rod system.
D. Posterior wire/cable techniques or rod-clamps should be complementary in every case.

Response (**A**) C1–C2 screw rod systems can be used in cases where transarticular screws are contraindicated (e.g., vertebral artery anomalies, severe kyphosis). Screw rod systems are more versatile and allowing for different screw placement (laminar, pars, pedicle etc.) when compared to transarticular screws. C1–C2 joints can be reduced intraoperatively. Preoperative reduction is not a prerequisite nor is it always possible. Posterior wire/cable techniques or rod-clamps are not complementary in every case and can be used alone when other techniques are not feasible [13].

Question 16

Regarding subaxial cervical spine instrumentation, all of the followings are true, **EXCEPT**:

A. C3–6 pedicle screw placement is not widely practiced owing to the relatively high risk of vertebral artery injury.
B. Compared to posterior wiring or cable fixation, cervical lateral mass fixation significantly increases rotation and extension stability.
C. Loss of wire fixation due to bony pullout or wire failure is the most common complication associated with wire/cable techniques.
D. Rigid external postoperative cervical immobilization should be done with screw fixation techniques.

Response (**D**) Rigid postoperative external cervical immobilization is not mandatory with screw fixation techniques. Screw fixation techniques are an internal brace making additional rigid external cervical immobilization unnecessary [14].

Question 17

Which one of the following regarding L5–S1 fixation is true?

A. 60% of axial load is transmitted through the anterior spinal column, and the remaining 40% is transmitted through the posterior column.
B. The oblique orientation of the L5–S1 disc results in decreased shear forces across this level.
C. The sacrum is composed of cancellous bone and possesses multiple sites for screw fixation.
D. Long-segment fusion constructs (e.g. T10–S1) have a higher failure rate than short-segment constructs (e.g. L4–S1).

Response (**D**) Pseudarthrosis rate increases as the number of levels undergoing fusion increases. Increasing the number of instrumented levels proximal to the sacrum increases the lever arm exerted by the proximal spine on the distal sacral implants. The other options are incorrect because 80% of axial load is transmitted through the anterior spinal column, and the remaining 20% is transmitted through the posterior column. The oblique orientation of the L5–S1 disc results in increased shear forces across this level. The sacrum is composed of cancellous bone and possesses limited sites for screw fixation [15].

Question 18

All of the following structures are at risk when a screw is placed through the anterior cortex of the sacrum, **EXCEPT**:

A. Straight Ventral S1 screw placed without medial angulation, the S1 nerve root is at risk of injury as it crosses the anterior sacrum.
B. Screws placed laterally at the S1 level have greater potential of injuring the lumbosacral trunk or the internal iliac vein.
C. Laterally directed screws at the S2 level can injure the colon.
D. Medially directed S1 screws directed parallel to the upper S1 endplate or toward the sacralpromontory may cause injury to the middle sacral artery and vein.

Response (**A**) Straight Ventral S1 screw placed without medial angulation, the L5 nerve root is at risk of injury where it crosses the anterior sacrum, not the S1 nerve root. All other answers are correct [16].

Question 19

Which of the following is not a contraindication for anterior odontoid screw fixation?

A. Type 3 odontoid fracture.
B. Barrel-shaped chest.
C. Long oblique fracture line that positioned from anterior-caudal to posterior-cranial.
D. Combined 5-mm overhang of the lateral masses of C1 on C2.
E. Disruption of the transverse atlantal ligament.

Response (**D**) Odontoid screw fixation is useful for patients with widely displaced type II odontoid fracture nonunions, fractures (6 mm or more), or patients who are unable to wear a halo brace. There are a variety of contraindications to odontoid screw fixation, including fractures that extend deeply into the body of the dens (type III), severe osteoporosis, irreducible fractures, large chest, short neck, oblique fracture line that positioned from anterior-caudal to posterior-cranial, and fixed cervical flexion deformities. The most significant absolute contraindication is disruption of traverse ligament (defined by the sum of the overhang of C1 lateral mass on C2 exceeds 7 mm) because C1-2 stability cannot be restored by odontoid screw, even if the dens is fixated solidly [17].

Question 20

The following necessitates an occipitocervical fusion **EXCEPT**:

A. Congenital absence of complete Cl arch.
B. Basilar invagination.
C. Congenital anomalies of occipitocervical joints.
D. Type II odontoid fracture.

Response (**D**) Type II odontoid fractures can be treated by an odontoid screw if the TAL is still intact. It is a problem of the atlantoaxial joint and does not necessitate fusion to the occiput. All other answers are indications for occipital cervical fusion [18].

Question 21

In the transoral approach, the patient must be able to open the mouth at least

A. 25 mm.
B. 35 mm.
C. 45 mm.
D. 20 mm.

Response (**A**) The patient needs to be able to open his mouth at least 25 mm; if not, then other approaches such as trans-nasal or trans-labio-mandibular should be considered.

Question 22

In the transoral approach, which anatomical structure can the surgeon palpate to identify the midline?

A. The odontoid process.
B. The arch of C1.
C. The C1 tubercle.
D. None of the above.

Response (**C**) The C1 tubercle can be palpated through the posterior pharynx to locate the midline and for craniocaudal orientations (see Fig. 3.1) [19].

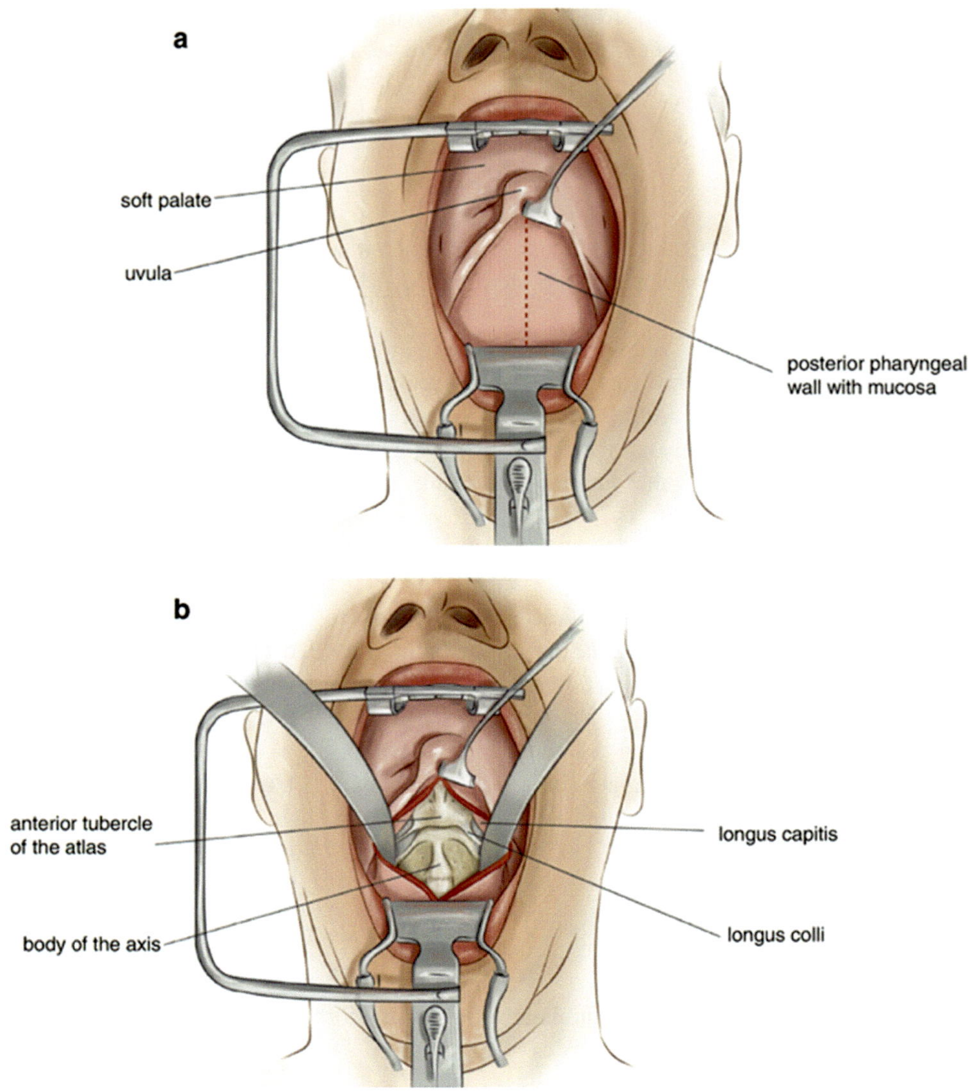

Fig. 3.1 Artist's rendering of transoral approach. The C1 tubercule can be palpated along the posterior pharynx and used to locate midline (Jeszenszky et al. [19])

Question 23

Absolute contraindication of odontoid screw include all of the following **EXCEPT**:

A. Rule of Spence > 7 mm.
B. Type 3 fracture when the fracture line is through the body portion of the body of C2.
C. Fracture line in oblique orientation to frontal plane.
D. If the fracture is greater than six months old.

Response (**D**) The age of fracture is controversial; fusion rates in fractures more than 18 months old were 25% fractures, while fractures less than six months old have 90% fusion rates. The Rule of Spence > 7 mm suggests an TAL disruption which is unstable. This would not be appropriately treated and stabilized with an odontoid screw because of the instability at the C1–C2 joint. An oblique fracture line from posterosuperior to anteroinferior that would parallel screw trajectory is another contraindication to anterior fixation. A shallow Type 3 fracture is unstable, Type II like fracture, and may be treated with an odontoid screw, unlike one with a fracture deeper through the C2 vertebral body.

Question 24

When considering entry point for C3–6 lateral mass screws, which one is correct?

A. In the An method, the screw is placed 1 mm medial to the midpoint and a trajectory of 15° in the cephalad direction and 30° in the lateral direction.

B. In the Magerl method, the screw is placed 2 mm medial to the midpoint and 2 mm cranial to the midpoint in the crania-caudal direction with a trajectory of 20–25° lateral and parallel to the facet joint.
C. In the Roy-Camille method, the screw is placed at the midpoint in the mediolateral direction and craniocaudal direction with a trajectory of 0–10° lateral and 0° craniocaudal.
D. All of the above.

Response (**D**) All of the above are methods for lateral mass screw placement.

Question 25

During anterior lumbar interbody fusion (ALIF) procedure at LS-51 level, which artery has to be sacrificed?

A. Median sacral artery.
B. Artery of Adamkiewicz.
C. Paraspinal artery.
D. Posterior sacral artery.

Response (**A**) The median sacral artery runs inferiorly in the midline over the anterior aspect of the vertebral body of the lumbar vertebrae and sacrum towards the apex of the coccyx and has to be sacrificed while doing an ALIF for the operative corridor.

Question 26

A twenty-six-year-old patient presented with right upper limb brachialgia. MRI showed a C4–5, C5–6, and C6–7 cervical disc prolapse. An anterior cervical discectomy and fusion was planned using a zero profile interbody device. Which of the following is wrong about the zero profile devices?

A. Often easier to place adjacent to a previously placed anterior plate.
B. Often avoid blades that are not parallel to the long axis of the spine.
C. Posterior migration of the cage is reduced once the screws are placed.
D. Biomechanical stability is inferior to that with a plate.

Response (**D**) The zero profile interbody devices offer equivalent biomechanical stability as plates. The four screw devices is as stable as three screw devices [20].

Question 27

Complications after lateral lumbar interbody fusion (LLIF) include:

A. Thigh numbness.
B. Retrograde ejaculation.
C. Weakness in thigh extension.
D. All of the above.

Response (**A**) In the transpsoas LLIF, injury to the lumbar plexus may cause thigh numbness. Direct damage to the psoas muscle that may also cause weakness in the thigh flexion. Anterior dissection of the superior hypogastric sympathetic plexus can result in retrograde ejaculation which is seen more in anterior lumbar interbody fusion.

Question 28

Twenty-five-year-old male patient presented after a fall from standing found to have an acute type II odontoid fracture. Good spinal alignment is maintained and the patient is neurologically intact. However, an MRI reveals disruption of the transverse ligament. Which of the following is the most appropriate treatment?

A. C-collar immobilization.
B. Occiput to C2 posterior fusion.
C. Odontoid screw placement.
D. Posterior C1–C2 instrumented fusion.

Response (**D**) Type II odontoid fractures have a high rate of nonunion, and therefore, surgical intervention is usually recommended. Odontoid screw placement and posterior C1–C2 fusion are two acceptable options, but disruption of the transverse ligament is a contraindication of the odontoid screw.

Question 29

45-year-old male patient with a history of rheumatoid arthritis presented with C2 pannus. The patient was planned for transoral odontiodectomy. All the following are recommended postoperative orders **EXCEPT**:

A. Intravenous hyperalimentation.
B. Nasogastric feeding.
C. Early removal of the endotracheal tube.
D. Halo-vest immobilization.

Response (C) Intubation should be maintained until the swelling subsides. Initial removal of an endotracheal tube over a tube changer facilitates reintubation. If needed, nasogastric feeding or intravenous hyperalimentation are used initially to avoid disruption of the mucosal closure. If immediate stabilization is not possible, then it is recommended to halo-vest immobilize the patient until stabilization is completed.

Question 30

Which suture type has been demonstrated to have evidence-based superiority at creating water-tight closure when repairing a spinal cord durotomy?

A. 5-0 surgilon.
B. 3-0 vicryl.
C. 6-0 prolene.
D. 4-0 neurolon.
E. 4-0 monocryl.

Response (C) A study by Dafford et al. compared CSF flow leaks following durotomy repair when completed using either 6-0 prolene or 5-0 surgilon. There was a statistically significant decrease in flow rate when the prolene sutures were used. The suturing technique (interrupted vs. continuous locking) was not found to have a significant role in the dural healing rate [21].

Question 31

Which of the following is not considered a benefit of anterior plating during anterior cervical discectomy and fusion (ACDF)?

A. Improved fusion rates for multilevel ACDFs.
B. Increased graft stability.
C. Decreased risk of dysphagia.
D. Decreased kyphosis.
E. Reduction in graft dislodgement.

Response (C) All answers except answer C are beneficial for using anterior plating during an ACDF. Though still somewhat controversial, several studies have demonstrated decreased incidence of dysphagia following ACDF when zero-profile cages are used [22].

Question 32

When using the Magerl technique for sub-axial cervical lateral mass screw placement, what is the direction and degree of angulation taken for screw placement?

A. 40–60° of lateral angulation.
B. 25–30° of medial angulation.
C. 40–60° of medial angulation.
D. 25–30° of lateral angulation.
E. 10° of lateral angulation.

Response (D) The Magerl technique is often used to guide lateral mass screw placement in the sub-axial cervical spine. In this technique, the lateral mass is divided into four quadrants. The entry point is 1–2 mm superior and medial to the mid-point of the quadrants. The screw is angled 25–30° laterally and 40–60° in the cranial direction (parallel to the facet joint).

Question 33

Which of the following corresponds with the correct description of the Roy-Camille technique for placement of lateral mass screws?

A. The screw insertion site is 2 mm medial and 1–2 mm cranial to the center of the lateral mass, and the orientation of the screw is aimed 20–30° laterally and parallel to the adjacent facet.
B. The screw insertion site is 1 mm medial to the midpoint of the lateral mass and the midpoint of the mass in the craniocaudal axis, and the orientation of the screw is aimed 30° laterally and 15° cephalad with the cortical surface.
C. The screw insertion site is located at the midpoint of the mediolateral and craniocaudal axes of the lateral mass, and the orientation of the screw is aimed perpendicularly to the posterior vertebral plane and 10° lateral to the sagittal plane.
D. The screw insertion site is located at the mid–facet line where the superior facet joins the transverse process, and the orientation of the screw is aimed 5–10° medially and 10–20° caudally.

Response (C) In the Roy-Camille technique, the screw is inserted at the midpoint of the mediolateral and craniocaudal axes of the lateral mass, aiming 0–10° laterally and 0° in the craniocaudal axis. Choice A is the Magerl technique. Choice B is the An technique. Choice D is used for the placement of a thoracic spine pedicle screw [23].

Question 34

What are the three landmarks used to guide the placement of pedicle screws in the lumbar spine?

A. Transverse process, superior articulating facet, and pars interaricularis.
B. Transverse process, inferior articulating facet, and pars interaricularis.
C. Transverse process, mamillary process, and lamina.
D. Transverse process, mamillary process, and pars interarticularis.
E. Spinous process, mamillary process and pars interarticularis.

Response (**D**) It is suggested pedicle screws be placed at the point at which the mamillary process, transverse process, and pars interarticularis join.

Question 35

Where is the entry point for a C1–2 transarticular screw?

A. 3 mm medial to the junction of the C2 lamina and inferior articulating process; 3 mm superior to the caudal border of the inferior articulating process.
B. 3 mm lateral to the junction of the C2 lamina and inferior articulating process; 3 mm inferior to the caudal border of the inferior articulating process.
C. 3 mm medial to the junction of the C2 lamina and inferior articulating process; 3 mm inferior to the caudal border of the inferior articulating process.
D. 3 mm lateral to the junction of the C2 lamina and inferior articulating process; 3 mm superior to the caudal border of the inferior articulating process.
E. 3 mm lateral to the junction of the C2 lamina and inferior articulating process; 3 mm inferior to the caudal border of the superior articulating process.

Response (**D**) The entry location for C1–2 transarticular screws is 3 mm lateral to the junction of the C2 lamina and the inferior articulating process. In terms of the cranial/caudal direction, the entry point is 3 mm superior to the caudal border of the inferior articulating process of C2. Typically, the screw is placed straight into the bone through 5° of medial angulation has been suggested as well.

Question 36

Pedicle violation during screw placement in which anatomic planes is most likely to result in neurologic injury?

A. Inferior-medial.
B. Inferior-lateral.
C. Superior-lateral.
D. Superior-medial.
E. Anterolateral.

Response (**A**) Anatomic studies using human cadavers have demonstrated that the distance to the nerve root adjacent to the pedicle is shortest in the inferior and medial planes (0.8–2.8 mm and 0.9–2.1 mm, respectively). Based upon these dimensions, damage to a nerve root due to violation of the pedicle is most likely to occur if the screw violates the pedicle in the inferomedial direction [24].

Question 37

Which of the following statements regarding polyether-ether-ketone (PEEK) cages is false?

A. PEEK is a hydrophobic polymer which in theory limits its contact with bone.
B. PEEK is radiolucent.
C. PEEK has been reported to have decreased rates of endplate subsidence owing to an elastic modulus that is similar to that of bone.
D. PEEK cages have demonstrated decreased hardware failure rates when used in stand-alone cages to treat spondylolisthesis.
E. PEEK spacers have been shown to have higher stress forces within bone grafts compared to titanium implants.

Response (**D**) All of the above answers are true statements about PEEK except statement D. In fact, studies have demonstrated that when stand-alone PEEK cages are used to treat spondylolisthesis, they are associated with an increased rate of hardware failure. One study done by Lastfogel et al. [25] demonstrated three patients who underwent anterior lumbar interbody fusion using stand-alone PEEK cages, which were complicated with anterior sacral fractures.

Question 38

Cervical pedicles with a width less than which of the following are considered unsafe for cervical pedicle screw fixation?

A. 5.5 mm.
B. 5 mm.
C. 4.5 mm.
D. 4.0 mm.
E. 3.5 mm.

Response (E) If the cervical pedicle width is less than 3.5 mm, it is suggested that cervical pedicle screws not be placed at that level and can be replaced by lateral mass screw.

Question 39

Which of the following choices best explains the concept of stress shielding in terms of spinal instrumentation of cervical spine?

A. The implantation of a prosthesis removes the normal physiologic stress on the bone, thus decreasing osteoblastic activity.
B. Implantation of anterior cervical cages decreases the stress on the anterior column, thus preventing pseudoarthrosis.
C. The innate property of implanted hardware to resist biomechanical stress.
D. The use of nanoparticle coating on implanted hardware to shield the implant from the immune system.
E. Dynamic anterior cervical plates are superior to static cervical plates because they shield the graft from biomechanical forces thus decreasing the screw pullout rate.

Response (A) Stress shielding is a concept first identified to be important in orthopedic literature in terms of bone instrumentation. Bone formation is stimulated by biomechanical stress on the bone, and implantation of a prosthesis removes this stress by acting as a force sump. Unfortunately, this has been found to result in focal osteopenia. This has proved to be a major issue in the setting of tibial fractures. However, in terms of spinal instrumentation, this concept has been important in developing dynamic cervical plating systems. In theory, static plates are too rigid and allow micromotions within the operative level. These micromotions are thought to induce stress on the bone touching the graft and promote osteogenic fusion. Dynamic plates have been shown to allow for this; however, much of the benefit is theoretical, with few studies demonstrating a significant difference in pseudoarthrosis rates between the two plate types.

Question 40

What is the location for the placement of transarticular screws in the thoracic spine?

A. Cranial to the transverse process.
B. Inferior and lateral border of the facet joint.
C. Inferior and medial border of the facet joint.
D. Superior and lateral border of the facet joint.
E. Superior and medial border of the facet joint.

Response (E) Transarticular screws may need to be placed in cases of abhorrent anatomy or pedicle fractures in the setting of trauma. The correct location for placement of transarticular screws in the thoracic spine is found at the intersection of the following lines: a horizontal line at the superior border of the facet joint and a vertical line at the medial border of the facet joint. The screw trajectory is 20° lateral in the coronal plane and 45° downwards in the sagittal plane [26].

Question 41

Which of the following is not considered a potential biomechanical benefit of cervical pedicle screws compared to lateral mass screws?

A. Higher pullout resistance.
B. Increased stiffness when undergoing lateral bending.
C. Increased resistance to axial rotation.
D. Increased stiffness when used in a construct spanning two unstable levels.
E. Greater construct stability when used at C7.

Response (C) Although cervical pedicle screws are thought to offer increased resistance to lateral bending after cyclic loading (fatigue testing), they do not offer increased resistance to axial rotation when compared to lateral mass screws [27].

Question 42

A 49-year-old male presents to the clinic with a 3-year history of bilateral lower extremity radicular symptoms and buttock pain. He had tried multiple conservative treatments, including epidural steroid injections and physical therapy, but none of them provided him with adequate symptom relief. Which of the following neurological complications is more likely to occur if this patient undergoes posterolateral fusion at the L5–S1 level?

A. Weakness to knee extension.
B. Decreased patellar reflexes.
C. Weakness to big toe dorsiflexion.
D. Loss of bowel/bladder control.
E. Decreased Achilles reflexes.

Response (C) L5–S1 posterolateral fusion is indicated for low-grade spondylolisthesis that failed non-operative treatment. However, this surgery places L5 nerve roots at risk for injury, which can manifest as a weakness to big toe dorsiflexion. Weakness to knee extension and decreased patellar reflexes are caused by L4 nerve injury. Loss of bowel/bladder control and decreased Achilles reflexes would result from S1 nerve injury [28].

Question 43

When performing anterior cervical discectomy and fusion (ACDF), what is the benefit of slightly oversizing the graft?

A. Directly reduces pullout strength of the construct.
B. Prevents subsidence of the graft into the endplate.
C. Prevents fatiguing of the implant.
D. Improves incorporation of the graft with the surrounding bone.
E. Avoids fibrous healing.

Response (**D**) According to Wolff's law, compressive loads increase the success of a bone graft incorporating with the surrounding bone. As such, sizing grafts slightly larger than the discectomy defect and using distraction to enlarge the disc space temporally is often used in order to achieve a larger compressive load.

Question 44

What is the preferred location for occipital plates and screws?

A. Superior to the superior nuchal line along midline ridge above the external occipital protuberance.
B. Inferior to the superior nuchal line along midline ridge below the external occipital protuberance.
C. Inferior to the inferior nuchal line along midline ridge below the external occipital protuberance.
D. Inferior to the superior nuchal line lateral to the midline ridge below the external occipital protuberance.
E. Superior to the superior nuchal line lateral to the midline ridge below the external occipital protuberance.

Response (**B**) Occipital plating and its associated screws are best placed inferior to the superior nuchal line along the midline ridge below the external occipital protuberance. At this location, bone is thick, allowing for good screw purchase, and overlying soft tissue is thick, decreasing the likelihood of hardware eroding through the skin. Additionally, the transverse sinus is superior to the nuchal line; therefore, this structure is avoided when the aforementioned location is used.

Question 46

Which fracture line orientations is/are considered amendable to odontoid screw fixation?

A. Horizontal.
B. Anterior–superior to posteroinferior.
C. Anteroinferior to posterosuperior.
D. A and B.
E. All of the above.

Response (**D**) Horizontally-oriented fractures and fractures oriented in an anterosuperior to posteroinferior direction are considered to be amendable to odontoid screw fixation. In particular, diagonal fractures oriented in an anterosuperior to posteroinferior fashion are considered excellent candidates for this technique as the screw will enter perpendicular to the fracture line promoting the edges to come together. Conversely, fractures with an orientation from anteroinferior to posterosuperior are contraindicated as the screw will enter parallel to the fracture line, which may promote anterior translation of the odontoid.

Question 46

When placing thoracic translaminar screws, which of the following answer choices regarding entry point or trajectory are correct?

A. Entry at the junction of the contralateral lamina and spinous process.
B. Trajectory should approximate the intersection of the ipsilateral transverse process and superior articulating process.
C. Trajectory should approximate the intersection of the ipsilateral transverse process and inferior articulating process.
D. A and B.
E. A and C.

Response (**D**) In the upper thoracic spine, pedicle diameter is sometimes unfavorable for pedicle screw placement. In this case, laminar screws can be used. The entry point is at the junction of the contralateral lamina and spinous process. The screw is aimed along the angle of the ipsilateral lamina, with a target trajectory approximating the intersection of the ipsilateral transverse process and superior articulating process.

Question 47

Which of the following is not considered an advantage of cortical trajectory screws compared to traditional pedicle screws?

A. Minimal lateral muscular dissection is required given the medial starting point of the screws.
B. Screws are directed away from the neural elements.
C. Has been shown to have increased insertional torque compared to traditional pedicle screws.
D. Has the equivalent safety when placed at S1.
E. Can be placed at the same level as previously placed pedicle screws to aid in fixation.

Response (**D**) All of the above statements except D are correct. The cortical trajectory is not applicable at S1. The cortical trajectory screws are theorized to have increased pullout strength and load-bearing properties compared to pedicle screws due to their placement in cortical bone, large-scale studies have not consistently demonstrated higher fusion rates. However, preliminary biomechanical and small-scale in-vivo studies are promising and have shown that cortical trajectory screws are at least equivalent to pedicle screws in their resistance to pullout and their screw-rod construct stability. It has also been shown to have less screw loosening and pullout in patients with diagnosed osteopenia and osteoporosis when compared to traditional pedicle screw insertion.

Question 48

Where is the entry point for a cortical trajectory screw?

A. The junction of the inferior articulating process and transverse process.
B. The center of the pars interarticularis at the level of the inferomedial border of the pedicle.
C. The junction of the transverse process and the superior articulating process.
D. The center of the pars interarticularis at the level of the superomedial border of the pedicle.
E. The junction of the lamina and the base of the spinous process.

Response (**B**) Cortical trajectory screws are placed at the center of the pars interarticularis at the level of the inferior border of the transverse process or inferomedial border of the pedicle. The screws are angled superiorly and laterally.

Question 49

Which of the following results from using stiffer instrumentation in spinal arthrodesis?

A. Increased risk for pseudarthrosis.
B. Increased vascularization.
C. Decreased elasticity modulus.
D. Decreased bone mineral density.

Response (**B**) Rigid spinal instrumentation, which allows for stronger fusion mass to form, is associated with significantly greater amounts of fusion mass and transverse processes vascularization. In the process of osteogenesis, early vascularization is essential in providing nutrition to the surviving cells of the peripheral portions of the graft. As a result, bone mineral density is high at the fusion mass level but decreases with increasing distance from the fusion level [29].

Question 50

Comparing C1 lateral mass—C2 pedicle screw fixation to posterior C1–C2 transarticular screw placement, which of the following is true?

A. C1 lateral mass—C2 pedicle screw fixation has a higher risk for vertebral artery injury and C2 neuralgia than C1–C2 transarticular screw placement.
B. C1–C2 transarticular screw placement has a higher risk for vertebral artery injury and C2 neuralgia than C1 lateral mass—C2 pedicle screw fixation.
C. C1 lateral mass—C2 pedicle screw fixation has a higher risk for vertebral artery injury but a lower chance of C2 neuralgia than C1–C2 transarticular screw placement.
D. C1–C2 transarticular screw placement has a higher risk for vertebral artery injury, but a lower chance of C2 neuralgia than C1 lateral mass—C2 pedicle screw fixation.
E. Both C1 lateral mass—C2 pedicle screw fixation and C1–C2 transarticular screw placement have an equal amount of risk for vertebral artery injury and C2 neuralgia.

Response (**D**) Atlantoaxial stabilization with C1 lateral mass—C2 pedicle screws provide comparable stability to C1–C2 transarticular screw. One advantage of C1 lateral mass—C2 pedicle screw fixation is reduced risk of vertebral artery injury. This is because the C2 pedicle screw has a more superior and medial trajectory, while the vertebral artery loops and turns lateral to ascend into the transverse foramen starting from C2. However, C1 lateral mass—C2 pedicle screw fixation tends to have more C2 neuralgia than C1–C2 transarticular screw placement [30].

Question 51

Which of the following is not a landmark that can be used to identify the entry point for the L3 pedicle screw?

A. The confluence of the mid transverse process and mamillary process.
B. The inferolateral aspect of the L2–3 facet joint.
C. The inferolateral aspect of the L3–L4 facet joint.
D. The confluence of the lateral margin of the superior articulating process and the mid traverse process.

Response (C) The entry point for lumbar pedicle screw is defined as the junction of the confluence of any of the four lines: mamillary process, pars interarticularis, lateral border of the superior articular facet, and mid transverse process. The inferolateral aspect of the L3–L4 facet joint is the landmark for the L4 pedicle screw (see Fig. 3.2) [31].

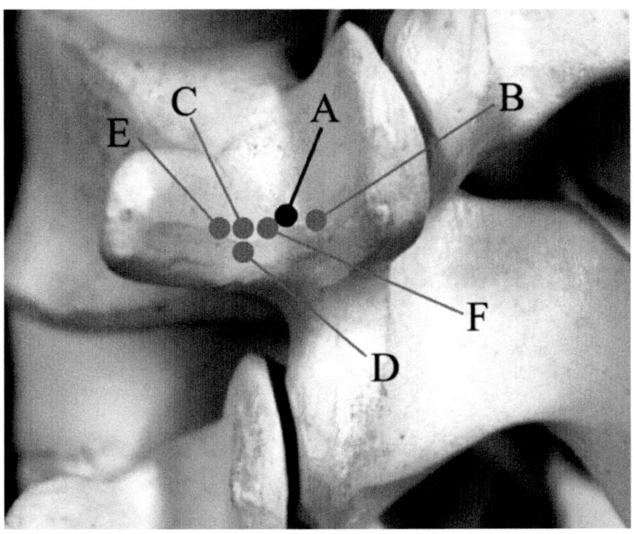

Fig. 3.2 Lateral photograph of spinal bone anatomy. The optimal point of pedicle screw entry is at the junction of the pars interarticularis, the midpoint of the transverse process and the inferior point of the superior articular facet: the point A indicates the entry point of current study with the junction of the proximal edge of the transverse process and lamina; the point B indicates Roy-Camille's screw entry point; the point C indicates Magerl's method; the point D indicates Levin and Edwards method; the point E indicates Weinstein's method; and the point F indicates the D and Zhao method (Oh et al. [31])

Question 52

Which of the following is the most appropriate trajectory for placing a C2 pedicle screw?

A. Caudal and lateral.
B. Rostral and lateral.
C. Caudal and medial.
D. Rostral and medial.
E. Parallel to the spinous process.

Response (D) The pars interarticularis of the C2 vertebra is located between the superior articular facet and the inferior articular process, while the C2 pedicle is located medially beneath the superior articular facet and anteromedially to the transverse foramen. The entry point of the C2 pedicle screw is usually 5 mm rostral and 1 mm medial to the inferomedial aspect of the inferior articulating surface of the C2 vertebra. The screw is then placed with 15–25° of medial angulation and approximately 20–30° craniocaudal angulation to the bottom half of the tubercle of the C1 vertebra.

References

1. Eldin MM, Hassan ASA. Free hand technique of cervical lateral mass screw fixation. J Craniovertebr Junction Spine. 2017;8(2):113–8.
2. Dhawale AA, Shah SA, Yorgova P, Neiss G, Layer DJ Jr, Rogers KJ, Gabos PG, Holmes L Jr. Effectiveness of cross-linking posterior segmental instrumentation in adolescent idiopathic scoliosis: a 2-year follow-up comparative study. Spine J. 2013;13(11):1485–92. https://doi.org/10.1016/j.spinee.2013.05.022. Epub 2013 Jun 22. PMID: 23800823.
3. Wang T, Zhao Y, Liang Y, Zhang H, Wang Z, Wang Y. Risk factor analysis of proximal junctional kyphosis after posterior osteotomy in patients with ankylosing spondylitis. J Neurosurg Spine. 2018;29(1):75–80.
4. Lutters B, Groen RJM, Koehler PJ. Myelography and the 20th century localization of spinal cord lesions. Eur Neurol. 2020;83(4):447–52. Published online 2020 Sep 1.
5. Karnaze MG, Gado MH, Sartor KJ, Hodges FJ III. Comparison of MR and CT myelography in imaging the cervical and thoracic spine. AJNR Am J Neuroradiol. 1987;8(6):983–9. https://doi.org/10.3109/13813457809069903.
6. Makhni MC, Shillingford JN, Laratta JL, Hyun SJ, Kim YJ. Restoration of sagittal balance in spinal deformity surgery. J Korean Neurosurg Soc. 2018;61(2):167–79. https://doi.org/10.3340/jkns.2017.0404.013.
7. Noh T, Zakaria H, Massie L, Ogasawara CT, Lee GA, Chedid M (2021). Bone marrow aspirate in spine surgery: case series and review of the literature. Cureus. 2021;13(12):e20309. Published online 2021 Dec 9. https://doi.org/10.7759/cureus.20309.
8. Kim Y-H, Ha K-Y, Rhyu K-W, Park H-Y, Cho C-H, Kim H-C, Lee H-J, Kim S-I. Lumbar interbody fusion: techniques, pearls and pitfalls. Asian Spine J. 2020;14(5):730–41. Published online 2020 Oct 14. https://doi.org/10.31616/asj.2020.0485.

9. Schmoelz W, Huber JF, Nydegger T, Claes L, Wilke HJ. Dynamic stabilization of the lumbar spine and its effects on adjacent segments: an in vitro experiment. Spine. 2003;1(28):418–23.
10. Dobbs MB, Lenke LG, Kim YJ, Luhmann SJ, Bridwell KH. Anterior/posterior spinal instrumentation versus posterior instrumentation alone for the treatment of adolescent idiopathic scoliotic curves more than 90. Spine. 2006;31(20):2386–91.
11. Eleraky M, Papanastassiou I, Tran ND, Dakwar E, Vrionis FD (2011) Comparison of polymethylmethacrylate versus expandable cage in anterior vertebral column reconstruction after posterior extracavitary corpectomy in lumbar and thoraco-lumbar metastatic spine tumors. Eur Spine J. 2011;20(8):1363–70. Published online 2011 Mar 10. https://doi.org/10.1007/s00586-011-1738-1.
12. Wright NM. Posterior C2 fixation using bilateral, crossing C2 laminar screws: case series and technical note. Clin Spine Surg. 2004;17(2):158–62.
13. Harms J, Melcher RP. Posterior C1–C2 fusion with polyaxial screw and rod fixation. Spine. 2001;26(22):2467–71.
14. Abumi K, Ito M, Sudo H. Reconstruction of the subaxial cervical spine using pedicle screw instrumentation. Spine. 2012;37(5): E349–56.
15. Tsuchiya K, Bridwell KH, Kuklo TR, Lenke LG, Baldus C. Minimum 5-year analysis of L5–S1 fusion using sacropelvic fixation (bilateral S1 and iliac screws) for spinal deformity. Spine. 2006;31(3):303–8.
16. Mirkovic S, Abitbol JJ, Steinman J, Edwards CC, Schaffler M, Massie J, Garfin SR. Anatomic consideration for sacral screw placement. Spine. 1991;16(6 Suppl):S289–94.
17. Cho DC, Sung JK. Is all anterior oblique fracture orientation really a contraindication to anterior screw fixation of type II and rostral shallow type III odontoid fractures? J Korean Neurosurg Soc. 2011;49(6):345–50. https://doi.org/10.3340/jkns.2011.49.6.345.
18. Zhu C, Wang L, Liu H, et al. Treatment of type II odontoid fracture with a novel technique: titanium cable-dragged reduction and cantilever-beam internal fixation. Medicine (Baltimore). 2017;96 (44): e8521. https://doi.org/10.1097/MD.0000000000008521.
19. Jeszenszky D, Loibl M. Transoral atlantoaxial and C2 corpectomy cage reconstruction techniques. In: Koller H, Robinson Y, editors. Cervical spine surgery: standard and advanced techniques. Cham: Springer; 2019. https://doi.org/10.1007/978-3-319-93432-7_27.
20. Barbagallo GM, Romano D, Certo F, Milone P, Albanese V. Zero-P: a new zero-profile cage-plate device for single and multilevel ACDF. A single institution series with four years maximum follow-up and review of the literature on zero-profile devices. Eur Spine J. 2013;22(Suppl 6):S868–78. https://doi.org/10.1007/s00586-013-3005-0.
21. Dafford EE, Anderson PA. Comparison of dural repair techniques. Spine J. 2015;15(5):1099–105.
22. Xiao S, et al. Zero-profile anchored cage reduces risk of postoperative dysphagia compared with cage with plate fixation after anterior cervical discectomy and fusion. Eur Spine J. 2017;26 (4):975–84.
23. Baek JW, Park DM, Kim DH. Comparative analysis of three different cervical lateral mass screw fixation techniques by complications and bicortical purchase: cadaveric study. J Korean Neurosurg Soc. 2010;48(3):193–8. https://doi.org/10.3340/jkns.2010.48.3.193.
24. Attar A, Ugur H, Uz A, et al. Lumbar pedicle: surgical anatomic evaluation and relationships. Eur Spine J. 2001;10:10–5. https://doi.org/10.1007/s005860000198.
25. Lastfogel JF, Altstadt TJ, Rodgers RB, Horn EM. Sacral fractures following stand-alone L5–S1 anterior lumbar interbody fusion for isthmic spondylolisthesis. J Neurosurg Spine. 2010;13(2):288–93.
26. Yu Y, Xie N, Song S, et al. A biomechanical comparison of a novel thoracic screw fixation method: transarticular screw fixation vs. traditional pedicle screw fixation. Neurosurgery 2011;69:141–6.
27. Wolfla C, MillerML (2011) Posterior subaxial and cervicothoracic instrumentation. In: Youmans and winn neurological surgery, vol 326, pp 2668–2674.e2
28. Inoue M, Inoue G, Ozawa T, Miyagi M, Kamoda H, Ishikawa T, Suzuki M, Sakuma Y, Oikawa Y, Yamauchi K, Orita S, Takaso M, Toyone T, Takahashi K, Ohtori S. L5 spinal nerve injury caused by misplacement of outwardly-inserted S1 pedicle screws. Eur Spine J. 2013;22(Suppl 3):S461–5. https://doi.org/10.1007/s00586-012-2634-z. Epub 2012 Dec 28. PMID: 23269529; PMCID: PMC3641263.
29. Johnston CE, Ashman RB, Baird AM, Allard RN. Effect of spinal construct stiffness on early fusion mass incorporation. Experimental study. Spine. 1990;15(9):908–12. PMID: 2259979. https://doi.org/10.1097/00007632-199009000-00013.
30. Lee SH, Kim ES, Sung JK, Park YM, Eoh W. Clinical and radiological comparison of treatment of atlantoaxial instability by posterior C1–C2 transarticular screw fixation or C1 lateral mass-C2 pedicle screw fixation. J Clin Neurosci. 2010;17 (7):886–92. https://doi.org/10.1016/j.jocn.2009.10.008. PMID: 20399666.
31. Oh CH, Yoon SH, Kim YJ, Hyun D, Park HC. Technical report of free hand pedicle screw placement using the entry points with junction of proximal edge of transverse process and lamina in lumbar spine: analysis of 2601 consecutive screws. Korean J Spine. 2013;10(1):7–13. https://doi.org/10.14245/kjs.2013.10.1.7.

Bone Biology and Bone Substitutes

4

Asham Khan, Moleca M. Ghannam, Ryan M. Hess, Slah Khan, Alexander O. Aguirre, Cathleen C. Kuo, Ali Y. Elkady, Ahmed H. Omar, Mohammad Elbaroody, and Mohamed A. R. Soliman

Question 1

Smoking significantly increases the risk of pseudarthrosis in patients undergoing spinal fusion surgery. Which of the following is not a correct statement regarding the effect of nicotine on vertebral bone healing?

A. Nicotine reduces type I and type II collagen levels within the fusion mass.
B. Nicotine upregulates VEGF expression to increase angiogenesis.
C. Nicotine reduces the expression of BMPs within the inner mass, particularly BMPs 2, 4, and 6.
D. Nicotine upregulates cortisol levels to inhibit periosteal cell proliferation.

A. Khan · M. M. Ghannam · R. M. Hess · S. Khan · A. O. Aguirre · C. C. Kuo · M. A. R. Soliman (✉)
Neurosurgery Department, University at Buffalo, Buffalo, NY, United States
e-mail: msolim8@uwo.ca

A. Khan
e-mail: akhan@ubns.com

M. M. Ghannam
e-mail: mghannam@ubns.com

R. M. Hess
e-mail: rhess@ubns.com

S. Khan
e-mail: slahkhan@buffalo.edu

A. O. Aguirre
e-mail: aa284@buffalo.edu

C. C. Kuo
e-mail: ckuo9@buffalo.edu

A. Y. Elkady · A. H. Omar · M. Elbaroody · M. A. R. Soliman
Neurosurgery Department, Cairo University, Cairo, Egypt
e-mail: ayousri54@gmail.com

A. H. Omar
e-mail: a.hussein.omar1990@gmail.com

M. Elbaroody
e-mail: mohammad.elbaroody@kasralainy.edu.eg

Response (B) Adequate blood supply, proper levels of gene expression, and mechanical stability are of paramount importance for bone healing to progress naturally. Smoking exerts a detrimental effect on fusion healing mainly because it disrupts angiogenesis and interferes with signaling molecules involved with osteoprogenitor cell differentiation. The reduction of angiogenesis is best supported by the decreased expression of VEGF, which is a mitogen for endothelial cells that increases vascular permeability and improves tissue oxygenation and nutrient delivery [1].

Question 2

Each type of bone graft below is only osteoconductive EXCEPT:

A. Allograft
B. Autograft
C. Synthetic ceramic
D. A and B.

Response (D) Osteoconductive materials simply provide structural support for cell growth. Solely osteoconductive materials will not include cellular components or growth factors that can stimulate differentiation. Autografts will have significant cellular and bioactive components. Allografts may contain some retained cellular and bioactive components, but not to the same degree that autografts will. Synthetic ceramics solely provide a structural support for cell growth but will not directly provide cells to the graft space or directly stimulate cells with the use of growth factors [2].

Question 3

Which signaling pathway is required for bone morphogenic protein (BMP) to stimulate bone formation?

A. SMAD (Suppressor of Mothers against Decapentaplegic)

C. Gragnaniello et al. (eds.), *MCQs in Spine Surgery*,
https://doi.org/10.1007/978-3-031-69332-8_4

B. CDK (cyclin-dependent kinase)
C. FOXO1 (Forkhead Box O1)
D. SHH (Sonic hedgehog).

Response (A) BMP protein stimulates bone formation through the SMAD pathway to transduce the signal into the nucleus, activating transcription factors to stimulate bone growth. The other signaling pathways listed do not play a role in BMP osteoinduction [3].

Question 4

Which of the following is considered an advantage of transforaminal lumbar interbody fusion (TLIF) compared to posterior lumbar interbody fusion (PLIF)?

A. Increased rates of fusion
B. Lower blood loss
C. Need for less retraction of the neural elements resulting in lower rates of iatrogenic nerve injury
D. Decreased operative time
E. Decreased hospital stay.

Response (C) Based on studies by Mehta et al. and Humphreys et al., TLIF is associated with lower rates of complications such as iatrogenic nerve injury or durotomy. This is believed to be due to decreased need for retraction of neural elements given the anatomy of the approach. These studies did not find differences in fusion rates, operative time, hospital length of stay or blood loss [4–6].

Question 5

What is the term to describe osteoblasts that have matured and are surrounded by bone matrix?

A. Osteocyte
B. Osteoclast
C. Osteon
D. Canaliculi
E. Chondroblast.

Response (A) As osteoblasts become surrounded by bone matrix, their metabolic production of bone decreases and they are then termed osteocytes. They possess long stellate cellular processes that travel through small channels in the bone called canaliculi, which allow for communication between cells [7].

Question 6

How does Denosumab decrease the rate of bone reabsorption?

A. Binds to the calcium phosphate ions within the bone matrix to decrease reabsorption of bone
B. Increases the secretion of parathyroid hormone
C. It reduces the survival of osteoclasts, thereby decreasing bone reabsorption
D. Increases the reabsorption of vitamin D
E. Binds to and stimulates the parathyroid hormone receptor.

Response (C) Denosumab is a monoclonal antibody that targets the receptor activator of nuclear factor kappa-beta ligand (RANKL) on osteoblasts in disrupts its ability to bind with RANK on osteoclasts. Normally, this interaction facilitates the survival of osteoclasts; thus, the inhibition of this pathway results in a decrease in survival rate. Decreased numbers of osteoclasts result in an overall decrease in the reabsorption of bone. When used in the treatment of osteoporosis, it was found to decrease the rate of vertebral fracture formation in post-menopausal women by 68% [8].

Question 7

Which of the following is the recommendation for using human recombinant bone morphogenic proteins (rhBMP) in posterior interbody lumbar fusion?

A. No difference between rhBMP-2 and iliac crest bone graft. However, an iliac crest bone graft requires additional surgical site operation. When an autograft is unavailable or procedure is not desired, rhBMP-2 is a reliable alternative.
B. An FDA warning has been issued not to use rhBMP-2 due to inflammation causing airway compromise.
C. The use of rhBMP-2 has been associated with high rates of ectopic bone formation leading to neurological compromise.
D. The use of rhBMP-2 has been associated with seroma formation and neurological compromise. Further evidence is needed, but judicious use of rhBMP-2 is recommended due to complications.

Response (C) Using rhBMP-2 in posterior interbody lumbar fusion is associated with positive fusion results, but its usage has been found to increase the risk of heterotopic bone formation and cage migration. Meta-analysis data from

Yale University Open Data Access further suggests clinicians to avoid rhBMP-2 use in posterior interbody lumbar fusion due to concern about the ectopic bone formation and neurological compromise [9].

Question 8

Which of the following is a property that alloplast graft and xenograft typically share?

A. Osteogenesis
B. Osteopromotion
C. Osteoconduction
D. Osteoinduction
E. Osseointegration.

Response (C) There are four major types of bone graft material: autografts, allografts, alloplasts, and xenografts. The origin and composition are the primary determinants of the mechanisms by which the grafts act. Xenografts and alloplasts are typically only osteoconductive. Autografts harvested from patients have the capacity to form new bone by osteogenesis, osteoinduction, and osteoconduction. Allografts from cadavers are also primarily osteoconduction but have some osteoinductive potential [10].

Question 9

Grafted autogenous bone can be trabecular, cortical or corticotrabecular. Which of the following is an advantage of cortical bone over the trabecular bone?

A. Faster process of revascularization and remodeling
B. Contain higher percentage of endothelial growth factor
C. Provides most of the bone morphogenetic protein
D. Inhibits soft tissue ingrowth into the graft site
E. Confers higher osteogenic potential.

Response (C) Cortical bone forms the external layer of all bones and is found predominantly in the appendicular skeleton, while the trabecular bone is found mainly in the axial skeleton. In general, trabecular bone has more osteogenic potential than cortical bone due to the presence of hematopoietic marrow and a greater amount of pluripotential cells in cancellous bone. On the other hand, the cortical graft provides the most bone morphogenetic protein, which renders resistance to the graft structure absorption and prolongs the time needed for blood vessels to infiltrate the graft [11].

Question 10

Regarding the properties of the graft material, which one of the following is true:

A. Osteoinduction means that the graft should provide a framework or scaffold (bone mineral and collagen) to induce new bone formation.
B. Osteoconduction means that the graft should contain growth factors that conduct the process of mature bone-forming cells.
C. Osteogenesis means that the graft should contain osteoblast, which can induce new bone formation.
D. All of the above.
E. None of the above.

Response (E) Osteoinduction means that the graft should contain growth factors (non-collagenous bone matrix proteins) that can induce osteoblast precursors to differentiate into mature bone-forming cells. Osteoconduction means that the graft should provide a framework or scaffold (bone mineral and collagen) onto which new bone can form. Osteogenesis means that the graft should contain viable progenitor stem cells that can form new bone matrix and remodel bone as needed [12–15].

Question 11

Common autograft donor sites include:

A. Iliac crest.
B. Rib.
C. Fibula.
D. Bone removed during decompression.
E. All of the above.

Response (E) Autografts may retain some cell viability and are considered to promote bone healing mainly through osteogenesis and/or osteoconduction. All of the above can be used as an autograft [16].

Question 12

For spine fusions, osteoinductive components of bone graft include:

A. Non-collagenous proteins that promote differentiation
B. Cellular components that form new bone
C. Structure of graft for new bone to grow on
D. None of the above.

Response (A) Osteoinductive components are non-collagenous proteins such as growth factors that will activate intracellular signaling pathways to promote osteodifferentiation in osteoprogenitor cell lines. Cellular components that form new bone are the osteogenic components. Structure of graft for new bone to grow on describes osteoconductive components [16].

Question 13

A sixty-six-year-old female patient was diagnosed with L5-S1 pseudo-spondylolisthesis and was operated by interbody cage fusion, and electrical stimulation was used to enhance bony fusion. The mechanism of action of capacitive coupling electrical stimulation is:

A. Direct activation of osteoblastic membrane-bound voltage-gated Ca2+ channels.
B. Increase in cytosolic Ca2+.
C. Inducing downstream phospholipase-A2—and calmodulin-mediated bone formation.
D. All of the above.

Response (D) The capacitive coupling electrical stimulation is a non-invasive method to enhance bony fusion. It activates Ca2+ channels and increases the cytosolic Ca2+ and upregulation of osteoinductive growth factors (e.g., BMP-2, 4, 5, 6, and 7; and TGF-β1) [17].

Question 14

All of the following nerves are at risk of injury during iliac crest harvesting EXCEPT:

A. Ilioinguinal
B. Lateral cutaneous nerve of the thigh
C. Posterior femoral cutaneous nerve of the thigh
D. Iliohypogastric.

Response (C) Iliac crest bone graft is harvested from a point at least 3 cm behind the anterior superior iliac spine to avoid ilioinguinal ligament disruption. Nerves at risk during this procedure (from lateral to medial) include the iliohypogastric, ilioinguinal and lateral femoral cutaneous nerves. In contrast, the posterior cutaneous nerve of the thigh is deep in the subgluteal region [18].

Question 15

All of the following are true regarding the direct current stimulation (DCS) in bony fusion EXCEPT:

A. DCS involves the implantation of negative and positive electrodes.
B. A continuous electrical current is delivered to the fusion site via a subcutaneously implanted electric generator.
C. Electrochemical reaction at the cathode lowers the oxygen tension and raises the pH, favoring net bone formation.
D. It is noninvasive and employs two capacitive plates placed on the skin on opposite sides of the fusion site.

Response (D) DCS involves the implantation of cathodes (negative and positive electrodes) into the prospective fusion mass and an anode (positive electrode) into the adjacent soft tissue; the current is supplied by a subcutaneous electric generator. The capacitive coupling stimulation (CCS), in contrast to DCS, is completely noninvasive and employs two capacitive plates placed on the skin on opposite sides of the fusion site [17].

Question 16

Which of the following are true regarding electrical stimulation for bone fusion EXCEPT:

A. The inductive coupling stimulation (ICS) is a non-invasive and theoretically painless modality.
B. The recommended usage of ICS is 30 minutes to 2 hours per day.
C. Direct current stimulation (DCS) is a non-invasive technique.
D. The DCS increases the pH of the favoring net bone formation.

Response (C) The DCS needs surgical implantation for the electric generator. Both ICS and capacitive coupling stimulation (CCS) are non-invasive and theoretically painless devices. The recommended usage of ICS is 30 minutes to 2 hours per day compared to the CCS, which is wearable 24 hours/day [17].

Question 17

The 2nd stage of osseous healing includes:

A. Recruiting various inflammatory cells and fibroblasts to the site of injury.
B. Secretion of growth factors and inflammatory mediators.
C. Expansion of vascular-rich granulation tissue into a fibrous callus and immature bone.
D. All of the above.

Response (D) During the 2nd stage of healing, the release of VEGF leads to angiogenesis at the site, fibrin-rich granulation tissue begins to develop. Other mesenchymal stem cells are recruited to the area and differentiate (driven by BMPs) into fibroblasts, chondroblasts, and osteoblasts. As a result, chondrogenesis begins, laying down a collagen-rich fibrocartilaginous network spanning the fracture ends, with a surrounding hyaline cartilage sleeve [19].

Question 18

Bone Marrow Aspirate (BMA) is a cell-based bone graft characterized by all the following EXCEPT:

A. Osteoconductive
B. Can be harvested from the vertebral body
C. Osteogenic
D. High variability between preparations.

Response (A) Bone Marrow Aspirate (BMA) is a cell-based bone graft. It provides an autogenic source of osteogenic precursor cells that have the potential to differentiate into osteoblasts to synthesize new bone tissues. Furthermore, BMA possesses other pluripotent mesenchymal stem cells and less donor site morbidity than iliac crest bone graft [20].

Question 19

Demineralized Bone Matrix (DBM) is a human allograft-derived bone graft characterized by all the following EXCEPT:

A. Osteoconductive
B. High variability between preparations
C. Osteogenic
D. Osteoinductive.

Response (C) The organic matrix (collagens and noncollagenous proteins) provides osteoconductive properties while the growth factors, which consist of bone morphogenetic proteins (BMP), transforming growth factor-β, and fibroblast growth factors among other GFs, contribute to its osteoinductive potential, it can be harvested from the pedicle of vertebral body, however the DBM lack osteogenic properties. DBMs do NOT contain cells that can confer osteogenic properties to the material [21].

Question 20

A fifty-six-year-old male patient presented with left brachialgia. MRI showed C5-6 cervical disc prolapse, which was treated by ACDF. Four months later, the patient presented with axial neck pain increase with motion. All of the following radiological findings would suggest the diagnosis of pseudoarthrosis EXCEPT:

A. Lack of bridging trabeculae between the host bone and graft
B. Motion exceeding 1 mm or 2 mm between spinous processes on maximal flexion–extension
C. Change in Cobb angle of at least <2°.
D. Halo around the graft.

Response (C) Cobb's angle of > 2 degrees resulted in a specificity of 39% and a sensitivity of 82%. However, a change in Cobb angle of > 4 degrees significantly improve the specificity with a positive predictive value of 100% [22, 23].

Question 21

A patient undergoes spinal fusion. How many weeks after the operation would you expect to see an early fusion of bone?

A. 1–2 weeks
B. 2–3 weeks
C. 4–5 weeks
D. 6–8 weeks
E. 12+ weeks.

Response (C) Bone formation occurs in three distinct phases. The second phase includes calcification of cartilaginous tissue into the immature woven bone, which is characteristic of early fusion. This phase occurs typically around 4–5 weeks during healing. It is expected that 50% of fusion occurs by the conclusion of this phase [24].

Question 22

Which of the following graft properties can allow bone formation in any location of the body, including non-bony locations and soft tissue?

A. Osteogenesis
B. Osteoconduction
C. Osteoinduction
D. Osteopromotion
E. Osteodifferentiation.

Response (C) Osteoinduction takes advantage of endocrine and paracrine signaling pathways for cell recruitment and differentiation to promote bone formation. In this way, they can also promote bone formation in soft tissue. Osteogenesis implies the presence of cells that form bone or bony precursors in the graft material. Osteoconduction is the presence of scaffold material that can support bone growth and angiogenesis. Osteopromotion enhances existing bone growth or healing [24].

Question 23

A 65 years old woman undergoes a posterior lumbar interbody fusion to treat spondylolisthesis. An iliac crest bone graft (ICBG) is harvested during the procedure. What is the major expected postoperative complication from the ICBG harvesting?

A. Infection of the incision site
B. Chronic pain in the donor site
C. Paresthesia
D. Hematoma over the donor site
E. Permanent nerve injury.

Response (B) ICBG harvest can come with all of the above choices; however, the major complication of concern is pain from the donor site. This donor site pain occurs at far greater rates than the other complications listed above. Chronic pain from the donor site can affect day-to-day activities, including household activities, work, and recreational activities [24].

Question 24

A patient is being considered for spinal fusion. Unfortunately, this patient currently smokes, and you have concerns that their smoking will affect proper fusion after graft placement. Which of the following best describes the negative effect of smoking on fusion?

A. Inhibition of angiogenesis into the graft space.
B. Upregulation of osteoclast activity in the bone via calcitonin.
C. Increases fibroblast activity in the graft space leading to fibrosis of the graft.
D. Reduces osteoblast activity in the graft space preventing bone formation.

Response (A) The major adverse effect of smoking with bone graft technology is the prevention of angiogenesis. Nicotine inhibits the expression of bFGF and VEGF, which are crucial to new blood vessel formation. Without angiogenesis, the body is unable to provide an adequate blood supply to the graft space, and thus the graft has insufficient nutrients for bone formation [1].

Question 25

Of the following graft types, which is osteoconductive and weakly osteoinductive?

A. Autografts
B. Iliac crest bone graft (ICBG)
C. Hydroxyapatite
D. Allograft.

Response (D) Allografts maintain the microarchitecture of bone and may retain some growth factors making it osteoconductive but weakly osteoinductive due to lower than physiologic levels of growth factors. Autografts and ICBG are both osteoconductive and maintain physiologic levels of growth factors, making them very osteoinductive. Hydroxyapatite does not have growth factors and thus does not participate in paracrine or endocrine signaling. However, it does provide structural support for bone growth; therefore, it is osteoconductive but not osteoinductive [16].

Question 26

A 65 years old female with a history of a complete laminectomy at L4-S1 presents for a PLIF at L4-S1 and will require a bone graft for appropriate fusion. Which of the following graft material is least likely to be chosen?

A. Local graft
B. ICBG
C. Allograft
D. Xenograft
E. Ceramic (i.e. Hydroxyapatite, tricalcium phosphate, etc.).

Response (A) This patient had a PLIF procedure at multiple levels. She had a previous laminectomy that removed significant bone volume that may have contributed to a local graft. Thus, the local graft will not be appropriate in this situation [24].

Question 27

Bone marrow aspirates take advantage of the presence of nucleated cells in the bone marrow that can differentiate into osteogenic lineages. They are typically found in low numbers but can be concentrated in bone marrow concentrates. What are these cells?

A. Mesenchymal stem cells
B. Osteoblasts

C. Myelopoietic cells
D. Osteocytes.

Response (A) Mesenchymal stem cells (MSCs) are stem cells found in the bone marrow that can differentiate into many cell lineages, including osteogenic, chondrogenic, and adipogenic lineages. Bone marrow aspirates aim to remove the MSCs and can be concentrated in bone marrow concentrates [25].

Question 28

In what zone of endochondral bone formation will you find the presence of dead chondrocytes?

A. Zone 1 (Resting zone)
B. Zone 2 (Proliferative zone)
C. Zone 3 (Hypertrophic zone)
D. Zone 4 (Calcification zone).

Response (D) In endochondral bone formation, chondrocytes proliferate, hypertrophy, and then die in a cartilaginous extracellular matrix. This death occurs in the fourth and final zone of endochondral bone formation. As a result, this cartilage will be invaded by blood vessels and osteoprogenitor cells [26].

Question 29

In what zone of endochondral bone formation will you find large chondrocytes arranged into columns?

A. Zone 1 (Resting zone)
B. Zone 2 (Proliferative zone)
C. Zone 3 (Hypertrophic zone)
D. Zone 4 (Calcification zone).

Response (C) Chondrocytes enlarge and organize into ordered columns in the hypertrophic zone. These columns will later be permeated by metaphyseal blood vessels, and bone will form on the residual columns to calcify the cartilage [26].

Question 30

Which of the following bone product is not primarily an osteoconductive agent?

A. Hydroxyapatite
B. Bone morphogenic protein
C. Tricalcium phosphate
D. Demineralized bone matrix
E. Calcium sulfate.

Response (B) Modern bone grafts, bone substitutes, and bioactive factors facilitate and enhance the healing process via osteoconductive (implanted scaffold for bone growth), osteoinductive (exogenous growth factors promote differentiation into osteoblastic cells), and osteogenic (synthesis of new bone by donor cells). Bone morphogenic protein is primarily an osteoinductive and osteogenic material. Demineralized bone matrix, which is prepared from cadaveric bone, has some osteoinductive potential, but it is mainly considered an osteoconductive agent [16, 27].

Question 31

Bone undergoes constant remodeling throughout a person's lifetime. What is the primary stimulus that guides this remodeling?

A. Mechanical stresses on the bone
B. Growth factors released by marrow cells
C. Changes in perfusion of the bone
D. Fibrosis of bone tissue from age.

Response (A) Bone is placed under mechanical stresses daily. These stresses will guide the remodeling of bone as coupled osteoblast and osteoclast activity will remove the microdamaged bone matrix and replace it with new bone [26].

Question 32

A 55-year-old male underwent an anterior cervical discectomy and fusion ten years ago. The patient had a titanium cage placed in the intervertebral disc space during the procedure. Radiologic assessment of the implant showed increased radiolucency around the implant but otherwise normal. What is a potential mechanism for this?

A. Fracture of the vertebral body
B. Hyperthyroidism
C. Rheumatoid arthritis
D. Stress-shielding around the implant.

Response (D) Metal implants have a higher stiffness compared to the surrounding bone. This will lead to decreased loads acting on the bone and less mechanical stimuli to the bone. This will ultimately result in bone loss around the implant after chronic cyclic loading of the bone leads to remodeling over several months [28].

Question 33

Food and Drug Administration (FDA) has issued a warning on bone morphogenetic proteins in which of the following spinal fusion surgeries?

A. Transforaminal Interbody Fusion
B. Posterolateral Fusion
C. Posterior Interbody Lumbar Fusion
D. Anterior Cervical Fusion
E. Anterior Lumbar Interbody Fusion.

Response (D) In 2008, the FDA issued a warning that the "off-label" use of bone morphogenetic proteins in anterior cervical spine surgery contributed to marked dysphagia, hematoma, seroma, swelling, and the need for intubation/tracheostomy. As such, current clinical recommendations to physicians are to avoid using bone morphogenetic proteins in anterior cervical fusion [9].

Question 34

A patient is undergoing an anterior cervical discectomy and fusion (ACDF), and graft material is being considered for the fusion. You decide to use a graft material that is osteo-conductive and osteo-inductive but has limited to no osteo-genic potential. Which of the following graft materials fit these criteria?

A. Cancellous allograft
B. Cancellous autograft
C. Cortical allograft
D. Tricalcium phosphate.

Response (C) Allografts will provide both osteoconductive and osteoinductive properties. However, the preparation of these materials tends to affect cell viability and thus will have limited osteogenic potential [16].

Question 35

Bone morphogenetic protein (BMP) is a growth factor that promotes osteoblast differentiation and osteogenesis. All but one of the twenty known BMPs is part of the TGF-β family. Which of the following is not a part of the TGF-β family?

A. BMP-1
B. BMP-2
C. BMP-7
D. BMP-14.

Response (A) BMP-1 is a metalloproteinase and is the only known BMP that is not a part of the TGF-β family. This protein may induce cartilage formation in vivo [16].

Question 36

A 50 years old male is undergoing an anterior lumbar interbody fusion and will have a titanium cage loaded with rh-BMP2 placed in the space as a part of the procedure. What major complication of bone morphogenetic proteins should be considered in this patient?

A. Disease transmission
B. Neurovascular complications
C. Unproven efficacy of BMPs
D. Rapid resorption and metabolism of BMPs.

Response (B) BMPs are difficult to contain to a certain space and may deviate from the site they are applied to initially. In addition, recent studies in BMP use have shown evidence that ectopic bone formation from BMPs can result in painful nerve compression and inflammatory reactions near vital structures [16].

Question 37

Synthetic grafts such as tricalcium phosphate can provide structural support for bone growth. Which of the following is true regarding synthetic bone grafts?

A. Rapid resorption of some bone grafts can be faster than bone growth which will not be ideal for supporting bone formation in fusion.
B. Synthetic grafts are often formed from biological serums and carry the risk of disease transmission.
C. Synthetic grafts can have osteoinductive and osteogenic capabilities.
D. Synthetic grafts are extremely expensive when compared to allografts.

Response (A) Resorption rates can be highly variable amongst synthetic grafts. While some may show slow biodegradability, others will be rapidly resorbed. Rapid resorption will often lead to improper bone formation or unstable bone formation in such situations [16].

Question 38

Of the following BMPs, which is the only BMP that is FDA approved for anterior lumbar interbody fusion (ALIF)?

A. BMP-1
B. BMP-2
C. BMP-6
D. BMP-14.

Response (B) BMP-2 is the only BMP FDA approved for orthopedic applications such as ALIF. Currently, the rh-BMP2 is marketed as Infuse for application in ALIF [16].

Question 39

Assessment of fusion is crucial to determining the success of spinal fusion. Which of the following is the best option for assessing successful fusion?

A. Assessment of flexion and/or extension at the site of fusion
B. Plain film radiography
C. MRI
D. Axial CT with reconstruction.

Response (D) Newer instrumentation is often radiopaque and makes fusion challenging to assess on plain radiography. Assessment of range of motion may also be difficult as instrumentation may provide rigid fixation. Therefore, axial CT with reconstruction is the standard of evaluation [24].

Question 40

Which of the following graft material is osteoinductive but lacks osteoconductive and osteogenic capabilities?

A. Platelet-rich plasma
B. Bone marrow aspirate
C. rhBMP
D. Demineralized bone matrix.

Response (A) Platelet-rich plasma is a highly concentrated platelet formulation rich in various growth factors but lacks structural support and osteogenic capabilities [16].

Question 41

Platelet-rich plasma is a formulation of concentrated platelets formed from whole blood. Which of the following is false?

A. Platelet-rich plasma needs to be activated using calcium chloride.
B. Platelet-rich plasma contains large concentrations of growth factors.
C. There is strong evidence in the literature suggesting the efficacy of platelet-rich plasma.
D. Once activated, it can be applied to a site of injury to promote bone growth.

Response (C) While animal studies have shown benefit from platelet-rich plasma, it has been inconclusive in human fracture healing and shows little evidence in the setting of fusion [16].

Question 42

Of the following BMPs, which has shown to have angiogenic properties?

A. BMP-1
B. BMP-3
C. BMP-7
D. BMP-14.

Response (C) BMP-2 and BMP-7 have both been shown to not only have osteogenic properties but are also highly capable of local neovascularization [16].

Question 43

Platelet-rich plasma contains a wide variety of growth factors. Of the growth factors found in platelet-rich plasma, which of the following promotes differentiation of mesenchymal stem cells (MSCs) into osteoblasts?

A. VEGF
B. BMP-7
C. PDGF
D. BMP-2.

Response (D) BMP-2 is the only BMP that has been shown to differentiate MSCs to osteoblasts. VEGF plays a role in angiogenesis. PDGF has a role in inflammation, cellular proliferation, and angiogenesis. BMP-7 does not induce osteoblastic differentiation of MSCs but is still osteogenic [16].

Question 44

A patient that had just undergone spinal fusion decides to take ibuprofen for postoperative pain. However, there is concern that the medication may interfere with bone healing. When in the healing process is the medication most likely to affect healing?

A. 1 to 3 weeks

B. 4 to 5 weeks
C. 6 to 10 weeks
D. 12+ weeks.

Response (A) Callus formation, release of growth factors, and inflammatory cytokines mediate the early phases of bone healing. This occurs in the first 1–3 weeks of healing. This inflammatory phase may be affected by the use of NSAIDs such as ibuprofen. This can delay bone healing and result in poorer outcomes [24].

Question 45

Demineralized bone matrix (DBMs) is formed from ground cadaveric bone processed via acid extraction. Which of the following is true regarding DBMs?

A. The efficacy of DBMs is variable as processing methods are highly variable between various DBM products.
B. Disease transmission is not of concern with DBMs.
C. Demineralization processes retain BMP function in final products.
D. Cellular components are intact in DBMs.

Response (A) Demineralizing is a highly proprietary process, and as such, these processes are not typically published. Thus, it isn't easy to regulate these processes. DBMs retain a high level of variability from one product to the next. DBMs are formed from cadaveric bone; so, still capable of disease transmission. Demineralization can inactivate BMPs in DBMs. DBMs are typically acellular [16].

Question 46

Which of the following grafts has a large supply of viable cells, including osteocytes and osteoprogenitor cells that confers osteogenic properties?

A. Cortical bone autograft
B. Vascularized bone autograft
C. Cancellous bone allograft
D. Demineralized bone matrix.

Response (B) Vascularized bone grafts retain large amounts of viable cells in their structure that confer osteogenic properties. Cortical bone autografts still contain viable cells; however, their supply is limited. Cancellous bone and demineralized bone matrix lose cellularity in their processing methods [16].

Question 47

The surgeon decided to utilize calcium phosphate cement in the intervertebral space during spinal surgery to augment the fusion. Which of the following is not a property of calcium phosphate?

A. Slow biodegradation
B. Osteointegration capability
C. Ability to withstand tensile and shear forces
D. Good compressive strength.

Response (C) Ceramic cement is typically very brittle under tensile and shear forces. While they can withstand compressive forces in vitro, they may fail when subjected to these other forces in vivo. These properties are crucial to why calcium phosphate materials are not popular amongst surgeons [16].

Question 48

Which of the following BMPs has shown no osteoinductive properties?

A. BMP-2
B. BMP-3
C. BMP-4
D. BMP-7.

Response (B) BMP-3 has no demonstrated osteoinductive activity and, as such, is not implicated in osteogenesis. Specifically, BMP-2, -4, -6, -7, -9, and -14 have significant osteogenic properties [16].

Question 49

Endochondral ossification is crucial in the process of bone formation. This requires neovascularization of hyaline cartilage. Which of the following growth factors plays a role in inducing vascular invasion of cartilage?

A. PDGF
B. BMP-1
C. VEGF
D. PTH.

Response (C) Vascular endothelial growth factor is released by platelets and chondrocytes in calluses to promote angiogenesis to vascularize hyaline cartilage [16].

Question 50

Recombinant human parathyroid hormone (rhPTH) can be used to increase bone mineral density and reduce overall fracture risk. Which of the following is true regarding the cellular action of PTH?

A. PTH has a direct effect on osteoblasts and indirect on osteoclasts.
B. PTH has an indirect effect on both osteoblasts and osteoclasts.
C. PTH has a direct effect on osteoclasts and osteoblasts.
D. PTH has a direct effect on osteoclasts and indirect on osteoblasts.

Response (A) PTH has a direct effect on osteoblasts, increasing their activity through PTH receptors on osteoblasts. Increased osteoblast activity will, in turn, activate osteoclast activity through cell-to-cell interactions, specifically pathways involving RANKL and osteoprotegerin [29].

Question 51

Which of the following factors could affect spinal fusion:

A. Type of graft material, e.g., autograft or synthetic biomaterials
B. Patient age
C. NSAIDs
D. Smoking status
E. All of the above.

Response (E) All of the following are factors that can contribute to the healing process of bone graft. These factors can each contribute to fusion failure or pseudoarthrosis. Each must be taken into account when counseling patients on expectations and post-operative procedures [30–33].

Question 52

Which of the following factors could affect spinal fusion:

A. Method of preparation of the graft recipient site
B. Mechanical stability of the spine segment
C. Spinal region
D. A and B
E. All of the above.

Response (E) The cervical region is considered a more favorable environment for fusion versus the thoracic or lumbar regions. Proper curettage of the endplate and proper stabilization of the spine after placement of the graft also affect the spinal fusion [30–33].

Question 53

Which of the following is the most abundant protein in the organic matrix of bone?

A. Type I collagen
B. Type II collagen
C. Type III collagen
D. Type IV collagen
E. Type V collagen.

Response (A) Type I collagen is a fibrillar type collagen. It forms 90% of the organic mass of bone and tendon and is the major collagen of skin, ligaments, cornea, and many interstitial connective tissues. Type II collagen is the main collagenous component of cartilage. Type III collagen forms reticulate, commonly found alongside type I collagen. Type IV collagen forms the basal lamina, and type V collagen is found within the dermal/epidermal junction and the placental tissues [34].

Question 54

Regarding Demineralized Bone Matrix (DBM), all of the following statements are true, EXCEPT:

A. It is an allograft bone that underwent the process of acid extraction.
B. It lacks osteoinductive properties.
C. It is devoid of bone minerals.
D. It contains collagen and non-collagenous proteins.

Response (B) Allograft bone may undergo processing by acid extraction to remove bone minerals while retaining collagen and non-collagenous proteins. The end product is DBM, an allograft form with osteoinductive activity. It is important to note that osteoinductive properties are highly dependent on the preparation method of the material so not all DBMs are equal in osteoinductive properties [35–37].

Question 55

Regarding Bone Morphogenetic Proteins (BMPs), all of the following statements are true, EXCEPT:

A. They are osteo-conductive proteins.
B. They are soluble proteins.

C. They are members of the transforming growth factor-beta (TGF-β) superfamily of growth factors.
D. The use of a carrier is a must to maintain an effective local concentration and prevent their diffusion away from the operative site.

Response (A) BMPs are osteoinductive proteins. The other statements are all true [38–40].

Question 56

Regarding the properties of the graft material, which one of the following is true:

A. Allografts have osteoconductive properties and lacks osteogenic properties.
B. Ceramics lack osteoinductive and osteogenic properties.
C. Composite grafts have both osteoinductive and osteoconductive properties.
D. Autograft have osteoconductive, osteoinductive and osteogenic properties.
E. A and C.
F. All of the above.

Response (F) Osteoinduction takes advantage of endocrine and paracrine signaling pathways for cell recruitment and differentiation to promote bone formation. In this way, they can promote bone formation in soft tissue as well. Osteogenesis implies the presence of cells that form bone or bony precursors in the graft material. Osteoconduction is the presence of scaffold material that can support bone growth and angiogenesis. Allografts will provide structure but do not typically contain cells within the material to provide osteogenic properties. Ceramics are only structural and have no growth factors or cells. Composite grafts may provide a variety of osteoinductive and osteoconductive properties based on the composition of the composite. Autografts provide all crucial properties for bone growth and are the most effective [12–15].

Question 57

Which one of the following statements regarding the classification of graft materials according to the intention of their use?

A. Extender is a type of graft material used in combination with autograft bone.
B. Enhancer is a type of graft material used in conjunction with autograft bone to increase the rate of successful arthrodesis above the rate of fusion achieved using autograft alone.
C. Substitute is a type of graft material used as an alternative to autograft bone and is intended to provide equivalent or superior fusion success compared with autograft bone.
D. All of the above.

Response (D) Extender is a type of graft material used in combination with autograft bone. Enhancer is a type of graft material used in conjunction with autograft bone to increase the rate of successful arthrodesis above the rate of fusion achieved using autograft alone. Substitute is a type of graft material used as an alternative to autograft bone and is intended to provide equivalent or superior fusion success compared with autograft bone [12–15].

Question 58

Regarding the difference between nonstructural grafts and structural grafts, which one of the following is false?

A. Nonstructural grafts are also termed morselized grafts.
B. Structural grafts consist of particles of bone, e.g., cancellous bone from the iliac crest.
C. Nonstructural grafts do not provide structural stability when used by themselves, and spinal instrumentation is used to facilitate bony union.
D. Structural grafts provide mechanical support during the process of fusion consolidation.

Response (B) Nonstructural grafts consist of particles of bone, e.g., cancellous bone from the iliac crest [41–43].

Question 59

Regarding anterior column structural grafts, which one of the following is true:

A. Strut grafts reconstruct the anterior spinal column following discectomy.
B. Interbody grafts reconstruct the anterior spinal column after corpectomy.
C. Trans-vertebral grafts are not across an intervening disc space.
D. None of the above.

Response (D) Strut grafts reconstruct the anterior spinal column following corpectomy. Interbody grafts reconstruct the anterior spinal column following discectomy; Trans-vertebral grafts are used to stabilize adjacent vertebrae and achieve fusion across an intervening disc space [44–47].

Question 60

Which of the following complications has been reported following the use of recombinant bone morphogenic protein-2 (rhBMP-2) during spinal fusion procedures?

A. Ectopic bone formation
B. Postoperative radiculitis
C. Increased rates of cage migration
D. Increased rates of postoperative seroma formation
E. All of the above.

Response (E) Although the FDA initially approved rhBMP-2 for use in anterior lumbar interbody fusion, it has seen much off-label use. Given its extensive use, there have been concerns regarding potential complications of its use. These complications are known to include: ectopic bone formation with compression of nearby structures, inflammation of the nerve roots due to local inflammatory reactions, increased rates of cage migration due to early osteolytic changes, and seroma formation [48].

References

1. Berman D, Oren JH, Bendo J, Spivak J. The effect of smoking on spinal fusion. Int J Spine Surg. 2017;11(4):29. https://doi.org/10.14444/4029.
2. Albrektsson T, Johansson C. Osteoinduction, osteoconduction and osseointegration. Eur Spine J. 2001;10(Suppl 2).
3. Miyazono K, Kusanagi K, Inoue H. Divergence and convergence of TGF-β/BMP signaling. J Cell Physiol. 2001;187(3):265–76.
4. Humphreys SC, Hodges SD, Patwardhan AG, Eck JC, Murphy BR, Covington LA. Comparison of posterior and transforaminal approaches to lumbar interbody fusion. Spine. 2001;26(5):567–71.
5. Mehta VA, McGirt MJ, Garcés-Ambrossi GL, et al. Transforaminal versus posterior lumbar interbody fusion: comparison of surgical morbidity. Neurol Res. 2011;33(1):38–42. https://doi.org/10.1179/016164110X12681290831289.
6. El-Ghandour N, Sawan M, Goel A, et al. A prospective randomized study of the safety and efficacy of transforaminal lumbar interbody fusion versus posterior lumbar interbody fusion in the treatment of lumbar spondylolisthesis: a cost utility from a lower-middle-income country perspective and review of literature. Open Access Maced J Med Sci. 2021;9(B):636–45. https://doi.org/10.3889/oamjms.2021.6569
7. Florencio-Silva R, Sasso GR, Sasso-Cerri E, Simões MJ, Cerri PS. Biology of bone tissue: structure, function, and factors that influence bone cells. Biomed Res Int. 2015;2015: 421746. https://doi.org/10.1155/2015/421746.
8. Jacob RP, Decker M. Bone metabolism and osteoporosis. In: Youmans, Winn, editors. Neurol. Surg. 2017;279:2315–21.e1.
9. Hustedt JW, Blizzard DJ. The controversy surrounding bone morphogenetic proteins in the spine: a review of current research. Yale J Biol Med. 2014;87(4):549–61. Published 2014 Dec 12.
10. Kumar P, Vinitha B, Fathima G. Bone grafts in dentistry. J Pharm Bioallied Sci. 2013;5(Suppl 1). https://doi.org/10.4103/0975-7406.113312
11. Liu J, Kerns DG. Mechanisms of guided bone regeneration: a review. Open Dent J. 2014;8:56–65. https://doi.org/10.2174/1874210601408010056.
12. Albrektsson T, Johansson C. Osteoinduction, osteoconduction and osseointegration. Eur Spine J. 2001;10(2).
13. Harris CT, Cooper LF. Comparison of bone graft matrices for human mesenchymal stem cell-directed osteogenesis. J Biomed Mater Res A. 2004;68(4):747–55.
14. Yuan N, Rezzadeh KS, Lee JC. Biomimetic scaffolds for osteogenesis. Receptors Clin Invest. 2015;2(3).
15. Helm GA, Dayoub H, Jane JA. Bone graft substitutes for the promotion of spinal arthrodesis. Neurosurg Focus. 2001;10(4):1–5.
16. Roberts TT, Rosenbaum AJ. Bone grafts, bone substitutes and orthobiologics: the bridge between basic science and clinical advancements in fracture healing. Organogenesis. 2012;8(4):114–24. https://doi.org/10.4161/org.23306.
17. Park P, Lau D, Brodt ED, Dettori JR. Electrical stimulation to enhance spinal fusion: a systematic review. Evid Based Spine Care J. 2014;5(2):87–94. https://doi.org/10.1055/s-0034-1386752.
18. Arrington ED, Smith WJ, Chambers HG, Bucknell AL, Davino NA. Complications of iliac crest bone graft harvesting. Clin Orthop Relat Res. 1996;329:300–9. https://doi.org/10.1097/00003086-199608000-00037. PMID: 8769465.
19. Morgan EF, De Giacomo A, Gerstenfeld LC. Overview of skeletal repair (fracture healing and its assessment). Methods Mol Biol. 2014;1130:13–31.
20. Li C, Kilpatrick CD, Smith S, et al. Assessment of multipotent mesenchymal stromal cells in bone marrow aspirate from human calcaneus. J Foot Ankle Surg. 2017;56(1):42–6. https://doi.org/10.1053/j.jfas.2016.09.006.
21. Zhang H, Yang L, Yang XG, et al. Demineralized bone matrix carriers and their clinical applications: an overview. Orthop Surg. 2019;11(5):725–37. https://doi.org/10.1111/os.12509.
22. Cannada LK, Scherping SC, Yoo JU, Jones PK, Emery SE. Pseudoarthrosis of the cervical spine: a comparison of radiographic diagnostic measures. Spine (Phila Pa 1976). 2003;28(1):46–51. https://doi.org/10.1097/00007632-200301010-00012. PMID: 12544955.
23. Soliman MA, Alkhamees AF, Khan A, Shamisa A. Instrumented Four-level anterior cervical discectomy and fusion: long-term clinical and radiographic outcomes. Neurol India. 2021;69(4):937–43.
24. Grabowski G, Cornett CA. Bone graft and bone graft substitutes in spine surgery: current concepts and controversies. JAAOS. 2013;21(1):51–60.
25. Abjornson C, Brecevich A, Callanan T, et al. ISASS recommendations and coverage criteria for bone graft substitutes used in spinal surgery. Int J Spine Surg. 2018;12(6):757–71.
26. Buck DW, Dumanian GA. Bone biology and physiology: part I. The fundamentals. Plast Reconstr Surg. 2012;129(6):1314–20.
27. Fernandez de Grado G, Keller L, Idoux-Gillet Y, et al. Bone substitutes: a review of their characteristics, clinical use, and perspectives for large bone defects management. J Tissue Eng. 2018;9:2041731418776819. https://doi.org/10.1177/2041731418776819.
28. Teles AR, Yavin D, Zafeiris CP, et al. Fractures after removal of spinal instrumentation: revisiting the stress-shielding effect of instrumentation in spine fusion. World Neurosurg. 2018;116.
29. Mannstadt M. Parathyroid hormone secretion and action. In: Rosen CJ, Mulder J, editors. UpToDate. 2021.
30. Boden SD. Overview of the biology of lumbar spine fusion and principles for selecting a bone graft substitute. Spine. 2002;27(16S).
31. Boden SD. Biology of lumbar spine fusion and use of bone graft substitutes: present, future, and next generation. Tissue Eng. 2000;6(4):383–99.

32. Gupta A, Kukkar N, Sharif K, et al. Bone graft substitutes for spine fusion: a brief review. World J Orthop. 2015;6(6):449.
33. Khan SN, Cammisa FP Jr, Sandhu HS, et al. The biology of bone grafting. JAAOS. 2005;13(1):77–86.
34. Sroga GE, Vashishth D. Effects of bone matrix proteins on fracture and fragility in osteoporosis. Curr Osteoporos Rep. 2012;10 (2):141–50. https://doi.org/10.1007/s11914-012-0103-6.
35. Gruskin E, Doll BA, Futrell FW, et al. Demineralized bone matrix in bone repair: history and use. Adv Drug Deliv Rev. 2012;64 (12):1063–77.
36. Lee KJ, Roper JG, Wang JC. Demineralized bone matrix and spinal arthrodesis. Spine J. 2005;5(6).
37. Zhang M, Powers RM Jr, Wolfinbarger L Jr. Effect(s) of the demineralization process on the osteoinductivity of demineralized bone matrix. J Periodontol. 1997;68(11):1085–92.
38. Cheng H, Jiang W, Phillips FM, et al. Osteogenic activity of the fourteen types of human bone morphogenetic proteins (BMPs). JBJS. 2003;85(8):1544–52.
39. Chen D, Zhao M, Mundy GR. Bone morphogenetic proteins. Growth Factors. 2004;22(4):233–41.
40. Sykaras N, Opperman LA. Bone morphogenetic proteins (BMPs): how do they function and what can they offer the clinician? J Oral Sci. 2003;45(2):57–73.
41. Yoon ST, Konopka JA, Wang JC, et al. ACDF graft selection by surgeons: survey of AOSpine members. Global Spine J. 2017;7 (5):410–6.
42. Spivak JM, Hasharoni A. Use of hydroxyapatite in spine surgery. Eur Spine J. 2001;10(2).
43. Bostrom MP, Seigerman DA. The clinical use of allografts, demineralized bone matrices, synthetic bone graft substitutes and osteoinductive growth factors: a survey study. HSS J. 2005;1(1):9–18.
44. Bridwell KH, Lenke LG, McEnery KW, et al. Anterior fresh frozen structural allografts in the thoracic and lumbar spine. Do they work if combined with posterior fusion and instrumentation in adult patients with kyphosis or anterior column defects? Spine. 1995;20(12):1410–8.
45. Molinari RW, Bridwell KH, Klepps SJ, Baldus C. Minimum 5-year follow-up of anterior column structural allografts in the thoracic and lumbar spine. Spine. 1999;24(10):967–72.
46. Singh K, DeWald CJ, Hammerberg KW, DeWald RL. Long structural allografts in the treatment of anterior spinal column defects. Clin Orthop Relat Res. 2002;1(394):121–9.
47. Lewandrowski KU, Hecht AC, DeLaney TF, et al. Anterior spinal arthrodesis with structural cortical allografts and instrumentation for spine tumor surgery. Spine. 2004;29(10):1150–8.
48. Murar J, Schroeder GD, Hsu WK. Complications of osteobiologics in spine surgery. In: Spinal instrumentation: challenges and solutions. 2020.

Intraoperative Neuromonitoring

5

Asham Khan, Moleca M. Ghannam, Ryan M. Hess, Slah Khan, Alexander O. Aguirre, Cathleen C. Kuo, Ali Y. Elkady, Ahmed H. Omar, Mohammad Elbaroody, and Mohamed A. R. Soliman

Question 1

Motor evoked potentials (MEPs) during spinal deformity surgery is a sensitive monitor of:

A. Corticospinal tract
B. Dorsal column
C. Medial lemniscus
D. Lateral spinothalamic tract.

Response (A) MEPs directly monitor the function of the motor pathways in the anterior/central portions of the spinal cord and the nerve roots. These are very sensitive indicators of corticospinal tract injury and have proven to be very sensitive indicators of spinal cord ischemia during spinal deformity correction. Spinal cord motor function monitoring is based on muscle responses to intermittent stimulation of the motor cortex in real-time [1].

Question 2

Which of the following anesthesia agents can be used during motor evoked potentials (MEPs) intraoperative monitoring?

A. Halothane.
B. Sevoflurane.
C. Isoflurane.
D. Propofol.

Response (D) MEPs have high sensitivity (75–100%) and specificity (84–100%), but they require avoidance of halogenated anesthetics (halothane, sevoflurane, isoflurane, etc.) and neuromuscular blockades (vecuronium, rocuronium, etc.). Ketamine-based anesthesia allows for appropriate MEP recordings, but total intravenous anesthesia (TIVA) with propofol is the anesthetic of choice [1].

Question 3

The use of EMG during surgery is to monitor:

A. The nerve root function during surgery
B. The muscle tone during surgery
C. The muscle movement during surgery
D. The presence of impulses in muscles during surgery.

Response (A) EMG is a type of 'real-time' neuromonitoring modality, mostly employed in detecting nerve root injuries [2].

A. Khan · M. M. Ghannam · R. M. Hess · S. Khan · A. O. Aguirre · C. C. Kuo · M. A. R. Soliman (✉)
Neurosurgery Department, University at Buffalo, Buffalo, NY, United States
e-mail: msolim8@uwo.ca

A. Khan
e-mail: akhan@ubns.com

M. M. Ghannam
e-mail: mghannam@ubns.com

R. M. Hess
e-mail: rhess@ubns.com

S. Khan
e-mail: slahkhan@buffalo.edu

A. O. Aguirre
e-mail: aa284@buffalo.edu

C. C. Kuo
e-mail: ckuo9@buffalo.edu

A. Y. Elkady · A. H. Omar · M. Elbaroody · M. A. R. Soliman
Neurosurgery Department, Cairo University, Cairo, Egypt
e-mail: ayousri54@gmail.com

A. H. Omar
e-mail: a.hussein.omar1990@gmail.com

M. Elbaroody
e-mail: mohammad.elbaroody@kasralainy.edu.eg

C. Gragnaniello et al. (eds.), *MCQs in Spine Surgery*,
https://doi.org/10.1007/978-3-031-69332-8_5

Question 4

The nerve impulses are actually:

A. ATP
B. Action potentials
C. Repolarization of nerves
D. Perception.

Response (B) Depolarization of the nerve cell leads to action potential formation, which propagates through the nerve body and axon to reach the target muscle [3].

Question 5

Regarding intraoperative somatosensory evoked potentials (SEPs) monitoring, all of the following is correct EXCEPT:

A. SEPs are more sensitive than motor evoked potentials (MEPs) to reduced blood flow secondary to vascular insult or hypotension.
B. SEPs were developed to monitor the posterior columns of the spinal cord.
C. SEPs monitoring does not provide any information on the descending corticospinal tract or spinal cord grey matter.
D. There is no difference between the SEPs monitoring between adults and infants.

Response (A) MEPs monitoring during spine surgery is both efficacious and safe. MEPs are more sensitive to reduced blood flow secondary to hypotension or vascular insult, compared to SEPs. Furthermore, MEPs change earlier than the SEPs signal, which facilitates quicker diagnosis of impending spinal cord injury [4].

Question 6

Which of the following is correct regarding somatosensory evoked potentials (SEPs) and motor evoked potentials (MEPs)?

A. SEPs are more sensitive to reduced blood flow secondary to vascular insult or hypotension.
B. SEPs change earlier than the MEPs signal, which facilitates quicker diagnosis of impending spinal cord injury.
C. There is no difference in monitoring MEPs between adults and infants.
D. The MEPs is elicited using a high-voltage short-duration stimulus applied to the scalp overlying the primary motor cortex.

Response (D) MEPs achieve motor specificity without the need for signal averaging. The MEPs is elicited using a high-voltage short-duration stimulus applied to the scalp overlying the primary motor cortex. The transcranial impulse generates multiple electrical waves that propagate down the spinal cord and synapse of the neuromuscular junction, leading to depolarization and muscle contraction. Monitoring the amplitude, latency, and morphology of the resultant compound muscle action potential assesses the motor pathway. Unlike SEPs, MEPs in pediatrics has some differences compared to adult patients. They require a greater charge delivered to obtain MEPs compared to adolescents, with decreased reliability in patients aged <6 years [4].

Question 7

A recording electrode was placed over the vastus lateralis muscle for EMG monitoring during a lumbar fusion surgery. Which root value corresponds to vastus lateralis?

A. L4-L5
B. L3-L4
C. S1-S2
D. T11-12.

Response (B) The vastus lateralis is supplied by muscular branches of the femoral nerve which is formed by contributions from L2, L3, and L4 [5].

Question 8

During thoraco-lumbar scoliosis correction surgery, the electrodes for intraoperative monitoring should be placed in all the following EXCEPT:

A. Intercostal
B. Rectus abdominus
C. Adductor pollicis
D. Vastus lateralis.

Response (C) Adductor pollicis is for C8-T1 root monitoring which is innervated proximal to the thoracolumbar levels involved in the surgery [6].

Question 9

All of the following decrease the amplitude of intraoperative somatosensory evoked potentials (SEPs) EXCEPT:

A. Propofol
B. Isoflurane

C. Nitrous oxide
D. Sevoflurane.

Response (A) All halogenated inhalational agents produce a dose-dependent decrease in amplitude and increase in latency for SEPs with cortical responses affected to a larger degree than subcortical and peripheral nerve responses. Nitrous oxide (N2O) causes a profound reduction in amplitude with increased latency in all neurophysiologic monitoring with suppression of cortical responses that mimic halogenated agents [7].

Question 10

During intraoperative scoliosis correction, the surgeon notes a decrease of >50% in the amplitude. According to the intraoperative neuromonitoring (IONM) checklist, which of the following should be considered?

A. Stop current manipulation.
B. Administration of steroids.
C. Check the depth of anesthesia.
D. All of the above.

Response (D) Decrease in the amplitude >50% means an affection to the neuronal tissue. All the above answers are actions done to avoid permanent neuronal injury [7].

Question 11

Intraoperative monitoring is highly recommended to be utilized in which of the following spinal procedures:

A. Correction of spinal deformities (e.g., scoliosis, kyphosis)
B. Insertion of spinal fixation devices (e.g., pedicle screw placement)
C. Decompression at the level of the spinal cord
D. Surgical treatment of spinal cord tumors
E. All of the above.

Response (E) In performing all of these spinal surgeries, intraoperative monitoring is highly recommended [8, 9].

Question 12

What is the most common mechanism responsible for neurologic injury during scoliosis surgery?

A. Direct injury due to surgical trauma (placement of spinal implants)
B. Traction and/or compression affecting neural structures (Spinal realignment and deformity correction)
C. Ischemia resulting in decreased perfusion of the spinal cord and/or nerve
D. Compressive neuropathy.

Response (C) Mechanisms that can cause neurologic injury during deformity surgeries are: (a) compression and/or traction of the neural structures, that could have occurred during spinal deformity correction and realignment using instrumentation or due to an epidural hematoma after corpectomy procedure; (b) iatrogenic direct neural injury, especially during spinal implant placement or neural decompression; (c) compressive neuropathy due to patient positioning before or during surgery (e.g. brachial plexus injury); (d) ischemia resulting in reduced perfusion of the neural structures, causing an ischemic injury to the spinal cord and/or nerve roots (e.g. following critical segmental vessels ligation that supplies the spinal cord or after sustained hypotension). Ischemia is the most common mechanism responsible for neurologic injury during scoliosis surgery [10, 11].

Question 13

Which one of the following statements regarding somatosensory evoked potentials (SEPs) is incorrect?

A. They are a modification of the basic EEG in which a cortical or subcortical response to repetitive stimulation of a peripheral mixed nerve is recorded at sites cephalad and caudad to the operative field.
B. They provide direct information about the status of the ascending spinal cord sensory tracts.
C. They can provide an indirect information about the status of the spinal cord motor tracts.
D. SEPs data provide real-time data regarding the intraoperative neurologic function.

Response (D) SEPs do not provide real-time data regarding neurologic function because there is a slight delay (usually, 1 min). The SEPs response is averaged for extraction from background noise [12–15].

Question 14

Which one of the following changes of somatosensory evoked potentials (SEPs) is incorrect?

A. A unilateral complete loss of amplitude mandates stopping of surgery.

B. A bilateral loss of amplitude 50% or greater relative to baseline amplitude mandates stopping of surgery.
C. Spinal cord injury is more likely to occur if the amplitude is unchanged.
D. Changes in latency are common and less significant.

Response (C) Spinal cord injury is unlikely if the amplitude is unchanged [12–15].

Question 15

Which of the following statements regarding the transcranial electric motor evoked potentials (tceMEPs) is false?

A. tceMEPs are neuroelectric impulses elicited by transcranial application of a high-voltage stimulus to electrodes placed over specific scalp regions to excite specific areas of the motor cortex.
B. tceMEPs can provide information about the functional integrity of the spinal cord motor tracts that cannot be obtained using somatosensory evoked potentials (SEPs).
C. tceMEPs are extremely sensitive to spinal cord blood flow alterations resulting from intraoperative hypotension or evolving vascular injury.
D. When evolving intraoperative injury occurs, the changes in tceMEPs appear delayed compared to SEPs changes.

Response (D) Alterations in tceMEPs present earlier than changes in SEPs in patients with evolving neurologic injury, which permits earlier initiation of corrective action to prevent permanent neurologic compromise. tceMEPs are not a replacement for SEPs but are used in combination with SEPs to directly measure both spinal cord sensory and motor tract function, thereby increasing the efficacy of spinal monitoring [16–18].

Question 16

Which of the following techniques are used for monitoring spinal cord function?

A. Stagnara wake-up test
B. Ankle clonus test
C. Somatosensory evoked potentials (SEPs)
D. Transcranial electric motor-evoked potentials (tceMEPs)
E. All of the above.

Response (E) Stagnara wake-up test, ankle clonus test, somatosensory-evoked potentials (SEPs), and transcranial electric motor-evoked potentials (tceMEPs) are all neuromonitoring techniques that can be used to assess the spinal cord function during spine surgery [19–20].

Question 17

Which one of the following regarding electromyographic monitoring during spinal procedures is false?

A. Electromyography (EMG) is used to assess the functional integrity of individual nerve roots.
B. Mechanically elicited electromyograms are used during the dynamic phases of surgery, such as pedicle screw insertion.
C. Mechanically elicited EMGs are termed stimulus-evoked EMG or triggered EMG.
D. Electrically elicited EMGs should be used during the static phases of surgery, such as immediately before or after pedicle screw placement.

Response (C) Mechanically elicited EMGs are termed spontaneous, or free-running EMGs. An electrically elicited EMG is termed a stimulus-evoked or triggered EMG [14, 21, 22].

Question 18

Regarding the effect of the anesthetic agents on neurophysiologic signals, all of the following statements are true, EXCEPT:

A. Inhalational agents depress signal amplitude, increase signal variability, and increase interpretative error.
B. All depolarizing and non-depolarizing paralytic agents should be avoided throughout the operation.
C. Inhalational agents should be avoided after induction and intubation.
D. A total intravenous anesthesia regimen (TIVA) is optimal when transcranial electric motor and somatosensory evoked potentials are recorded.

Response (B) All depolarizing and non-depolarizing paralytic agents should be avoided, except at the beginning of the procedure during spinal exposure, because these agents block neuromuscular junction transmission and preclude muscle contraction. Muscle relaxation allows for easier exposure and retraction [23–25].

Question 19

Which one of the following factors has an adverse effect on somatosensory evoked potentials (SEPs) recordings?

A. Halogenated anesthetic agents
B. Nitrous oxide
C. Hypothermia
D. Hypotension.
E. A, B, and C
F. All of the above.

Response (F) Halogenated anesthetic agents, nitrous oxide, hypothermia, and hypotension all have an adverse effect on SEPs recording [12–15].

Question 20

Why somatosensory evoked potentials (SEPs) are not considered a "real-time" intraoperative monitoring modality?

A. Need to use a stimulus frequency less than 60 Hz.
B. Low amplitude nature of the stimulus.
C. Slow conduction of electrical stimuli by the large fiber sensory nerves.
D. High number of stimulated responses in order to average out background noise.
E. Significant decrease in baseline SEPs is required to detect damage to the nervous system.

Response (D) SEPs are not considered to offer real-time monitoring as a significant number of trials of signal amplification are required in order to average out the background noise of other biologic stimuli and operating room equipment. It has been reported that 500–1000 stimuli are required, and the process of averaging these signals takes several minutes [26].

Question 21

Which of the following is considered an advantage of using motor evoked potentials (MEPs) for intraoperative monitoring compared to somatosensory evoked potentials?

A. Less disruption of surgical flow during obtaining signals.
B. Decreased risk of bite injuries.
C. Changes in patient positioning while obtaining stimulus are less likely.
D. Increased utility in patients with diabetic neuropathy.
E. Decreased risk of seizures.

Response (D) MEPs allow for a more accurate assessment of the cortical spinal tracts than somatosensory evoked potentials (SEPs). In addition, patients with polyneuropathies such as diabetic neuropathy have more difficulty conducting the low amplitude stimuli of SEPs compared to the higher amplitude stimuli seen in motor evoked potentials. However, there are downsides to the use of motor evoked potentials. These revolve mainly around the consequences of high-intensity stimulus used. The high amplitude of the signal causes jerking motions of the muscles, which can lead to damage from surgical instruments, tongue biting, position changes, and seizures in rare cases. As a result, all surgical activities are stopped to obtain motor evoked potentials. This can disrupt the operative flow [26].

Question 22

When performing an extreme lateral interbody fusion (XLIF), which of the following muscles is not commonly monitored via EMG?

A. Extensor hallucis longus
B. Vastus medialis
C. Biceps femoris
D. Tibialis anterior
E. Gastrocnemius.

Response (A) All of the following muscles except extensor hallucis longus are monitored via EMG during an XLIF. These muscles are easily palpable and are innervated by branches of the lumbar plexus, which is at risk of injury during the transpsoas approach used in this procedure [27].

Question 23

Which of the following is not a disadvantage of motor evoked potentials (MEPs)?

A. Long turn-around time for one stimulation.
B. Highly sensitive to neuromuscular blockade.
C. Highly vulnerable to inhalation anesthesia.
D. Highly intertrial variability in amplitude.
E. Possibility of seizure induction.

Response (A) MEPs monitor motor pathways by stimulating corticospinal tracts. This technique has some disadvantages, such as high sensitivity to inhalation agents and neuromuscular blockage and stimulation-related movement. However, the time required for any stimulation is relatively brief in MEPs. Meaningful monitoring information can be obtained in a minute or less, and multiple stimulations can be done without interrupting the ongoing flow of the surgery [28].

Question 24

A 54-year-old male with a history of a recent fall on his back after slipping on ice presents with diminished knee jerk reflex and has weakness in knee extension. The patient also has diminished sensation on the medial foot. The MRI of the lumbar spine has shown a single level central disc herniation. Which level of the lumbar spine does this patient most likely have a decreased baseline neuromonitoring EMG signal?

A. L2-3
B. L3-4
C. L4-5
D. L5-S1.

Response (B) This patient has all the symptomatology of someone who has a herniated disc at the L3-L4 level. This can be seen with weakness of knee extension, diminished patellar reflex, and diminished sensation in the medial aspect of the foot (L4) [29].

Question 25

If a disc herniation occurred at the C6-7 level, which motor evoked potentials (MEPs) would demonstrate increased amplitude after corrective spinal fusion?

A. Biceps
B. Deltoid
C. Triceps
D. Both A and C.

Response (C) Triceps will be the only MEPs that is diminished when a disc herniation occurs at this level since the C7 nerve root is compressed. The deltoid will be affected by a C4-5 herniation, and the biceps will be diminished with a C5-6 herniation [30].

Question 26

What is a limitation of the somatosensory evoked potentials (SEPs)?

A. Abrupt disturbance to the surgical procedure
B. Cannot be monitored constantly
C. Neuromuscular blocks alter the results
D. Only provides information about the posterior 2/3 of the spinal cord.

Response (D) Providing information about the posterior 2/3 of the spinal cord is the only limitation of SEPs among the above answers as it provides information from the sensory tracts and dorsal aspects of the cord. Somatosensory evoked potentials allow for limited disturbances during surgery, can be monitored constantly, and neuromuscular blocks do not impact the results [31, 32].

Question 27

Which of the following locations is not a placement for somatosensory evoked potentials in monitoring upper extremities?

A. Erb's point
B. Cz-A1 and Cz-A2
C. Over spinous process (CII)
D. Contralateral cortex (C3, C4).

Response (B) Erb's point, over spinous process (CII), and contralateral cortex (C3, C4) are all used for the monitoring of upper extremities. In contrast, Cz-A1/A2 are used to monitor lower extremities during an operation [33].

Question 28

Which of the following anesthesia gas agents cannot be used during transcranial motor evoked potential monitoring?

A. N2O
B. Halothane
C. Isoflurane
D. Sevoflurane.

Response (A) During transcranial motor evoked potential monitoring, N2O cannot be used as it disrupts the ability to stimulate motor evoked potentials. All the other gases are halogens, which do not interact with this monitoring approach [34, 35].

Question 29

Triggered electromyography (EMG) is used to detect:

A. Anterior spinal horn injury
B. Misplacement of spinal interbody
C. Pedicle screw breach
D. Inferior nerve injury.

Response (C) The triggered EMG is used to determine whether the pedicle screw has breached through the medial or lateral walls after their placement. The other choices cannot be monitored by the triggered EMG [36, 37].

Question 30

What is the accurate range of normal threshold potentials for a lumbar triggered EMG?

A. 6 to 8 mA
B. 7.6 to 10 mA
C. 7.6 to 11 mA
D. 15 to 20 mA.

Response (C) The range of 7.6–11 mA is the normal range for lumbar triggered EMG. The range of 6–8 mA is the normal range for thoracic thresholds, while 7.6–10 mA is the correct range for the normal cervical thresholds. 15–20 mA has a range that often strongly suggests a pedicle breach has occurred [36, 38].

Question 31

If the H reflex disappeared unilaterally during surgery, this represents which nerve roots compromise?

A. S4 and S5
B. L4 and L5
C. L1 and L2
D. S1 and S2.

Response (D) The H reflex is a monosynaptic reflex response that can be obtained from the soleus muscle after stimulation of the tibial nerve. Compromise of the S1 and S2 nerve roots would demonstrate a unilateral disappearance of the H reflex intraoperatively. The other answer choices do not have any association with the H reflex [37].

Question 32

If a surgeon wants to isolate the root of a nerve injury to a singular spinal level, which neuromonitoring modality should be added?

A. Dermatomal somatosensory evoked potentials (SEPs)
B. Pudendal SEPs
C. Transcranial motor evoked potentials
D. Triggered EMG.

Response (A) The dermatomal SEPs provide detailed sensory information to isolate a single nerve root dysfunction, which is a limitation of the other answer choices [39].

Question 33

During an L4-5 posterior lumbar interbody fusion, a decreased amplitude on dermatomal somatosensory evoked potentials (SEPs) due to nerve injury while performing the interbody cage placement can be demonstrated by loss of sensation to which anatomical location of the lower limb, most commonly?

A. Lateral foot
B. Posterior Calf
C. Lateral Calf
D. Medial Calf.

Response (D) The L4 nerve root exits at the L4-5 level to innervate the lateral thigh, patellar region, and medial calf to the medial foot and big toe. The posterior calf and lateral foot are innervated by the S1 nerve, while the L5 nerve innervates the lateral calf [40].

Question 34

Which of the following is NOT A TRUE statement regarding Spinal Cord Injury without Radiographic Abnormality (SCIWORA)?

A. SCIWORA is more commonly seen in the pediatric age group, with a predilection for the cervical spine.
B. The most important factor in SCIWORA prognosis is age.
C. Cord hemorrhage is not an expected finding on MRI of patients with SCIWORA.
D. The mainstay treatment for SCIWORA is cervical brace or collar and restriction of high-risk activities.
E. Within the diagnostic algorithm of SCIWORA, somatosensory evoked potentials are considered a special rather than routine test.

Response (B) In general, most SCIWORA patients show remarkable improvement in neurological status after the injury, and operative management is rarely justifiable. The most significant predictor of prognosis after SCIWORA is the initial neurological status. Pediatric patients with complete spinal cord injury rarely improve, and those with severe but incomplete spinal cord injury often improve but seldom regain normal function. Patients with mild to moderate initial neurological deficits, on the other hand, have a higher chance of attaining full recovery [41].

Question 35

Which of the following is NOT a consensus-based best practice guideline for Intraoperative Neurophysiological Monitoring in pediatric and adult spine deformity surgery in the United States?

A. Transcranial motor evoked potentials and/or descending neurogenic evoked potentials should be used in all spine deformity cases.
B. A 50% decrease in somatosensory evoked potentials (SEPs) signal amplitude from baseline and/or a sustained decrease in transcranial motor evoked potentials signal amplitude, and/or a decrease in descending neurogenic evoked potentials signal of >60% constitutes “significant warning criteria” in spine deformity surgery.
C. Spontaneous and triggered electromyography should be used in all spine deformity cases.
D. Intraoperative neuromonitoring is best performed with a team approach: surgeon, anesthesiologist, and qualified neuromonitoring personnel should all be involved in identifying and communicating neuromonitoring changes.
E. A wake-up test should always be considered in spine deformity cases with persistent signal degradation or in all patients who cannot be monitored.

Response (C) Somatosensory evoked potentials, not spontaneous and triggered electromyography, should be used in all spinal deformity surgeries. The consensus-based checklist for intraoperative neurophysiological monitoring was developed to improve patient care quality and minimize the risk of the neurological deficit through optimization of clinical decision-making. This checklist also contains several prompts for items that could be easily overlooked during a crisis response, such as checking limb positioning and anticipating the need for future actions such as a wake-up test [42].

Question 36

During an anterior cervical discectomy and fusion, the neurophysiologist notices a sudden change in the waveform at Erb’s point. Which of the following structure is most likely affected?

A. P14: cervico-medullary junction
B. N22: ulnar nerve
C. N13: radial nerve
D. N9: brachial plexus
E. N8: popliteal fossa.

Response (D) Somatosensory evoked potentials are recorded from the upper and/or lower extremity nerve to identify impending permanent damage to neurologic structures. N9, also known as Erb’s point, reflects the sensory contributions of the brachial plexus. Ulnar nerve and radial nerve are typically not monitored. N22 is the nomenclature for the post-synaptic dorsal horn of the lumbar spinal cord, and N13 refers to the post-synaptic dorsal horn of the cervical spinal cord [43].

Question 37

Which of the following is NOT a relative contraindication for intraoperative motor evoked potentials?

A. Increased intracranial pressure
B. Presence of pacemaker
C. Cochlear prosthesis
D. History of epilepsy
E. Morbid obesity.

Response (E) There is no absolute contraindication for any of the techniques of intraoperative neurophysiological monitoring. However, some relative contraindications for motor evoked potentials exist, including a history of seizure disorder, increased intracranial pressure or cortical lesions, defects of the skull or skull convexity, implanted deep brain stimulator leads, cardiac pacemakers, and other implanted devices (i.e. cochlear prosthesis) [44].

Question 38

A 15-year-old girl was scheduled to undergo an anterior and posterior fusion of her lumbar spine. The patient has a history of thoracic laminectomy and spinal cord astrocytoma resection three years prior. Bilateral lower extremity weakness and minimal sensation and proprioception on the left leg were noted on preoperative evaluation. A device was placed to monitor the central nervous system’s response to various surgical stimuli. Administering which of the following anesthetic agents during the surgery would increase the response amplitude?

A. Propofol
B. Ketamine
C. Midazolam
D. Clonidine
E. Tubocurarine.

Response (B) The described device in this vignette is somatosensory evoked potentials (SEPs). It directly assesses spinal cord sensory tracts while providing indirect information about motor tracts. Anesthetics have varying effects on SEPs. Ketamine is an N-methyl D-aspartate receptor and glutamate receptor antagonist that affects the amplitude of cortical SEPs without affecting the latency. Propofol and midazolam increase SEPs latency and decrease amplitude. As an alpha-2 agonist, Clonidine does not affect SEPs; however, it severely interferes with motor pathways neuromonitoring. Tubocurarine also has no direct effect on SEPs [45].

Question 39

Which of the following is NOT a potential risk factor for electrophysiologic and neurologic deterioration during cervical surgery?

A. Long segment surgery
B. Use of instrumentation
C. Preexisting myelopathy
D. Surgery at the clivus, the atlas, or the axis
E. Surgery at lower cervical segment.

Response (E) Risk factors for electrophysiologic and neurologic deterioration during cervical surgery are preoperative myelopathy, multi-segmental surgery, upper cervical surgery, use of instrumentation, and application of corrective forces to the neck. Among them, myelopathy is the strongest predictor that overshadowed the effect of the other recognized factors [46].

Question 40

After placing an interbody cage from a lateral approach, there is an immediate drop in amplitude in motor evoked potentials for the quadriceps muscle; at which level did the surgery most likely occur?

A. L1
B. L3
C. L5
D. S1.

Response (B) The cage was placed too posteriorly in this patient and caused either transient or permanent damage to the nerve root at the index level. The femoral nerve originates from the dorsal divisions of the L2-L4 ventral rami. It innervates the quadriceps muscle. The L3 nerve root is the only one in this range, making it the correct answer.

References

1. Baumgart M, Wiśniewski M, Grzonkowska M, et al. Digital image analysis of ossification centers in the axial dens and body in the human fetus. Surg Radiol Anat. 2016;38(10):1195–203.
2. Biscevic M, Sehic A, Krupic F. Intraoperative neuromonitoring in spine deformity surgery: modalities, advantages, limitations, medicolegal issues—surgeons' views. EFORT Open Rev. 2020;5 (1):9–16. https://doi.org/10.1302/2058-5241.5.180032.
3. Kress GJ, Mennerick S. Action potential initiation and propagation: upstream influences on neurotransmission. Neuroscience. 2009;158 (1):211–22. https://doi.org/10.1016/j.neuroscience.2008.03.021.
4. Levin DN, Strantzas S, Steinberg BE. Intraoperative neuromonitoring in paediatric spinal surgery. BJA Educ. 2019;19(5):165–71. https://doi.org/10.1016/j.bjae.2019.01.007.
5. Anloague PA, Huijbregts P. Anatomical variations of the lumbar plexus: a descriptive anatomy study with proposed clinical implications. J Man Manip Ther. 2009;17(4). https://doi.org/10.1179/106698109791352201.
6. Park JH, Hyun SJ. Intraoperative neurophysiological monitoring in spinal surgery. World J Clin Cases. 2015;3(9):765–73. https://doi.org/10.12998/wjcc.v3.i9.765.
7. Pajewski TN, Arlet V, Phillips LH. Current approach on spinal cord monitoring: the point of view of the neurologist, the anesthesiologist and the spine surgeon. Eur Spine J. 2007;16 (Suppl 2). https://doi.org/10.1007/s00586-007-0419-6.
8. Stecker MM. A review of intraoperative monitoring for spinal surgery. Surg Neurol Int. 2012;3(Suppl 3).
9. Laratta JL, Ha A, Shillingford JN, Makhni MC, Lombardi JM, Thuet E, Lehman RA, Lenke LG. Neuromonitoring in spinal deformity surgery: a multimodality approach. Global Spine J. 2018;8(1):68–77.
10. Buchowski JM, Bridwell KH, Lenke LG, Kuhns CA, Lehman RA Jr, Kim YJ, Stewart D, Baldus C. Neurologic complications of lumbar pedicle subtraction osteotomy: a 10-year assessment. Spine. 2007;32(20):2245–52.
11. Schwartz DM, Auerbach JD, Dormans JP, Flynn J, Drummond DS, Bowe JA, Laufer S, Shah SA, Bowen JR, Pizzutillo PD, Jones KJ. Neurophysiological detection of impending spinal cord injury during scoliosis surgery. JBJS. 2007;89(11):2440–9.
12. Neuloh G, Schramm J. Monitoring of motor evoked potentials compared with somatosensory evoked potentials and microvascular Doppler ultrasonography in cerebral aneurysm surgery. J Neurosurg. 2004;100(3):389–99.
13. Toleikis JR. Intraoperative monitoring using somatosensory evoked potentials. J Clin Monit Comput. 2005;19(3):241–58.
14. Uribe JS, Vale FL, Dakwar E. Electromyographic monitoring and its anatomical implications in minimally invasive spine surgery. Spine. 2010;35(26S).
15. Avila EK, Elder JB, Singh P, Chen X, Bilsky MH. Intraoperative neurophysiologic monitoring and neurologic outcomes in patients with epidural spine tumors. Clin Neurol Neurosurg. 2013;115 (10):2147–52.
16. Schwartz DM, Sestokas AK, Dormans JP, Vaccaro AR, Hilibrand AS, Flynn JM, Li PM, Shah SA, Welch W, Drummond DS, Albert TJ. Transcranial electric motor evoked potential monitoring during spine surgery: is it safe? Spine. 2011;36(13):1046–9.
17. Hilibrand AS, Schwartz DM, Sethuraman V, Vaccaro AR, Albert TJ. Comparison of transcranial electric motor and somatosensory evoked potential monitoring during cervical spine surgery. JBJS. 2004;86(6):1248–53.
18. Pastorelli F, Di Silvestre M, Vommaro F, Maredi E, Morigi A, Bacchin MR, Bonarelli S, Plasmati R, Michelucci R, Greggi T.

Intraoperative monitoring of somatosensory (SSEPs) and transcranial electric motor-evoked potentials (tce-MEPs) during surgical correction of neuromuscular scoliosis in patients with central or peripheral nervous system diseases. Eur Spine J. 2015;24(7):931–6.
19. Møller AR, Ansari S, Cohen-Gadol AA. Techniques of intraoperative monitoring for spinal cord function: their past, present, and future directions. Neurol Res. 2011;33(4):363–70.
20. Kalkman CJ, Been HD, Visser BW. Intraoperative monitoring of spinal cord function: a review. Acta Orthop Scand. 1993;64 (1):114–23.
21. Holland NR. Intraoperative electromyography. J Clin Neurophysiol. 2002;19(5):444–53.
22. Epstein NE. The need to add motor evoked potential monitoring to somatosensory and electromyographic monitoring in cervical spine surgery. Surg Neurol Int. 2013;4(Suppl 5).
23. Chen Z. The effects of isoflurane and propofol on intraoperative neurophysiological monitoring during spinal surgery. J Clin Monit Comput. 2004;18(4):303–8.
24. Hans P, Bonhomme V. Why we still use intravenous drugs as the basic regimen for neurosurgical anaesthesia. Curr Opin Anaesthesiol. 2006;19(5):498–503.
25. Wang AC, Than KD, Etame AB, La Marca F, Park P. Impact of anesthesia on transcranial electric motor evoked potential monitoring during spine surgery: a review of the literature. Neurosurg Focus. 2009;27(4).
26. Bartol SW. Intraoperative monitoring. In: An anatomic approach to minimally invasive spine surgery.
27. Pimenta L, Amaral R, Marchi L, Oliveira L. Extreme lateral interbody fusion. In: An anatomic approach to minimally invasive spine surgery.
28. Kim SM, Kim SH, Seo DW, Lee KW. Intraoperative neurophysiologic monitoring: basic principles and recent update. J Korean Med Sci. 2013;28(9):1261–9. https://doi.org/10.3346/jkms.2013.28.9.1261.
29. Baaj AA, Mummaneni PV, Uribe JS, Vaccaro AR, Greenburg MS. In: Baaj AA, Mummaneni PV, Uribe JS, Vaccaro AR, Greenburg MS, editors. Handbook of spine surgery, 2nd ed. New York; 2016.
30. Bryndal A, Wojtysiak M, Moskal J, Lipiec-Kowalska J, Borowczyk M, Tańska M, Grochulska A, Huber J, Majchrzycki M. Motor evoked potentials after supraspinal stimulation in pre- and postoperative evaluations of patients with cervical radiculopathy. Biomed Res Int. 2019;2019:4576493. https://doi.org/10.1155/2019/4576493.
31. Restuccia D, Valeriani M, Di Lazzaro V, Tonali P, Mauguière F. Somatosensory evoked potentials after multisegmental upper limb stimulation in diagnosis of cervical spondylotic myelopathy. J Neurol Neurosurg Psychiatry. 1994;57(3):301–8. https://doi.org/10.1136/jnnp.57.3.301.
32. Veilleux M, Daube JR. The value of ulnar somatosensory evoked potentials (SEPs) in cervical myelopathy. Electroencephalogr Clin Neurophysiol. 1987;68(6):415–23. https://doi.org/10.1016/0168-5597(87)90053-0.
33. Yue Q, Hale T, Knecht A. A comparison of interside asymmetries of lower extremity somatosensory evoked potentials in anesthetized patients with unilateral lumbosacral radiculopathy. Asian Spine J. 2017;11(1):99–104. https://doi.org/10.4184/asj.2017.11.1.99.
34. Ubags LH, Kalkman CJ, Been HD, Koelman JH, Ongerboer de Visser BW. A comparison of myogenic motor evoked responses to electrical and magnetic transcranial stimulation during nitrous oxide/opioid anesthesia. Anesth Analg. 1999;88:568–72. https://doi.org/10.1213/00000539-199903000-00019.
35. Kempton LB, Nantau WE, Zaltz I. Successful monitoring of transcranial electrical motor evoked potentials with isoflurane and nitrous oxide in scoliosis surgeries. Spine (Phila Pa 1976). 2010;35:E1627–9.
36. Kassis SZ, Abukwedar LK, Msaddi AK, Majer CN, Othman W. Combining pedicle screw stimulation with spinal navigation, a protocol to maximize the safety of neural elements and minimize radiation exposure in thoracolumbar spine instrumentation. Eur Spine J. 2016;25:1724–8. https://doi.org/10.1007/s00586-015-3973-3.
37. Makovec M, Benedičič M, Bošnjak R. H wave and spinal root potentials in neuromonitoring of S1 root function during evacuation of herniated disc: preliminary results. Croat Med J. 2006;47 (2):298–304.
38. Mikula AL, Williams SK, Anderson PA. The use of intraoperative triggered electromyography to detect misplaced pedicle screws: a systematic review and meta-analysis. J Neurosurg Spine. 2016;24:624–38. https://doi.org/10.3171/2015.6.SPINE141323.
39. Jo NG, Ko MH, Won YH, Park SH, Kim GW, Seo JH (2021) Diagnostic implication and clinical relevance of dermatomal somatosensory evoked potentials in patients with radiculopathy: a retrospective study. Pain Res Manag. 2021;2021:8850281. https://doi.org/10.1155/2021/8850281.
40. Liyew WA. Clinical presentations of lumbar disc degeneration and lumbosacral nerve lesions. Int J Rheumatol. 2020;2020:2919625. https://doi.org/10.1155/2020/2919625.
41. Konovalov N, Peev N, Zileli M, Sharif S, Kaprovoy S, Timonin S. Pediatric cervical spine injuries and SCIWORA: WFNS spine committee recommendations. Neurospine. 2020;17(4):797–808. https://doi.org/10.14245/ns.2040404.202.
42. Vitale MG, et al. Best practices in intraoperative neuromonitoring in spine deformity surgery: development of an intraoperative checklist to optimize response. Spine Deform. 2014;2(5):333–39. https://doi.org/10.1016/j.jspd.2014.05.003. Epub 2014 Aug 27.
43. Draughn LR, Swanson TH. Axillary somatosensory evoked potential response: an alternate peripheral recording site. J Clin Neurophysiol. 1998;15(1):64–8. https://doi.org/10.1097/00004691-199801000-00008.
44. MacDonald DB. Safety of intraoperative transcranial electrical stimulation motor evoked potential monitoring. J Clin Neurophysiol. 2002;19(5):416–29. https://doi.org/10.1097/00004691-200210000-00005.
45. Stoicea N, Versteeg G, Florescu D, et al. Ketamine-based anesthetic protocols and evoked potential monitoring: a risk/benefit overview. Front Neurosci. 2016;10:37. https://doi.org/10.3389/fnins.2016.00037.
46. Cheung JP, Luk KD. Complications of anterior and posterior cervical spine surgery. Asian Spine J. 2016;10(2):385–400. https://doi.org/10.4184/asj.2016.10.2.385.

Minimally Invasive Spine Surgery

6

Asham Khan, Moleca M. Ghannam, Ryan M. Hess, Slah Khan, Alexander O. Aguirre, Cathleen C. Kuo, Ali Y. Elkady, Ahmed H. Omar, Mohammad Elbaroody, and Mohamed A. R. Soliman

Question 1

During a minimally invasive lumbar microdiscectomy, what complication often occurs but should be avoided when introducing the initial dilators?

A. Penetration of the interlaminar space
B. Tear of the Ligamentum Flava
C. Vascular injury
D. Nerve root retraction

Response (A) Penetration of the interlaminar space occurs when placing the initial dilator tube and should be avoided in this procedure. A tear of the ligamentum flavum is not seen in this procedure while vascular injury and nerve root injury from retraction happen in less than 1% of cases [1, 2].

Question 2

The trajectory of the minimally invasive transforaminal lumbar interbody fusion (MIS TLIF) avoids the need to perform which of the following?

A. Laminectomy/laminotomy
B. Remove the ipsilateral facet joint
C. Retraction of the nerve root and dura
D. Remove a part of the Ligamentum Flava

Response (C) The retraction of the nerve root and the dura are minimal compared to other approaches such as the PLIF. All the other answers are still required during an MIS TLIF [1, 2].

Question 3

Damage to the psoas muscle during a minimally invasive lateral lumbar interbody fusion (LLIF) causes which of the following postoperative complications?

A. Abdominal viscera perforation
B. Quadriceps weakness
C. Thigh numbness
D. Hip flexor weakness

Response (D) The psoas muscle is one of the contributing muscles to flexion of the leg, which is weakened by the trans-psoas approach often used in LLIF approaches. The others are also complications of the LLIF approach but do not occur because of damage to the psoas muscle [3].

A. Khan · M. M. Ghannam · R. M. Hess · S. Khan · A. O. Aguirre · C. C. Kuo · M. A. R. Soliman (✉)
Neurosurgery Department, University at Buffalo, Buffalo, NY, United States
e-mail: msolim8@uwo.ca

A. Khan
e-mail: akhan@ubns.com

M. M. Ghannam
e-mail: mghannam@ubns.com

R. M. Hess
e-mail: rhess@ubns.com

S. Khan
e-mail: slahkhan@buffalo.edu

A. O. Aguirre
e-mail: aa284@buffalo.edu

C. C. Kuo
e-mail: ckuo9@buffalo.edu

A. Y. Elkady · A. H. Omar · M. Elbaroody · M. A. R. Soliman
Neurosurgery Department, Cairo University, Cairo, Egypt
e-mail: ayousri54@gmail.com

A. H. Omar
e-mail: a.hussein.omar1990@gmail.com

M. Elbaroody
e-mail: mohammad.elbaroody@kasralainy.edu.eg

C. Gragnaniello et al. (eds.), *MCQs in Spine Surgery*,
https://doi.org/10.1007/978-3-031-69332-8_6

Question 4

Damage to what nerve can cause thigh numbness after a minimally invasive lateral lumbar interbody fusion?

A. Anterior femoral cutaneous nerve
B. Common peroneal nerve
C. Obturator nerve
D. Genitofemoral nerve

Response (A) The anterior femoral cutaneous nerve is a branch of the femoral nerve that causes thigh numbness. No transient weakness is seen as this branch is only isolated to respond to sensory information [3].

Question 5

Which of the following is not a complication of the thoracoscopic approach to a thoracic corpectomy?

A. Cerebrospinal fluid leak
B. Chyle leak
C. Wrong level surgery
D. Decreased pulmonary function

Response (D) The risk of wrong level surgery is high due to limited field exposure; while CSF and Chyle leaks are less commonly observed, the risk during this approach is still present. There are no changes in pulmonary function after thoracoscopic approach to thoracic corpectomy; rather, this is seen in scoliosis correction surgery [4].

Question 6

Which of the following is not a benefit of a minimally invasive approach for spine surgery?

A. Less blood loss
B. Decreased operative time
C. Diminished amount of postoperative opioid use
D. Reduced risk of infection

Response (B) Less blood loss, diminished amount of postoperative opioid use and reduction in risk of infection are all proven benefits to the use of minimally invasive spine surgeries [3].

Question 7

What is NOT an accepted minimally invasive approach for spinal decompression surgery?

A. Tubular dilators
B. Microscope
C. Endoscopic approach
D. All of the above are accepted approaches

Response (D) Tubular dilators, microscopes, and endoscopes are all accepted instruments for minimally invasive spine surgery [6].

Question 8

A 60-year-old male presents to the spine clinic with low back pain, left radicular leg pain, and numbness along the sciatic region to the calf. He reports that these symptoms started after carrying heavy loads a week ago. His surgical history was significant for a successful microdiscectomy at the L4-L5 level ten months ago. Physical examination reveals 3/5 left big toe dorsiflexion strength, mild sensory loss in the left lateral lower leg, and 45 degrees on the right straight leg raising test. MRI shows left-sided L4-L5 paracentral disc herniation. Conservative therapy was initiated, but the effect was poor. What is the most appropriate next step in management?

A. Decompression with transforaminal lumbar interbody fusion
B. Microdiscectomy through a far lateral approach
C. Microdiscectomy through a midline approach
D. Extreme lateral lumbar interbody fusion
E. Anterior lumbar interbody fusion

Response (C) The vignette is consistent with single-level recurrent lumbar disc herniation. Nonoperative treatment is usually the first-line therapy for most patients. However, when it fails, revision microdiscectomy is indicated. A midline approach is suggested because this patient has a paracentral disc herniation [5].

Question 9

What is an indication for the use of minimally invasive transforaminal lumbar interbody fusion?

A. >3 levels degenerative disc disease
B. Spondylolisthesis with Meyerding grade < III
C. Recurrent lumbar disc herniation
D. All of the above are correct indications for this approach

Response (C) Recurrent lumbar disc herniation is an appropriate indication for the use of MIS TLIF. A single-level or 2-level surgery is an indication for the minimally invasive (MIS) approach; anything more is considered a contraindication for MIS. Meyerding grade < III is also an indication for MIS [7, 8].

Question 10

Which of the following outcomes is NOT TRUE regarding the percutaneous pedicle screw insertion (PPSI) approach performed by an experienced surgeon?

A. Reduced radiation exposure
B. Increased blood loss
C. Decreased operative time
D. None of the following are true

Response (B) A decrease in radiation exposure is seen in the PPSI approach due to a shorter duration of fluoroscopy, in experienced hands, needed to place the screws accurately. PPSI does not increase blood loss, while it does decreases operative time in general [9].

Question 11

All of the following are boundaries of the Kambin's triangle EXCEPT:

A. Superior endplate of the inferior vertebral body
B. Inferior endplate of the superior vertebral body
C. Superior articulating facet
D. Exiting nerve root (ENR)

Response (B) Kambin's triangle is a three-dimensional anatomical triangle located over the dorsolateral intervertebral disc of the lumbar spine. This concept is widely accepted for not only percutaneous endoscopic lumbar discectomy (PELD) but also epidural injection, discography and interbody fusion techniques. Kambin's safety zone is the area surrounding the superior endplate of the inferior vertebral body, superior articulating facet, and exiting nerve root (ENR) [10, 11].

Question 12

After moving his parents' heavy furniture out of their house, a 38-year-old man experiences lower back pain. He presented to his doctor with tingling numbness radiating in his right lower limb down to the medial part of his foot. A T1-weighted MRI revealed L4-L5 intervertebral disc herniation. The patient was operated on with percutaneous endoscopic lumbar discectomy through the Kambin's triangle. Which nerve root is at high risk of injury during this approach?

A. S1 spinal nerve roots
B. L5 spinal nerve roots
C. L4 spinal nerve roots
D. All of the above

Response (C) In an L4-L5 disc herniation, the L4 nerve root, exiting nerve root, forms the hypotenuse of the Kambin's triangle, which may be at potential risk for injury [12].

Question 13

A 60-year-old female presented with lower extremity ataxia and back pain. Workup revealed T9-10 calcified thoracic disc herniation with severe spinal cord compression. She underwent a minimally invasive transthoracic decompression and removal of the calcified disc. Her symptoms resolved, and she was discharged in an improved condition. Removal of the head of which rib is necessary during this approach?

A. 9th
B. 10th
C. 11th
D. None of the above

Response (B) The rib articulates and projects from the superior aspect of the T10 level and would obstruct access to the T9-T10 foramen. Therefore, removal of the 10th rib head is necessary for identification of the ventral aspect of the dura above the pedicle [13].

Question 14

The entry point of the percutaneous iliac screw is:

A. PSIS
B. Midway between S1 and S2
C. Superior facet of S1
D. Superior facet of L5

Response (A) The entry point of iliac screws is the posterior superior iliac spine, and the trajectory is toward the acetabulum and passes approximately 1 cm superior to the sciatic notch. The midway between S1 and S2 is the entry point of the S2 alar iliac screws [14].

Question 15

Relative contraindications of stand-alone anterior lumbar interbody fusion (ALIF) include:

A. Significant prior abdominal retroperitoneal surgery with adhesions
B. Severe osteoporosis
C. Isthmic spondylolisthesis at L5/S1
D. Solitary kidney on the side of exposure
E. High-grade spondylolisthesis

Response (C) Significant prior abdominal retroperitoneal surgery with adhesions, severe osteoporosis, solitary kidney on the side of exposure, and high-grade spondylolisthesis are an absolute contraindication for ALIF. Isthmic spondylolisthesis at L5/S1 is considered relative contraindications for stand-alone ALIF and should be posteriorly supplemented [3].

Question 16

The anterior lumbar interbody fusion (ALIF) approach is suitable for all the following levels EXCEPT:

A. L4/L5
B. L5/S1
C. L2/3
D. None of the above

Response (C) The ALIF approach is suitable for levels L4/L5 and L5/S1, primarily the latter due to vascular anatomy. Although rare, the ALIF approach is limited for L2/3 and L3/4 secondary to extensive peritoneal and kidney (L2/3) retraction and the risk of superior mesenteric artery thrombosis [3].

Question 17

Lateral lumbar interbody fusion (LLIF) is suitable for all levels EXCEPT:

A. L3/4
B. T12/L1
C. L4/5
D. L5/S1

Response (D) This technique is not suitable for the L5/S1 level due to the location of the iliac crest that obstructs lateral access. Furthermore, at more caudal levels of the lumbar spine, the lumbar plexus courses more anteriorly, and the iliac vessels course more laterally. This increases the risk of injury via a lateral approach [3].

Question 18

Which one of the following MIS approaches uses the trans-psoas approach?

A. Oblique lateral interbody fusion (OLIF)
B. Anterior lumbar interbody fusion (ALIF)
C. Lateral lumbar interbody fusion (LLIF)
D. Posterior lumbar interbody fusion (PLIF)

Response (C) The OLIF approach involves an MIS access to the disc space via a corridor between the peritoneum and psoas muscle. The ALIF approaches the disc space anteriorly. The PLIF is a posterior approach not related to the psoas muscle, while the LLIF uses a transposes approach [3].

Question 19

All of the following are true regarding cervical posterior keyhole foraminotomy EXCEPT:

A. Can be used for soft lateral disc herniation
B. Patient selection includes singer or speaker profession
C. The first bone to be removed is the superior facet of the vertebrae below
D. The success rate ranges from 90 to 96%

Response (C) The first bone to be removed is the inferior facet of the vertebrae above. The approach is best indicated for soft lateral disc, patients with risk of injury of recurrent laryngeal nerve and short neck patients [15].

Question 20

45-years-old female patient was diagnosed with L4-L5 spondylolisthesis. The decision was made to do minimally invasive retroperitoneal trans-psoas interbody fusion. Which of the following is a contraindication for this approach?

A. Pinpoint central canal stenosis
B. Disc space height is > 12 mm
C. Osteoporosis
D. All of the above

Response (D) Contraindications to this approach include cases requiring direct decompression like pinpoint central canal stenosis and tall disk space of more than 12 mm, implying that further distraction may be challenging. Furthermore, osteoporosis is a relative contraindication to lateral plates [16].

Question 21

All of the following are general principles of minimally invasive spine surgery (MISS), EXCEPT:

A. Does not necessitate small surgical incisions
B. Minimal disruption of musculature
C. Requirement for specialized equipment, retractor systems, and implants
D. Use of intraoperative imaging modalities, e.g., fluoroscopy

Response (A) Small surgical incisions are one of the main principles of minimally invasive spine surgery [17–20].

Question 22

Which one of the following goals can be achieved with minimally invasive spine surgery (MISS)?

A. Adequate neural decompression
B. Stabilization and arthrodesis
C. Balanced correction of spinal deformity
D. Relief of axial and/or radicular pain
E. All of the above

Response (E) Adequate neural decompression, stabilization and arthrodesis, balanced correction of spinal deformity and relief of axial and radicular pain are all goals that can be achieved via MISS [17–20].

Question 23

Which one of the following nerves may be encountered in the thoracoscopic operative field?

A. Sympathetic chain
B. Greater and lesser splanchnic nerves
C. Vagus nerve
D. B & C
E. All of the above

Response (E) Sympathetic chain, greater and lesser splanchnic nerves, vagus nerve, and/or phrenic nerve can be encountered in the thoracoscopic operative field [21, 22].

Question 24

Which of the following is true of video-assisted thoracoscopic spinal fusion and instrumentation compared with traditional open thoracotomy?

A. Reduced postoperative pain
B. Reduced amount of blood loss
C. Improved skin incisions cosmeses
D. Diminished length of hospital stay

Response (B) Video-assisted thoracoscopic spinal fusion and instrumentation is associated with significantly reduced blood loss, but there were no differences between video-assisted thoracoscopic spinal fusion and instrumentation and traditional open thoracotomy in terms of the length of stay, postoperative pain, and skin incision cosmeses [23–26].

Question 25

Regarding the lateral trans-psoas approach, all of the following are true, EXCEPT:

A. The approach is most commonly performed from the left side.
B. The patient is usually positioned in the left lateral decubitus position.
C. Dissection through the psoas is performed to expose the disc space, or the psoas may be dissected, mobilized, and retracted to expose the disc space.
D. This approach was developed as a less invasive option for achieving anterior fusion from L1 to L5.

Response (B) The patient is usually positioned in the right lateral decubitus position to allow for a left-sided approach. This allows access to the zone between the left lateral border of the aorta and the anterior medial border of the psoas muscle. A left-sided approach is preferred in patients without a coronal plane deformity because of the relatively anterior position of the vasculature on the left side [27–31].

Question 26

Regarding the lateral trans-psoas approach, all of the following are true, EXCEPT:

A. This approach avoids the need to mobilize the iliac vessels or sympathetic plexus.
B. The genitofemoral nerve, lateral femoral cutaneous nerve, and femoral nerve are at risk of injury due to their intimate relationship with the psoas muscle.

C. The approach is feasible at L5–S1 level.
D. The approach is challenging at L4–L5 and may not be possible in some patients.

Response (C) The approach is not feasible at L5–S1 due to the location of the iliac crest and iliac vessels. The approach is challenging at L4–L5 and may not be possible in some patients due to obstruction by the iliac crest or due to the relationship of the lumbosacral plexus to the lateral aspect of the disc space [27–31].

Question 27

Regarding the presacral surgical approach to the lumbosacral junction, all of the following statements are true, EXCEPT:

A. The patient is usually placed in the prone position, and the incision is made lateral to the coccyx.
B. The blunt trocar is advanced into the presacral space while maintaining contact with the anterior surface of the sacrum.
C. At first, the guide pin is inserted into the sacrum at the S1–S2 level and then advanced across the L5–S1 disc space into the L5 vertebral body.
D. Mobilization of the iliac vessels is required to reach the presacral space.

Response (D) The presacral approach is intended to provide an option for minimally invasive surgical access to the lumbosacral junction that does not require mobilization of the iliac vessels, limits muscle dissection, and avoids disruption of the autonomic nerves overlying the lumbosacral disc [32–34].

Question 28

All of the following procedures could be done using minimally invasive spine surgery (MISS), EXCEPT:

A. Lumbar discectomy
B. Transforaminal lumbar interbody fusion (TLIF)
C. Spinal canal stenosis
D. Pedicle screw-rod placement
E. None of the above

Response (E) Lumbar discectomy, TLIF, spinal decompression and pedicle screw and rod placement can all be done using minimally invasive techniques [17–20].

Question 29

Regarding the extreme lateral mini-thoracotomy approach, which one of the following statements is FALSE:

A. It is used for pathologies in the anterior portion of the spinal canal between T4 and L1/2.
B. It is used for pathologies located in the posterior part of the spinal canal or spinal stenosis.
C. Previous surgery in the same area is a contraindication for this approach.
D. The risk of injury to the thoracic cavity and lung tissues is not eliminated.

Response (B) Pathologies located in the posterior portion of the spinal canal, or spinal stenosis, cannot be addressed via the extreme lateral mini-thoracotomy approach [35–38].

Question 31

Which of the following is NOT considered an advantage of the minimally invasive transforaminal interbody fusion (TLIF) compared to anterior lumbar interbody fusion (ALIF) or traditional TLIF and posterior lumbar interbody fusion (PLIF)?

A. Minimizes retraction of great vessels when done above the L5-S1 level
B. Allows for pedicle screw placement in the same setting
C. Less retraction on traversing nerve roots and thecal sac
D. Limited visualization of the target anatomy
E. Decreased rates of retraction induce neuropraxia

Response (D) Although minimally invasive transforaminal interbody fusion (TLIF) has many advantages, one of the main limiting factors is the limited visualization of anatomy due to the minimally invasive exposure. This makes adequate exposure to this technique in training paramount [39].

Question 32

Which of the following statements is INCORRECT regarding the technique of minimally invasive laminotomy?

A. A CO_2 laser or CUSA can be used to thin the contralateral ligamentum flavum to allow for easy access with the Kerrison.

B. The table is tilted away from the surgeon during the contralateral laminotomy, and the tubular retractor is angled medially.
C. Removal of the ipsilateral ligamentum flavum is performed before contralateral laminotomy.
D. Before removing the ligamentum flavum, both ipsilateral and contralateral laminotomies are performed.
E. During the placement of serial dilators, rotation of the dilators reduces the need for downward pressure and thus decreases the risk of entry into the spinal canal.

Response (C) During minimally invasive laminotomy it is suggested that all bony drilling of the bilateral lamina is completed before removal of the ligamentum flavum. This allows the ligament to act as a cushion for the dura, thus decreasing the risk of durotomy or nerve root damage [40].

Question 33

Which of the following statements regarding minimally invasive cervical foraminotomy is FALSE?

A. Patients have decreased length of stay compared to patients undergoing open procedures.
B. Patients with unilateral foraminal stenosis due to lateral disc herniations are considered good candidates.
C. Patients with primarily central canal stenosis due to disc herniations are considered good candidates.
D. Patients have decreased postoperative opioid use compared to patients undergoing open procedures.
E. Patients with imaging findings that are concerning for instability are not considered good candidates for this approach.

Response (C) Given the minimally invasive nature of this approach, there is limited exposure of the bony anatomy and neural structures. As such, minimally invasive foraminotomy cannot adequately address central pathology given the laterality of the approach [41].

Question 34

Which of the following conditions is least suitable for spinal deformity patients to undergo minimally invasive decompression with or without fusion of the index level?

A. Lumbar lordosis–pelvic incidence mismatch: 15 degrees
B. Sagittal vertical axis: 5 cm
C. Pelvic tilt: 15 degrees
D. Coronal Cobb angle: 15 degrees
E. Thoracic kyphosis: 15 degrees

Response (A) Minimally invasive surgery with decompression only or with a focal fusion at the level of interest is most suitable for patients with minimal sagittal plane deformity such as sagittal balance less than 6 cm positive, lumbar lordosis–pelvic incidence mismatch less than 10 degrees, the pelvic tilt under 25 degrees, and coronal Cobb angle under 20 degrees. These patients should also have a non-fused or non-rigid spine, and their main complaints stem from spinal cord compression [42].

Question 35

Which one of the following minimally invasive surgical techniques for managing thoracic disc herniations has been largely abandoned with a sole indication of migrated disc lying ventral to the spinal cord?

A. Trans-facetal pedicle-sparing approach
B. Mini-thoracotomy approach
C. Microtubular interlaminar approach
D. Retro-pleural approach using a tubular retractor
E. Oblique paraspinal approach using tubular micro-endoscopic discectomy

Response (C) The interlaminar approach for thoracic disc herniations has been abandoned due to the high incidence of cord damage associated with the procedure. On top of this reason, the window of the thoracic region is either absent or very small, indicating that additional bone removal is required for entry into the canal. It is only indicated in migrated disc lying dorsal to the spinal cord [13].

Question 36

When comparing traditional open to minimally invasive (MIS) lumbar discectomy, which of the following statement is least appropriate?

A. There are similar complications and recurrence rates between open and MIS techniques.
B. MIS techniques can be used to revise recurrent lumbar disc herniation after either MIS discectomy or conventional open techniques.
C. MIS techniques may result in a shorter postoperative length of stay compared to open techniques.
D. Open techniques have reliably better immediate outcomes, though long-term disability rates postoperatively are inferior to MIS techniques.

Response (D) Level 1 evidence has demonstrated equivalently good outcomes for MIS technique compared with standard techniques. Likewise, Level I data has indicated similar safety profiles and may indicate lower blood loss for MIS techniques. Nevertheless, no definitive long-term conclusions can be made yet [43, 44].

References

1. Kai-Uwe L, José-Antonio SS, Xifeng Z, Jorge Felipe RL, Sergio Soriano S, José Gabriel RO, Carolina Ramírez M, Gabriel Oswaldo AC, Kaixuan L, Qiang F, Marlon Sudário de L, Paulo Sérgio T, Stefan H, Álvaro D, Nicholas P, Gun C, Girish D, Anthony Y. Regional variations in acceptance, and utilization of minimally invasive spinal surgery techniques among spine surgeons: results of a global survey. J Spine Surg. 2020;6(Suppl 1): S260–74. https://doi.org/10.21037/jss.2019.09.31 PMCID: PMC7063310
2. Nancy EE. More nerve root injuries occur with minimally invasive lumbar surgery, especially extreme lateral interbody fusion: a review. Surg Neurol Int. 2016;7(Suppl 3):S83–95. Published online 2016 Jan 25. https://doi.org/10.4103/2152-7806.174895. PMCID: PMC4743267
3. Mobbs RJ, Phan K, Malham G, Seex K, Rao PJ. Lumbar interbody fusion: techniques, indications and comparison of interbody fusion options including PLIF, TLIF, MI-TLIF, OLIF/ATP LLIF and ALIF. J Spine Surg. 2015;1(1):2–18. https://doi.org/10.3978/j.issn.2414-469X.2015.10.05.
4. Baaj AA, Mummaneni PV, Uribe JS, Vaccaro AR, Greenburg MS. Handbook of spine surgery. In: Ali AB, Praveen VM, Juan SU, Alexander RV, Mark SG, editors. Second edition. ed: New York; 2016.
5. Shepard N, Cho W. Recurrent lumbar disc herniation: a review. Global Spine J. 2019;9(2):202–9. https://doi.org/10.1177/2192568217745063.
6. Akinobu S, Hiroaki N. Microendoscopic lumbar posterior decompression surgery for lumbar spinal stenosis: literature review. Medicina (Kaunas). 2022; 58(3):384. Published online 2022 Mar 4. https://doi.org/10.3390/medicina58030384
7. Qing-Yi Z, Jie T, Kai H, Hui-Qi X. Minimally invasive transforaminal lumbar interbody fusion versus oblique lateral interbody fusion for lumbar degenerative disease: a meta-analysis. BMC Musculoskelet Disord. 2021;22:802. Published online 2021 Sep 18. https://doi.org/10.1186/s12891-021-04687-7
8. Gu G, Zhang H, Fan G, et al. Comparison of minimally invasive versus open transforaminal lumbar interbody fusion in two-level degenerative lumbar disease. Int Orthop. 2014;38:817–24.
9. Yang BP, Wahl MM, Idler CS. Percutaneous lumbar pedicle screw placement aided by computer-assisted fluoroscopy-based navigation: perioperative results of a prospective, comparative, multicenter study. Spine (Phila Pa 1976). 2012;37(24):2055–60
10. Kumari C, Gupta T, Gupta R, et al. Cadaveric anatomy of the lumbar triangular safe zone of Kambin's in North West Indian population. Anat Cell Biol. 2021;54(1):35–41. https://doi.org/10.5115/acb.20.243.
11. Fanous AA, Tumialán LM, Wang MY. Kambin's triangle: definition and new classification schema. J Neurosurg Spine SPI. 2020;32(3):390–8.
12. Hirayama J, Hashimoto M, Sakamoto T. J Neurol Surg A Cent Eur Neurosurg. 2020;81(4):302–9 Epub 2020 Jan 21.
13. Sharma SB, Kim JS. A review of minimally invasive surgical techniques for the management of thoracic disc herniations. Neurospine. 2019;16(1):24–33. https://doi.org/10.14245/ns.1938014.007.
14. Shin JK, Lim BY, Goh TS, et al. Effect of the screw type (S2-alar-iliac and iliac), screw length, and screw head angle on the risk of screw and adjacent bone failures after a spinopelvic fixation technique: a finite element analysis. PLoS One. 2018;13(8): e0201801. Published 2018 Aug 16. https://doi.org/10.1371/journal.pone.0201801
15. Terai H, Suzuki A, Toyoda H, et al. Tandem keyhole foraminotomy in the treatment of cervical radiculopathy: retrospective review of 35 cases. J Orthop Surg Res. 2014;9:38. Published 2014 May 16. https://doi.org/10.1186/1749-799X-9-38
16. Staub BN, Holman PJ. Lateral retroperitoneal transpsoas interbody fusion in a patient with achondroplastic dwarfism. J Neurosurg Spine. 2015;22(2):162–5. https://doi.org/10.3171/2014.10.SPINE14300. Epub 2014 Nov 21 PMID: 25415482.
17. Oppenheimer JH, DeCastro I, McDonnell DE. Minimally invasive spine technology and minimally invasive spine surgery: a historical review. Neurosurg Focus. 2009;27(3):E9.
18. McAfee PC, Phillips FM, Andersson G, Buvenenadran A, Kim CW, Lauryssen C, Isaacs RE, Youssef JA, Brodke DS, Cappuccino A, Akbarnia BA. Minimally invasive spine surgery. Spine. 2010;35(26S):S271–3.
19. Kim CW, Siemionow K, Anderson DG, Phillips FM. The current state of minimally invasive spine surgery. JBJS. 2011;93(6):582–96.
20. Jaikumar S, Kim DH, Kam AC. History of minimally invasive spine surgery. Neurosurgery. 2002;51(suppl_2): S2–1
21. Longo UG, Papapietro N, Maffulli N, Denaro V. Thoracoscopy for minimally invasive thoracic spine surgery. Orthopedic Clinics. 2009;40(4):459–64.
22. Johnson JP, Drazin D, King WA, Kim TT. Image-guided navigation and video-assisted thoracoscopic spine surgery: the second generation. Neurosurg Focus. 2014;36(3)
23. Lonner BS, Auerbach JD, Estreicher M, Milby AH, Kean KE. Video-assisted thoracoscopic spinal fusion compared with posterior spinal fusion with thoracic pedicle screws for thoracic adolescent idiopathic scoliosis. JBJS. 2009;91(2):398–408.
24. Cunningham BW, Kotani Y, McNulty PS, Cappuccino A, Kanayama M, Fedder IL, McAfee PC. Video-assisted thoracoscopic surgery versus open thoracotomy for anterior thoracic spinal fusion: a comparative radiographic, biomechanical, and histologic analysis in a sheep model. Spine. 1998;23(12):1333–40.
25. Regan JJ, Mack MJ, Picetti GD 3rd. A technical report on video-assisted thoracoscopy in thoracic spinal surgery. Preliminary Descript: Spine. 1995;20(7):831–7.
26. Al-Sayyad MJ, Crawford AH, Wolf RK. Early experiences with video-assisted thoracoscopic surgery: our first 70 cases. Spine. 2004;29(17):1945–51.
27. Arnold PM, Anderson KK, McGuire RA Jr. The lateral transpsoas approach to the lumbar and thoracic spine: a review. Surg Neurol Int. 2012;3(Suppl 3):S198.
28. Bergey DL, Villavicencio AT, Goldstein T, Regan JJ. Endoscopic lateral transpsoas approach to the lumbar spine. Spine. 2004;29(15):1681–8.
29. D'Mitri AS, Briseño MR, Abrams J, Patel AA. Complications of the lateral transpsoas approach for lumbar interbody arthrodesis: a case series and literature review. Clinic Orthopaed Relat Res®. 2012;470(6):1621–32
30. Graham RB, Wong AP, Liu JC. Minimally invasive lateral transpsoas approach to the lumbar spine: pitfalls and complication avoidance. Neurosurgery Clinic. 2014;25(2):219–31.
31. Park DK, Lee MJ, Lin EL, Singh K, An HS, Phillips FM. The relationship of intrapsoas nerves during a transpsoas approach to

the lumbar spine: anatomic study. Clinical Spine Surg. 2010;23 (4):223–8.
32. Marotta N, Cosar M, Pimenta L, Khoo LT. A novel minimally invasive presacral approach and instrumentation technique for anterior L5–S1 intervertebral discectomy and fusion: technical note and case presentations. Neurosurg Focus. 2006;20(1):1–8.
33. Tobler WD, Ferrara LA. The presacral retroperitoneal approach for axial lumbar interbody fusion: a prospective study of clinical outcomes, complications and fusion rates at a follow-up of two years in 26 patients. J Bone Joint Surg Br. 2011;93(7):955–60
34. Akesen B, Wu C, Mehbod AA, Transfeldt EE. Biomechanical evaluation of paracoccygeal transsacral fixation. Clinical Spine Surg. 2008;21(1):39–44.
35. Assaker R. Minimal access spinal technologies: state-of-the-art, indications, and techniques. Joint Bone Spine. 2004;71(6):459–69.
36. Falavigna A. Minimally invasive approaches for thoracic decompression from discectomy to corpectomy. J Neurosurg Sci. 2013;57(3):175–92.
37. Kossmann T, Jacobi D, Trentz O. The use of a retractor system (SynFrame) for open, minimal invasive reconstruction of the anterior column of the thoracic and lumbar spine. Eur Spine J. 2001;10(5):396–402.
38. Bouthors C, Benzakour A. Surgical treatment of thoracic disc herniation: an overview. Int Orthop. 2019;43(4):807–16.
39. Costa J, Silva PS, Cunha M, Almeida M, Vaz R, Pereira P. Predictors of poor outcome in patients submitted to minimally invasive transforaminal lumbar interbody fusion. World Neurosurg. 2018;119:488–93.
40. Minimally invasive laminectomy for lumbar stenosis. In: Mick JP, Ronnie IM, Patrick Jacob R, Richard GF, editors. An anatomic approach to minimally invasive spine surgery
41. Posterior cervical microforaminotomy and discectomy. In: Carter SG, Lee AT, Richard GF, editors. An anatomic approach to minimally invasive spine surgery
42. Mummaneni PV, Park P, Shaffrey CI, Wang MY, Uribe JS, Fessler RG, Chou D, Kanter AS, Okonkwo DO, Mundis GM, Eastlack RK, Nunley PD, Anand N, Virk MS, Lenke LG, Than KD, Robinson LC, Fu KM. International Spine Study Group (ISSG). The MISDEF2 algorithm: an updated algorithm for patient selection in minimally invasive deformity surgery. J Neurosurg Spine. 2019;32(2):221–8. https://doi.org/10.3171/2019.7.SPINE181104. PMID: 31653809
43. McClelland S 3rd, Goldstein JA. Minimally invasive versus open spine surgery: what does the best evidence tell us? J Neurosci Rural Pract. 2017;8(2):194–8. https://doi.org/10.4103/jnrp.jnrp_472_16.
44. Soliman MAR, Ali A. Decompression of lumbar canal stenosis with a bilateral interlaminar versus classic laminectomy technique: a prospective randomized study. Neurosurg Focus. 2019;46(5). https://doi.org/10.3171/2019.2.FOCUS18725

7 Degenerative Conditions of the Spine

Teresa Somma, Domenico Solari, Vincenzo Meglio, Lorenzo Ugga, Oreste de Divitiis, and Paolo Cappabianca

Introduction

1. **Among the following morphological parameters of cervical sagittal balance, which one is the most important in determining the lordosis of cervical spine?**
   a. C7 slope.
   b. C-Cobb.
   c. SCA.
   d. C-SVA.
   e. Sacral Slope.

A: C-7 slope is a key parameter for the static cervical sagittal balance. According to the literature, this is the only parameter affecting cervical lordosis. The median value is 20°. Patients presenting a value > 20° have a lordotic cervical spine, while patients with a value < 20° present a cervical flattening, with a neutral or even kyphotic curvature [1].

T. Somma (✉) · D. Solari (✉) · V. Meglio · O. de Divitiis · P. Cappabianca
Division of Neurosurgery, Dept of Neurosciences, Reproductive and Odontostomatological, Università degli studi di Napoli Federico II, Naples, Italy
e-mail: teresa.somma85@gmail.com

D. Solari
e-mail: domenico.solari@unina.it

V. Meglio
e-mail: vinmeglio790@gmail.com

O. de Divitiis
e-mail: oreste.dedivitiis@unina.it

P. Cappabianca
e-mail: paolo.cappabianca@unina.it

L. Ugga
Unit of Neuroradiology, Dept of Advanced Biomedical Sciences, Università degli Studi di Napoli Federico II, Naples, Italy
e-mail: lorenzo.ugga@unina.it

2. **Which is the best radiological exam for evaluating the cervical sagittal balance?**
   a. Cervical MRI.
   b. Long-standing radiographs.
   c. Whole spine column CT.
   d. Clinical examination is sufficient.
   e. Supine-positioned radiographs.

B: Sagittal Balance of the spine displays all its spectrum of proprieties only in situations where gravity is free to exert its effects on the human spine. In studying the sagittal balance of the spine, long-standing radiographs are the only available radiological exam which allows to evaluate the patient in an upright position [2].

3. **According to 2017 AO Spine Guidelines, in a patient affected by Degenerative Cervical Myelopathy (DCM):**
   a. A score < of 12 at mJOA scoring system is sufficient to define the myelopathy severity.
   b. A history of at least 12 months of cervical pain is necessary to define the myelopathy severe.
   c. A score of 3 at Nurick's Scale is necessary to define the myelopathy moderate.
   d. The development of strength deficit is a necessary and sufficient element in classifying the DCM as severe.
   e. Surgery is the only therapeutic accepted strategy in mild DCM treatment.

A: According to AO Spine guidelines for DCM classification, a mJOA score < 12 (0–11) is enough to define a DCM as severe, regardless the presence of cervical pain. Moderate DCM is defined by mJOA score system with a 12–14. Finally, mild DCM corresponds to an mJOA score ≥ 15 [3].

C. Gragnaniello et al. (eds.), *MCQs in Spine Surgery*,
https://doi.org/10.1007/978-3-031-69332-8_7

4. **Cervical spondylotic myelopathy (CSM) treatment includes a variety of surgical options, namely anterior, posterior, and combined approaches. When is a combined approach indicated?**
   a. Marked kyphosis.
   b. Extensive pathology requiring anterior multilevel cervical decompression.
   c. Fusion requiring supplemental fusion
   d. None of the mentioned situations.
   e. "a","b" and "c".

E: CSM is a pathological condition due to narrowing of the cervical tract of the spinal canal. Usually, this narrowing is consequent to an anterior compression, like a degenerative disc disease, or to a posterior one, such as ligamentum flavum hypertrophy. In cases of anterior and posterior cervical abnormalities, a combined approach is necessary. Moreover, in cases of anterior cervical pathology affecting 3 or more levels, an anterior approach with discectomy or corpectomy and fusion may lead to iatrogenic instability, requiring also a concurrent posterior instrumentation. As well as in cases of posterior compression but with an excessive kyphosis, a stand-alone posterior approach is not to consider because of the risk of worsening the kyphosis [4].

5. **According to the World Federation of Neurosurgical Societies (WFNS) guidelines for surgical management of cervical myelopathy:**
   a. Anterior approaches to the cervical spine are indicated only in cases of anterior cervical pathologies causing compression involving one level.
   b. Anterior approaches to the cervical spine are indicated only in cases of anterior cervical pathology causing compression involving less than three levels, with straightened or kyphotic spine.
   c. Anterior approaches to the cervical spine are indicated only in cases of anterior cervical pathologies causing compression involving less than three levels, with lordotic cervical spine.
   d. Anterior discectomy and fusion allow for better surgical outcomes than anterior corpectomy.
   e. Anterior corpectomy offers better surgical outcomes than anterior discectomy and fusion.

B: According to WFNS guidelines, anterior approaches to the cervical spine are indicated for straightened or kyphotic cervical spines with myelopathy involving less than three levels. Corpectomy and discectomy offer the same efficacy, except when a single-level disc and osteophyte excision are inadequate to decompress the cord [5].

6. **A 66 years old male patient presented with a long-history of cervical pain, with a six-months progressive manifestation of paresthesia to the upper and lower limbs, gait rigidity and postural instability, without recent referred trauma. Neurological examination showed stiff gait due to spastic hypertonia with clonus in both legs, tetra-hyperreflexia, Babinski sign in both sides and oscillations at Romberg test. Cervical spine MRI** (Fig. 7.1) **and cervical X-ray** (Fig. 7.2) **depicted the following:**

What is the best surgical option for this patient?

a. ACDF.
b. ACCF.
c. ACD.
d. Laminectomy.

D: The clinical picture was compatible with cervical spondylotic myelopathy (CSM), mainly due to posterior multilevel compression. In cases of multilevel DCM, many authors proved that anterior approach are less suitable than posterior ones. This is mostly due to the high rate of complications (pseudoarthrosis and non-fusion experimented with the anterior approaches) with similar outcomes as compared with posterior approaches. Moreover, anterior surgical techniques for multilevel cervical pathology are associated with a higher reoperation rate. For multilevel compression, anterior approaches are related with higher blood loss, operation time and surgical trauma than posterior ones [6]. Finally, pre-operative cervical x-ray is a fundamental tool in choosing the best surgical approach, since a physiological cervical lordotic curvature allows a posterior approach. Therefore, this patient should be treated by laminectomy.

7. **In a patient affected by rheumatoid arthritis (RA) with subluxation and, then pannus of the C2 involvement causing myelopathy and neurological deficits, surgical treatment is indicated. Which one of the following sentences is true?**
   a. A dorsal C1-C2 fusion is sufficient in every case.
   b. An occipitocervical fusion alone is sufficient in every case.
   c. In cases where rheumatoid pannus causes a subluxation of the C2 axis with compression of the spinal cord, a transoral or endoscopic endonasal decompressive approach coupled with dorsal upper cervical fusion may be necessary.
   d. A transoral decompressive approach is almost always not indicated in consideration of the increased post-operative complications risk and low efficacy rates.
   e. None among the reported sentences is true.

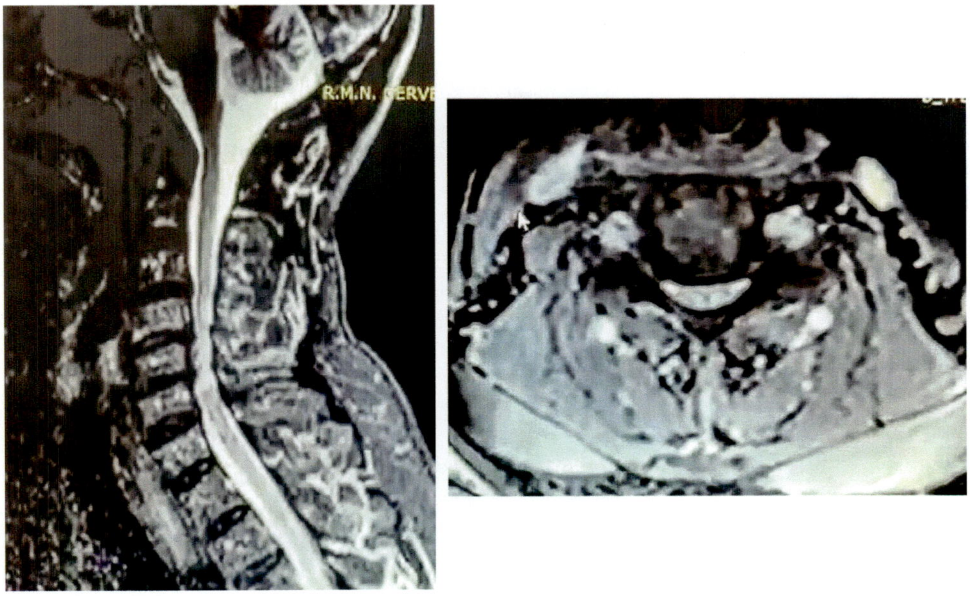

Fig. 7.1 Patient cervical sagittal and axial T2WI MRI

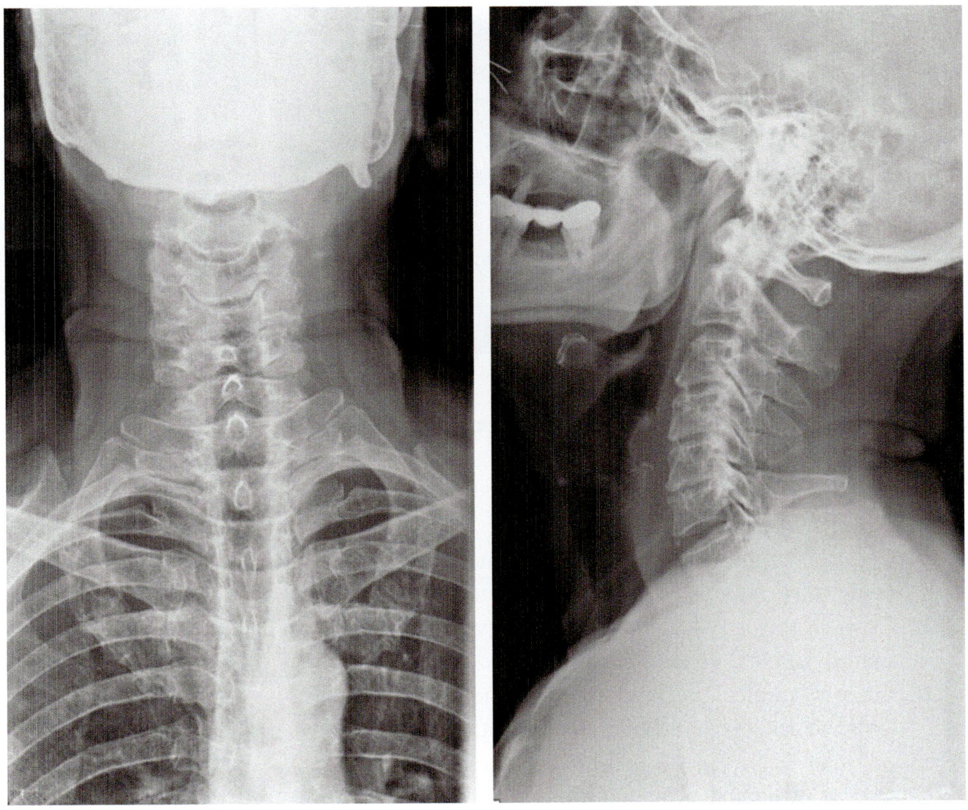

Fig. 7.2 Patient's cervical AP and lateral X-Ray

C: RA is an inflammatory disease which can involve cervical spine, causing atlantoaxial subluxation, vertical subluxation of the odontoid process and subaxial subluxation with consequent instability. In such cases, C1-C2 dorsal stabilization may be considered alone. Contrarywise, when spinal cord compression by rheumatoid pannus is present, transoral or endoscopic endonasal decompression may be necessary [7, 8].

8. **A 55 patient comes to your attention referring claudication. Neurological examination shows evidence of hyperreflexia in both legs, with spastic paraparesis and Hoffman sing, configuring the suspect of simultaneous presence of lumbar and cervical stenosis. Spine MRI (as in** Fig. 7.3) **confirms the clinical suspect of a tandem stenosis. Which one among the**

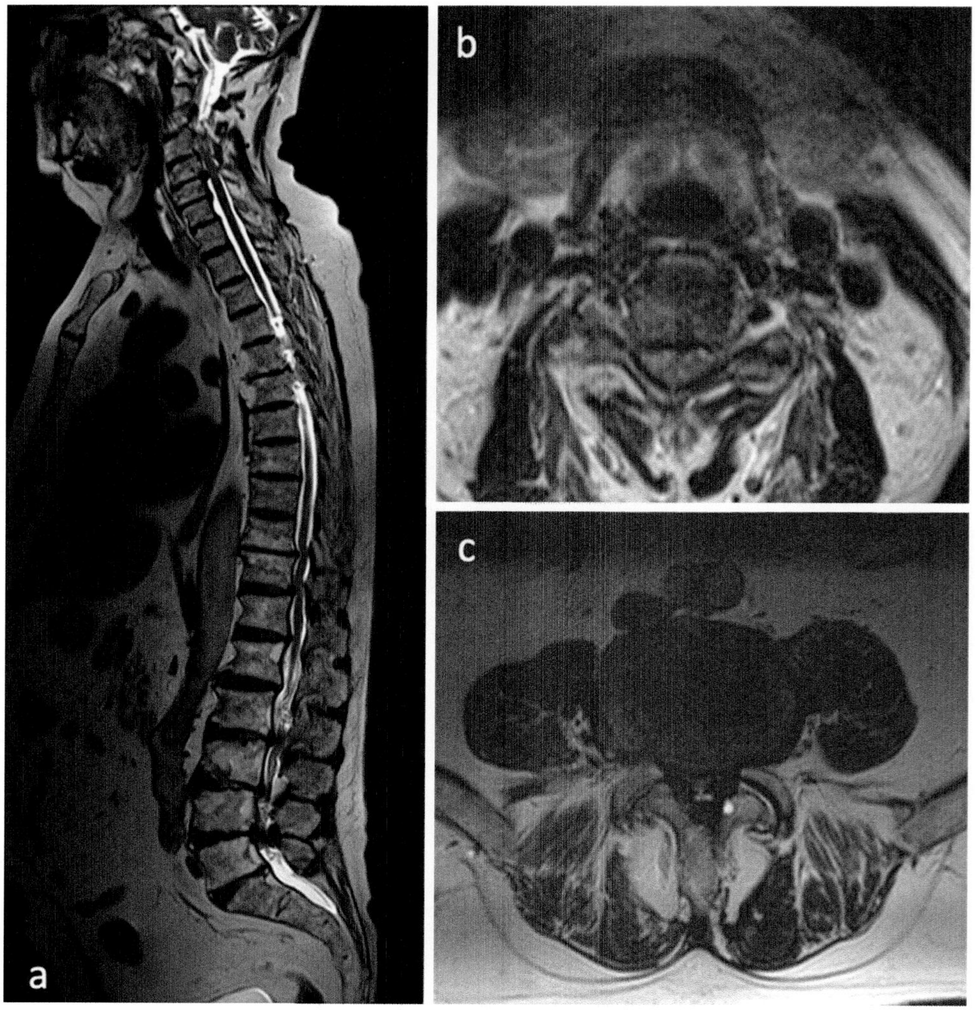

Fig. 7.3 From right to left and from the top down: figure a - full spine sagittal MRI of patient affected by tandem stenosis (cervical and lumbar). Figure b cervical stenosis and figure c lumbar stenosis of the same patient

following is the best therapeutic strategy in this situation?

a. Lumbar surgical decompression at first, followed by cervical surgical decompression.
b. Cervical surgical decompression alone, in order to avoid unnecessary risks for the patient.
c. Cervical surgical decompression at first, followed by lumbar surgical decompression.
d. Lumbar surgical decompression alone, in order to avoid unnecessary risks for the patient.

C: In cases of tandem stenosis, decompressing both, lumbar and cervical spinal cord is mandatory. However, doing both in the same surgical time is technically demanding and dangerous for the patient. Therefore, cervical decompression should be considered at first, a fortiori in cases of myelopathy. After cervical decompression lumbar release should be considered [9].

9. **Which one of the following sentences regarding the Ossification of Posterior Longitudinal Ligament (OPLL)'s Occupancy Ratio is true?**
   a. The OPLL's occupancy ratio is a parameter that defines the operability of a patient affected by OPLL and a value major than 30% indicate poor post-operative outcome.
   b. The OPLL's occupancy ratio major than 40% indicates an augmented risk of developing cervical myelopathy.
   c. The OPLL's occupancy ratio is a parameter that defines the risk of a patient affected by OPLL of developing CSF leak after cervical surgery: a value major than 30% indicates an augmented risk.
   d. The OPLL's Occupancy Ratio is assessed on CT imaging.
   e. The OPLL's Occupancy Ratio is assessed on MRI imaging.

B: OPLL's occupancy ratio is a parameter than defines the risk of a patient affected by OPLL of developing cervical myelopathy. A value major than 40% implies an augmented risk of developing myelopathy. It is calculated on 6-foot plain x-rays by dividing the thickness of the measured ossified lesion by the anterior/posterior developmental canal diameter [10].

10. **In which cases of cervical pathology, laminoplasty is not indicated?**
    a. Presence of kyphotic cervical spine.
    b. Presence of a large anterior lesion.
    c. a + b.
    d. Presence of herniated nucleus pulposus.
    e. None of the mentioned.

C: Cervical laminoplasty is one of the possible posterior surgical approaches to cervical pathology, first described by Hattori in 1973 and historically more diffused in Japan than in the Western World. It accounts various techniques with the same result of creating more space in the cervical canal, without removing the laminas, in the attempt of reducing the risk of iatrogenic instability and increased risk of adjacent-segment disease. In cases of cervical kyphosis > 5–10°, however, this procedure is strictly contraindicated because the spinal cord will not change his position, staying draped along the compressing anterior structures due to the vertebral channel morphology. The same happens in case of larger anterior lesions. Compression due to herniated cervical nucleus pulposus, instead, shows excellent neurological improvement after laminoplasty [11, 12].

11. **In a patient affected by prognathism, which one among the following cervical spine alterations would you expect?**
    a. Hyperlordosis.
    b. Hypolordosis.
    c. Mandibular malalignment does not affect cervical curvature.
    d. Mandibular malalignment causes variable effects on the cervical curvature.

A: Changes in mandibular position can induce dislocation of body's center of gravity, modifying the center of foot pressure. As a result, patients affected by prognathism present an excessively forward head position, leading to a lowering of the field of vision. In order to compensate this alteration, cervical lordosis increases leading to cervical hyperlordosis [13].

12. **In degenerative cervical myelopathy (DCM) patients older than sixty-five, which cervical level is affected most often?**
    a. The same as patients younger than sixty-five.: C5–C6.
    b. Higher than younger patients: C3–C4.
    c. Lower than younger patients: C6–C7.
    d. All levels have the same probability of being involved.

B: DCM presents some singular aspects in elderly patients being prevalent at C3–C4 levels.

The reduction in ROM (range of motion) of lower cervical segments in elderly patients induces an abnormal hyper-mobility at higher cervical levels, as C3–C4. This could be the cause of the preferential higher localization of myelopathy [14].

13. **Which one is the minimum cut off of pedicle diameter value for posterior cervical stabilization with pedicle screw fixation?**
    a. < 3.5 mm.
    b. < 4.5 mm.
    c. < 5.5 mm.
    d. < 6.5 mm.

B: Posterior cervical fixation is a valuable option for treating instability due to different cervical degenerative pathologies. Cervical pedicle screw fixation provides the higher strength among the existing techniques. However, a pedicle diameter inferior than 4.5 mm is considered a contraindication to this approach [15].

14. **Which of the following are possible etiological causes of degenerative cervical myelopathy?**
    a. DDD (discal degeneration disease).
    b. Spondylosis (cervical spondylotic myelopathy).
    c. Ligamentous alterations.
    d. Congenital pathologies.
    e. All of the above

E: Cervical Myelopathy is a progressive degenerative disease with multiple etiologies. It can be caused by different degenerative conditions like degenerative disc disease (DDD), cervical spondylotic myelopathy (CSM), ligamentous anomalies and congenital syndromes. Aging, along with excessive mechanical stress, leads to degeneration of the nucleus pulposus, with increased pressure on the annulus, starting a cascade of degenerative changes that ends with disc bulging or herniation. As a compensative mechanism, ligamentous aberrations develop, like hypertrophy or calcification, involving the posterior longitudinal ligament (PLL) or the ligamentum flavum (LF) in order to enlarge the vertebral weight-bearing surface. These processes, individually or combined, cooperate in the narrowing of the spinal canal and then in spinal compression. Some congenital disorders, like Down Syndrome or Ehlers-Danlos syndrome carry a major risk of CSM [16].

15. **Nonoperative treatment of patients with Degenerative Cervical Myelopathy (DCM):**
    a. Is not to consider for the inevitable progressive nature of the pathology.
    b. Is to take into account also in "milder" DCM as first line treatment, regardless to the number of involved levels, reserving surgery only for failed treatment.
    c. Is to take into account only in moderate to mild DCM as first line treatment with single level involvement, reserving surgery only for failed treatment.
    d. Is to consider as a valid option only for "milder" DCM cases (mJOA > / = 13 pts) with less than three-level myelopathy.
    e. Is to consider as a valid option only for "milder" DCM cases (mJOA > / = 13 pts) with single-level myelopathy.

D: According to the WFNS guidelines on DCM, nonoperative management results in similar outcomes as surgical treatment in patients with a "milder" DCM (mJOA 13) [17].

16. **Which one among the following conditions is not an urgent/emergent indication for anterior cervical fusion (ACF), with or without discectomy?**
    a. Documentation of progressive neurological deficit on two separate physical examinations.
    b. Severe o rapidly progressive symptoms of motor loss, bowel incontinence o bladder incontinence/retention due to a neurocompressive pathology.
    c. Infections.
    d. Non-traumatic occipitocervical instability due to rheumatoid arthritis.
    e. All the listed are indication for urgent/emergent surgical treatment.

E: According to the literature, all the listed conditions require an urgent/emergent ACF approach [18, 19].

17. **In an osteoporotic patient treated for degenerative cervical pathology with an anterior approach with fusion, which of the following risks is increased?**
    a. Vertebral fractures.
    b. Subsidence of the graft, but only in case of autogenous graft.
    c. Subsidence of the graft, but only in case of allogenous graft.
    d. Subsidence of the graft, but only in case of titanium mesh cage.
    e. Subsidence of the graft, regardless of its composition.

E: According to the literature, in patients with CSM and osteoporosis treated by anterior approaches with fusion, there is an augmented risk of graft subsidence and hardware failure [20]. Interestingly, the type of graft chosen does not affect the risk entity [21, 22]. Titanium mesh cages (TMC) filled with autogenous iliac cancellous bone graft helps in early fusion [23].

18. **Which of the following neurological signs is not indicative of cervical spondylotic myelopathy (CSM)?**
    a. The Babinski reflex.
    b. The Hoffman reflex.
    c. The Chaddock reflex.
    d. The Chvostek reflex.
    e. All the listed are indicative of cervical myelopathy.

D: In CSM motor deficits and reflex's alterations are the result of upper and lower motor neuron injury due to spinal cord compression. Hoffman sing, Babinski and Chaddock reflex could be positive [24]. The Chvostek reflex is a pathological sign present in cases of hypocalcemia and is not related to spinal pathology [25].

19. **In cases of cervical degenerative pathology treated by corpectomy:**
    a. Posterior fixation is always recommended.
    b. Posterior fixation is recommended only in case of two levels corpectomy.
    c. Posterior fixation is recommended in case of more than two levels corpectomy.
    d. Posterior fixation is never recommended.
    e. None of the listed sentences is true.

C: In cases of multiple level corpectomy and fusion, in particular with 2 or more levels involved, additional poster fixation should be used [26–28].

20. **Which of the following sentences is not true, regarding combined approaches for cervical spondylotic myelopathy (CSM)?**
    a. Combined approaches do not present a higher complication rate compared to a single approach.
    b. The most frequent minor complication associated to combined approaches is dysphagia.
    c. In other to perform a combined approach to the cervical spine a two-stage procedure is necessary.
    d. This type of cervical approaches comprises posterior-anterior–posterior, anterior–posterior and anterior–posterior-anterior procedures.
    e. All the listed sentences are true.

B: Combined approaches (also known as "circumferential") include posterior-anterior–posterior and anterior–posterior approaches. These approaches can be performed in a single- or two-stage procedures. According to the current literature, dysphagia is the most frequent minor complication of combined approaches [24]. It may be due to the longer operative time and cervical levels involved. [29, 30].

21. **The modified K-line method:**
    a. Is a method to predict the risk of instability after anterior cervical surgery.
    b. Is identified on mild- sagittal cervical TC, connecting the occipital plane to C6.
    c. Is identified on mild-sagittal cervical MRI, connecting the occipital plane to the middle point of C6 vertebral body.
    d. Is identified on mild-sagittal cervical MRI and consists in a line connecting all the sagittal midpoints of the cervical vertebras, from C2 to C7.
    e. Is identified on mild-sagittal cervical TC, connecting the vertebral body of C2 to the middle point of C7 vertebral body.

D: The modified-K line method is a measurement tool that predicts the residual anterior compression of the spinal cord after surgery for degenerative cervical myelopathy (DCM). This method consists in individuating a connecting line from the sagittal midpoints of the spinal canal at the levels of C2 and C7, on mid-sagittal cervical MRI (see Fig. 7.4). Its final aim is to individuate the minimum interval distance (mINT) which consists in the distance between the anterior compressive elements and the k-line. A mINT < 4 mm is considered a cutoff for an optimal neurological recovery in non-lordotic patients [16, 31, 32].

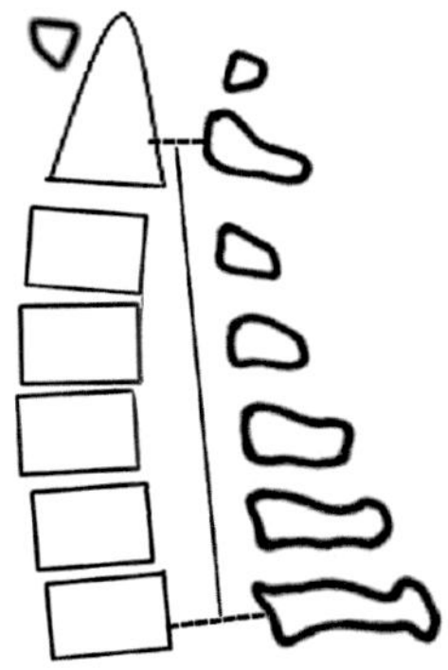

Fig. 7.4 Schematic representation of the modified k line as seen from a lateral view [16]

22. **In treating elderly patients affected by Cervical Spondylotic Myelopathy (CSM), which one is the most frequent complications?**
    a. Delirium.
    b. C-5 palsy.
    c. CSF leak.
    d. Pneumonia.
    e. Cervicalgia.

A: Surgery for CSM in elderly patients carries several post-operative complications such as C-5 palsy, CSK leak, pneumonia o cervicalgia. Among these, delirium has the most frequent [24, 33].

23. **Which sentence describes correctly the amount of lordosis, in an ascending order?**
    a. Anterior cervical discectomy and fusion (ACDF), C7 Pedicle Subtraction Osteotomy (PSO), Smith-Peters osteotomy (SPO), Anterior Osteotomy (ATO).
    b. ACDF, C7 PSO, ATO, SPO.
    c. SPO, ATO, ACDF, C7 PSO.
    d. C7 PSO, SPO, ATO, ACDF.
    e. ACDF, SPO, ATO, C7 PSO.

E: The average amount of lordosis gained with ACDF is 3–5° for a single level, 10° for a Smith-Petersen osteotomy (SPO), 17° for an Anterior Osteotomy (ATO) and up to 35° for a C7 pedicle subtraction osteotomy [26, 34].

24. **Chaddock sign consists in:**
    a. Dorsiflexion of the big toe and fanning of the other toes, after scratching the lateral plantar surface and the transverse arch with a blunt pointed object, stopping at the middle metatarsophalangeal joint.

b. Dorsiflexion of the big toe and fanning of the other toes, after stroking the lateral aspect of the foot with a dull instrument.
c. Abduction of the hand and flexion of the fingers when the distal radius is stroked.
d. Flexion and abduction of the thumb and other fingers, after nipping and snapping the nail of the patient's middle finger, with the relaxed hand
e. None of the description is correct.

B: Chaddock reflex is a clinical sign useful in testing the integrity of the corticospinal tract. It presents the same meaning of Babinski sign. Chaddock reflex, however, can be tested also In cases of significant withdrawal [35]. *Sentence "a"* describes the Babinski signs featured by toe extension instead of normal flexion, classically used to ascertain presence of pyramidal tract dysfunction [36]. *Sentence "c"* describes the Bekhterev-Jacobsohn reflex (also known as the "Jacobsohn finger flexion sign"), which is indicative of a lesion of the pyramidal tract of the upper limb and is useful in determining the localization of a lesion [37]. Sentence "d" describes the Hoffman sign used for testing corticospinal tract at the upper extremities [38].

25. **In practicing an Anterior Cervical Discectomy (ACD) approach:**
   a. The addition of an interbody graft for fusion has not shown to improve surgical outcomes.
   b. The addition of an interbody graft for fusion is suggested only in selected cases.
   c. The addition of an interbody graft for fusion is suggested in all cases, in order to improve sagittal alignment.
   d. The addition of an interbody graft for fusion has shown to be detrimental in terms of risk of complications.
   e. The addition of an interbody graft for fusion has shown to be detrimental in terms of sagittal imbalance.

C: According to the 2011 NASS guidelines for diagnosis and treatment of cervical radiculopathy from degenerative disorders, the addition of graft for fusion is suggested in all cases of ACD for improving spine sagittal alignment (grade B recommendation) [39]. The first description of the anterior approach for cervical discectomy was made by Smith-Robinson and Cloward. These pioneers of cervical surgery described the bony fusion as part of the procedure. During the following years, however, this step was questioned. Nowadays, several high quality studies have demonstrated that fusion is an essential step in order to obtain the best post-operative outcomes [40].

26. **In cases of cervical degenerative pathology treated by anterior cervical discectomy and fusion (ACDF) involving more than 3 levels, posterior fusion is advised mainly with the aim of:**
   a. Avoiding the developing of kyphosis deformity of the cervical spine.
   b. Reducing the risk of vertebral fractures.
   c. Reducing the risk of fusion graft subsidence.
   d. Reducing the pressure on adjacent disks.
   e. Reducing the risk of pseudoarthrosis.

E: Pseudoarthrosis is a complication of fusion. Precisely, this term indicates the presence of a false joint. Multilevel ACDF, 3 o more levels, has been associated to an incremented risk of this complication. This may be the result of a higher contact stress at the graft-body interface. Several aspects can interfere with the arthrodesis, concerning either the patient or the surgical approach or both, impairing vascularity, decreasing stability or increasing stress through a fusion site. Nevertheless, the real etiology of this complication is often not clear [26, 41, 42].

27. **Which one among the following criteria should not be considered in choosing the more suitable approach for the treatment of cervical degenerative disease?**
   a. Flexibility of the deformity.
   b. Presence of anterior or posterior ankylosis.
   c. Location of the deformity.
   d. Prior surgery.
   e. None of the above.

E: In surgical treatment of cervical degenerative pathology, many different surgical approaches are available. In choosing the most appropriate, many different aspects should be considered.

The ankylosis or the flexibility of the deformity are important elements for surgical planning.

History of prior cervical surgery is also important. In previously operated patients, the presence of prior fusion masses and eventual pseudoarthrosis must be ruled out. Moreover, it is advisable to operate through the opposite side of the prior cervical approach, in order to avoid scar tissue [26].

28. **In cases of kyphotic deformation located at the cervicothoracic junction, which one among the following surgical solutions is the most indicated?**
    a. ACDF and thoracic osteotomies.
    b. C7 Anterior corpectomy.
    c. C7 or T1 pedicle subtraction osteotomy (PSO) alone.
    d. C7 or T1 pedicle subtraction osteotomy (PSO) alone with simultaneous thoracic osteotomies.
    e. C7 Anterior corpectomy and T1 PSO.

C: The kyphotic deformation is an important element in the surgical planning for the treatment of cervical degenerative pathologies. In cases of a focal kyphotic deformity with cervical localization, a single cervical corpectomy is usually enough. If the kyphosis is at the cervicothoracic junction, C7 or T1 PSO should be performed. In cases of cervical spinal deformity coupled with severe thoracic kyphosis, additional osteotomies in the thoracic spine may be required to obtain the necessary correction. In cases of deformities located above and below T2, it is usually indicated to first correct the upper deformity in order to avoid overcorrection in case of lower deformity correction [26].

29. **Posterior approaches to cervical spine are indicated in cases of Cervical Spondylotic Myelopathy (CSM) but with preserved cervical lordosis. Which one is the limit for cervical sagittal orientation beyond which posterior-only cervical approaches are not considered effective?**
    a. Cervical lordosis of more than 13°.
    b. Cervical kyphosis of more than 13°.
    c. Cervical lordosis of more than 65°.
    d. Cervical lordosis or kyphosis more than 90°.
    e. Cervical kyphosis of more than 180°.

B: Posterior approaches for treating Cervical Degenerative Pathologies, especially Cervical Spondylotic Myelopathy (CSM), are indicated in specific cases, namely multilevel CSM, preserved cervical lordosis or ankylosed spines. Preservation of the cervical lordosis is a key point in choosing a posterior approach. In fact, the mechanism that underlies cervical spine cord decompression by posterior approaches is to obtain an indirect decompression by a "drift back" of the spinal cord far from the anterior pathology. If an excessive cervical kyphosis is present, greater than 13° grades, the posterior migration of the spinal cord is hindered. For this reason, posterior-only cervical approaches are usually not indicated in cases of cervical kyphosis greater than 13° [24].

30. **In degenerative cervical myelopathy (DCM) surgical management, which one among the following is the best timing in order to achieve the best clinical outcome?**
    a. 4 months.
    b. 6 months to 1 year.
    c. Surgery treatment has no efficacy in modifying DCM natural history.
    d. Immediately.
    e. Timing does not affect DCM natural history.

A: According to the literature, the majority of DCM patients worsen their mJOA score at least one point if not treated on time. Surgery proved to be an effective treatment, impacting on DCM natural history [43]. AOSpine in an international survey detected that spinal surgeons agree in considering a valid timing for treatment a range between 6 and 12 months. Nevertheless, this cut-off has not been statistically validated [44]. A recent study has shown that patient surgically treated within four months show a statistically significant better long-term mJOA outcome [45].

31. **When Spurling test can be considered positive?**
    a. When after neck extension and lateral flexion toward the involved side, applying an axial pressure to the head provokes pain.
    b. When lateral extension of the neck toward the affected side is able to provoke pain to the patient on the side opposite to the one affected by the cervical hernia.
    c. When applying pressure on the nail of the middle finger it provokes the involuntary contraction of the index and other fingers.
    d. When asking to the patient for positioning the hands flexed, with dorsal hand surfaces facing together, and to press one hand against the other, he feels an intensive pain at the wrist's level.
    e. All the listed descriptions are possible manifestations of spurling test's positivity.

A: Spurling test is a clinical test for cervical radiculopathy assessment first describe by Spurling and Scoville in 1844 [46]. This test has shown a moderate efficacy in terms of sensibility and specificity in detecting the presence of a cervical disc herniation in patients affected by cervical radiculopathy. In particular, this test proved its affordability in predicting the presence of soft discal herniations. This test is to consider positive when axial pressure applied on the neck when it is extended and laterally flexed toward the involved side evokes pain [47].

32. **In cervical ossification of the posterior longitudinal ligament:**
    a. The occupying ratio has no relevance for surgical and clinical outcomes.
    b. The occupying ratio is directly proportional to patients' mortality.
    c. The occupying ratio is indirectly proportional to patients' mortality.
    d. The occupying ratio is directly proportional to blood loss.
    e. None of the listed is true.

D: Surgical treatment of OPLL by posterior approaches has shown to carry high risk of blood loss, leading to an augmented risk of neurological deterioration and to a longer hospital stay. An important element that affects the entity of blood loss during posterior cervical approaches for OPLL treatment is the occupying ratio [48]. In fact, according to the literature a high occupying ratio, major than 60%, is associated to a greater amount of intraoperative blood loss. A possible explanation is that a thick OPLL, that corresponds to a higher occupying ratio, is able to obstruct local epidural venous drainage resulting in a major blood loss during the surgical decompression [49].

33. **Regarding posterior surgical approaches to the cervical spine:**
    a. Wiring techniques have been complete abandoned.
    b. In situ fusion has showed better clinical outcomes in terms of pseudoarthrosis, than the other posterior approaches to the cervical spine.
    c. Insertion of screws in the cervical lateral masses is not allowed, in contrast with lumbar screw fixation, because of the presence of the vertebral artery.
    d. Screw-rod constructs have shown to be biomechanically stronger than in situ or wiring techniques.
    e. None among the listed sentences is correct.

D: There are many different cervical pathologies requiring the implantation of cervical internal fixation, namely trauma, infections, neoplasms, congenital malformations and degenerative conditions. Many different techniques are available. In situ fusion is one of the first techniques developed for cervical internal fixation, consisting in application of autologous bone graft and postoperative external cervical fixation. However, this technique has been abandoned for the high rates of pseudoarthrosis [50]. Wiring techniques were developed with the aim of overcoming the limits of in situ fusion technique. Unfortunately, they present the limits of not providing immediate stability and conferring poor resistance against extension, side bending and rotational forces. Although presenting some limitations, this technique hasn't been completely abandoned since it results particularly precious in treating some categories of patients, such as pediatric patients that have spinal dimension making impossible the placement of screws for fixation. Currently, screw-rod constructs are considered the most effective in terms of biomechanical strength [51].

34. **Regarding the cervical spinal tract, which one among the following is false?**
    a. The vertebral artery enters the transverse foramen at the C6.
    b. At the C7 vertebra, the vertebral artery passes far from the lateral masses.
    c. Usually, vertebra's spinal processes are bifid from C3 to C5.
    d. Cervical vertebras from C3 to C7 composes the subaxial cervical spine.
    e. All the listed sentences are true.

B: Cervical tract of the vertebral artery usually passes through the transverses foramina, entering at the C6 one and running until the C2 transverse foramen. Otherwise, at the C7 level this artery passes anterior to the lateral mass of C7. This is an important aspect to considerate in C7 pedicle screw fixation. Spinous vertebral processes of cervical vertebras are usually bifid at the C3-C5 vertebras. In some patients this process starts to be monofid at C6 and it results almost always monofid at C7 level [52]. Vertebral artery usually enters the vertebral channel at C6 level. In some patients, however, it is also possible that it enters in the vertebral foramina at C5 or also at C7 level. This variability is always to take into account when planning cervical screw placement. For this reason, a preoperative magnetic resonance imaging must be carefully evaluated, looking for eventual vertebral artery anomalies, or even an angiography should be considered if necessary. In cervical spine segment, two different major cervical segments are individuated: the craniocervical junction (CCJ) and the subaxial spine. The first segment is made by the first two cervical vertebras that presents an anatomical aspect that make them different from the rest of the cervical vertebras, namely the atlas (C1) and the axis (C2). On the other hand, the vertebras of the subaxial cervical segment from C3 to C7 present similar anatomical characteristic. This distinction is important in deciding the best cervical posterior instrumentation technique [53].

35. **Which one among the following is a surgical technique of cervical lateral mass screw fixation?**
    a. Roy-Camille technique.
    b. Nazarian and Louis technique.
    c. Magerl technique.
    d. Anderson technique.
    e. All the listed are variations of cervical lateral mass screw fixation.

E: Cervical lateral mass screw fixation is a widely adopted surgical posterior approach to the cervical spine. It has been described for the first time by Roy-Camille in 1964 [54]. After that, several different strategies have been developed with different angulations, inclinations and entry points [55]. The Roy-Camille technique featured an entry point at the midpoint of the lateral mass [54]. Contrariwise, the Nazarian and Louis techniques described the entrance point at the intersection of a vertical line 5 mm medial to the lateral edge of the facet joint and an horizontal line 3 mm below the inferior edge of the underlying facet [56]. On the other hand, in the Magerl approach, the entry point is 1 mm medial and 1 mm cranial to the midpoint of the lateral mass [57]. Finally, according to the Anderson method, that is also called as the modified Magerl technique, the entry point is located 1 mm medial to the center of the lateral mass [58].

36. **In posterior approaches to the cervical spine:**
    a. Dissection of the muscles of the posterior compartment of the cervical spine can be done without much limitation considering that it doesn't' affects much cervical load-bearing capacity.
    b. In cases of degenerative posterior cervical spine compression, decompression should be made only at the involved level in order to reduce the traumatism for the patient and to improve the post-operative recovery course.
    c. Skin incision should be made on the left side, in order to reduce the risk of recurrent laryngeal nerve injury.
    d. Dissection of the muscles of the posterior compartment of the cervical spine should be made as much conservatively as possible, sparing dissection of the levels beyond the ones involved.
    e. None of the listed sentences is correct.

D: In posterior approaches to the cervical spine, caution must be made in muscle dissection, considering the importance of not interrupting the posterior tension band. It is important to avoid whenever is possible the dissection of C2 and C7 muscles [51]. Posterior cervical skin incision should be made on the midline, in an avascular plane [59]. In cases of degenerative posterior cervical spine compression, decompression made only at the involved level may be dangerous because it can cause bulging of the decompressed spinal cord tract, with cranial and caudal suffering of the rest of the spinal cord.

37. **In lateral masses placing of cervical screws:**
    a. Angling the screw trajectory laterally helps to reduce the risk of cervical nerve injury.
    b. Angling the screw trajectory medially helps to reduce the risk of vertebral artery injury.
    c. Angling the screw trajectory cranially helps to reduce the risk of facet joint violation.
    d. Angling the screw trajectory caudally helps to reduce the risk of cranial nerve injury.
    e. Angling the screw trajectory caudally helps to reduce the risk of vertebral artery violation.

C: Screw-rod constructs have become the most used method for cervical instrumentation in cervical degenerative pathologies. However, care must be taken in screw placement, especially regarding screws trajectory, in consideration of the risk of damaging important vascular and neurological structures. First of all, excessive laterally angling of the screw must be avoided in order to reduce the vertebral artery damaging risk. Moreover, excessive medial angling of the screw trajectory can make the spinal cord at risk, whilst an excessive cranial angulation of the screw increases the risk of facet joint violation. Finally, excessive medial direction of the screw may lead to exiting nerve root impingement [51].

38. **Among the different segments of the spine, which one is the most mobile one?**
    a. Cervical spine.
    b. Dorsal spine.
    c. Lumbar spine.
    d. b + c.
    e. All the segments have the same mobility.

A: The cervical spine tract shows the highest mobility compared to the others. This is particularly important considering that the main role of the cervical spine is to support the head. This a delicate role considering that the head, amongst its several functions, also serve as a platform that houses the sensory apparatus. For this reason, the cervical spine has assumed an anatomical conformation that allows an high mobility in order to confer the ability of moving and orientating the head in the three-dimensional space, scanning the environment and delivering it in direction of the objects of interest [51, 60].

39. **Regarding the Seventh Cervical Vertebra (C7):**
    a. All the surgical techniques developed for pedicle screw fixation of the other cervical vertebras are not applicable.
    b. Later masses are thicker compared to the other cervical vertebras.
    c. Considering its peculiar anatomy, compared to the other cervical vertebras, it is more difficult to violate the C7-T1 facet joint when placing the screws.
    d. While the vertebral body, the spinous process and the lateral masses present peculiar aspects while the facet joint are similar to the ones of the other cervical vertebras.
    e. If upper thoracic instrumentation is used, C7 fixation can often be omitted.

E: The C7 vertebra presents a unique anatomy in comparison to the other cervical vertebras. It presents the biggest vertebral body and spinous process, but it also has the thinnest lateral masses if compared with C3-C6 cervical vertebras. For this reason, there are higher odds of violating the C7-T1 facet joint during screws placement. Intra- and post-operative imaging evaluation is advised. Although all these peculiar aspects, all the surgical techniques developed for pedicle screw fixation of the other cervical vertebras are not applicable. However, if C7 is involved in an upper thoracic instrumentation, it can be omitted in consideration of the strong fixation points provided by the upper thoracic pedicles [51].

40. **In cervical syndrome:**
    a. Spinal cord damage is frequent.
    b. Spinal cord damage is rare but cervical nerves damage is even more rare.
    c. C8-T1 radiculopathies are the most frequent involved nerves, causing a peculiar syndrome (C8-T1 nerve palsies).
    d. Even if rare, spinal cord damage during cervical surgery irreversibly causes paraplegia.
    e. C5 nerve root palsy syndrome is associated with nearly all types of cervical procedures, regardless of the whether the surgery is performed anteriorly or posteriorly.

E: Damaging of cervical spine cord and cervical nerve roots injuries are among the possible complications associated to cervical spine surgery. Spinal cord damage is considerably rarer than nerve root injuries. Moreover, even in patients with a documented spine cord injury, neurological deficits are almost always transitory [61]. C8-T1 radiculopathies are relatively rare, representing only 6.2% of all cervical radiculopathies [62]. The C5 nerve palsy syndrome is the more frequently complication associated to cervical spine surgery, in both anterior and posterior approaches [63].

41. **Which one among the followings sentences is not true?**
    a. C5 root palsy syndrome is usually bilateral.
    b. Parsonnage-Turner syndrome presents with a sudden onset of pain.
    c. C8-T1 nerve palsies are often confused with cubital tunnel syndrome.
    d. Horner's syndrome is characterized by a clinical picture consisting in ipsilateral pupillary miosis, facial anhidrosis and ptosis.
    e. All the listed sentences are not true.

A: Although being infrequent, C5 root palsy syndrome is the most frequent complication associated with cervical spine surgery. It basically consists in deltoid and a biceps muscle weakness coupled to diminished biceps reflex. Only rarely both sides are involved [64].

Parsonnage-Turner Syndrome, instead, also known as idiopathic brachial plexopathy or neuralgic amyotrophy, is characterized by pain insurgence in a really brief period of time after cervical surgery, located at the neck, shoulder and arm. Sometimes, during the following hours or days, also motor weakness can occur involving the upper brachial plexus. Wining scapula can also manifest [65].

Among the possible root damage syndromes associated to cervical spine surgery, C8-T1 post-operative nerve palsies are also to take into account. These rare complications are often misdiagnosed as other nerve compression syndromes, namely the ulnar neuropathy at the elbow also called cubital tunnel syndrome. However there are some important clinical differences that can help in differential diagnosis [66].

Horner's syndrome is another rare but possible root damage due to cervical spine surgery. It is characterized by a clinical picture consisting in ipsilateral pupillary miosis, facial anhidrosis and ptosis. It is only associated to anterior cervical approaches and can cause serious discomfort and severe distress, mainly due to important cosmetic issues [67].

42. **Regarding posterior instrumentation techniques for the cervical spine:**
    a. Pedicle screw fixation is not possible in subaxial cervical spine due to the precedence of the vertebral artery.
    b. Pedicle screw fixation is not possible in subaxial cervical spine due to the small pedicle size, especially at C2 and C7 vertebras.
    c. Pedicle screw fixation in the subaxial cervical spine is more commonly used in C2 and C7 vertebras considering the wider pedicle diameters.
    d. Pedicle screw fixation is challenging but at C3 and C4 level are more commonly used due to the more favorable course of the vertebral artery.
    e. Pedicle screw fixation in the subaxial cervical spine is appliable only at the C7 vertebra, considering its wider pedicle diameters.

C: Pedicle screw fixation in cervical subaxial fixation is more challenging than in other spine regions due to the smaller size of the pedicles and also to the close proximity of the vertebral arteries. For C2 and C7 vertebrae, pedicle screws are used more frequently due to the higher pedicle dimensions the absence of the vertebral artery at C7 [51].

43. **For C7 pedicle screw placement, which one is the entry point?**
    a. A point located just below the inferior facet of C6 and slightly lateral (2–4 mm) to the center of the junction between C6 and C7 lateral masses.
    b. A point located just below the inferior facet of C6 and slightly medial (2–4 mm) to the center of the junction between C6 and C7 lateral masses.
    c. A point located at center of the C7 pedicle, between C6 and C7 lateral masses.
    d. A point located 2–4 mm below to the center of a crux that splits the pedicle of C7.
    e. None of the listed is correct.

A: Pedicle screw fixation is a challenging technique due to the small size of the pedicles and the close proximity of the vertebral arteries. However, C7 has some anatomical peculiarities that make it suitable for pedicle screw placement [51]. Albumi et al. popularized the use of this technique for cervical subaxial spine describing the entry point as slightly lateral to the center of the lateral mass and close to the inferior margin of the inferior facet joint of the cranially adjacent vertebra [68].

44. **In a patient with a clinical picture of lumbar radiculopathy, and absence of the Achilles reflex, which level is to consider involved?**
    a. L3-L4.
    b. L4-L5.
    c. L5-S1.
    d. L1-L2.
    e. it does not provide any clue to the level of lumbar disc herniation.

C: According to North American Spine Society guidelines (NASS), clinical examination has a primary role in providing clues regarding the level of a lumbar disc herniation. In particular, there is level I evidence that absence of Achilles reflex suggests the diagnosis of L5-S1 lumbar disc rupture [69, 70].

45. **According to NASS guidelines, in patients with lumbar disc herniation:**
    a. Electrodiagnostic studies are useless considering that they do not differentiate between lumbar disc herniation and other causes of nerve compression.
    b. Electrodiagnostic studies are contraindicated because they can be misleading regarding the diagnosis considering that they do not differentiate between different lumbar levels involved.
    c. Electrodiagnostic studies may be useful for the diagnosis of nerve root compression, with the same accuracy of cross-sectional imaging.
    d. Electrodiagnostic studies are sufficient alone in diagnosis of nerve root compression, in cases where lumbar disc hernia is strongly suspected.
    e. In the patient with suspected lumbar disc herniation and radiculopathy, electrodiagnostic studies may be useful only in detecting the presence of comorbid conditions, but cross-sectional imaging is the diagnostic test of choice.

E. According to NASS guidelines, electrodiagnostic studies may have utility in diagnosing nerve root compression although they do not to differentiate between lumbar disc herniation and other causes of nerve root compression. In particular, although cross-sectional imaging has to be considered as the test of choice, electrodiagnostic studies should be used to confirm the presence of comorbid conditions [69]. Somatosensory-evoked potentials are suggested as an adjunct to cross-sectional imaging to confirm the presence of nerve root compression but are not specific to the level of nerve root compression or the diagnosis of lumbar disc herniation with radiculopathy [71].

46. **In case of lumbar disc herniation, when is endoscopic treatment contraindicated?**
    a. In case of high lumbar level (L1-L2).
    b. In case of segmental instability.
    c. In case of soft disc herniation.
    d. In case of high iliac crest, for L5-S1 discal hernia treatment.
    e. All the sentences are contraindications.

B: Endoscopic spine discectomy is a minimally invasive spine surgery technique whose clinical application is gaining popularity. There are many different techniques for endoscopic lumbar spine discectomy, namely transforaminal percutaneous transforaminal lumbar discectomy (PELD), interlaminar PELD and others. In all these modalities, soft disc herniation is an unavoidable criterion and not a contraindication. High lumbar level is not a contraindication, considering that many cases have been described in the literature. In case of L5-S1 discal herniation in a patient with high iliac crest transforaminal PELD is contraindicated, but interlaminar PELD is suitable [72]. However, this minimally invasive technique is not safe if segmental instability is present [73].

47. **Which one is a false sentence among the following, regarding lumbar disc herniation risk factors?**
    a. Smoking history of more than 15 years increases the risk of developing lumbar disc hernia.
    b. Mental stress is a risk factor suspected of being involved in lumbar disc hernia
    c. According to the literature, genetic disposition is not a risk factor to consider in lumbar disc herniation predisposition.
    d. Patients involved in mainly sedentary activities have a major tendency in herniation of lumbar discs.

C: Identification of risk factors for lumbar disc herniation is not a simple task due to various technical issues. Smoking history has proved to increase the risk for lumbar disc herniation [74], as well as exposure to frequent heavy lifting [75] and sedentary activities. Moreover, many studies support the role of genetic disposition in the genesis of this pathology [76].

48. **A patient present to your attention with a clinical picture of radiculopathy and a lumbar MRI showing a lumbar disc herniation as in the picture. How do you would classify this herniation according to the Michigan State University (MSU) classification system?**
    a. 1-A.
    b. 1-B.
    c. 2-A.
    d. 2-B.
    e. 3-C.

B: MSU classification is a classification system developed for herniated lumbar disc, based on Axial T2 MRI. According to this classification, size and location of the hernia are measured in terms of grade of herniation and location of the hernia. The first aspect is described in respect to a line drawn transversely through the lumbar spinal canal, to and from the medial edge of the facet joint articulation (intra-facet line), defining 3 grades of herniation (grade 1, 2 or 3) on an antero-posterior direction. The herniated disc location is described as A, B or C, according to the position of the hernia in relation to three lines passing through the intra-facet line, dividing the intracanal space is in three different areas on the latero-lateral direction. Intersecting all these lines is possible to delineate two central areas (right area "A" and left area "A"), two lateral areas (Area "B" left and right) and two "far lateral" areas (Area "C" on the left and on the right) [77].

49. **Which one among the followings is a relative indication for surgical treatment of lumbar disc herniation?**
    a. Cauda equina syndrome.
    b. Severe paresis according to the medical research council scale (MRC < 3).
    c. Paraparesis/paraplegia (high lumbar disc herniation).
    d. Severe sciatica with large disc herniation non-responsive to analgesic and NSAIDs.
    e. All the listed are absolute indications.

D: Selection of the patient is a key point in surgical treatment of lumbar disc herniation and is mandatory for achieving favorable clinical outcomes. It is important to have a good correlation between clinical symptoms and radiological findings [78]. Severe sciatica non-responsive to conservative management should be surgically treated before three months of symptoms to avoid chronic pathologic alterations. Nevertheless, the latter is not an absolute indication [79].

50. **In a patient with a lumbar disc herniation, you expect:**

a. a worse clinical status in a patient with a paramedian and intraforaminal herniation, considering that the lateral aspects of the lumbar canal are narrower than the medial one.
b. a worse clinical status in a patient with a median herniation, considering that the median aspects of the lumbar canal is narrower than the lateral ones.
c. a better clinical status in a patient with a paramedian and intraforaminal herniation, considering that the lateral aspects of the lumbar canal have more room for the nervous structures than the medial one.
d. the position of the herniation does not affect the gravity of the clinical picture in the lumbar disc herniation.

A: The lumbar canal does not offer the same room for neurological structures along the latero-lateral axis. Indeed, its lateral aspects are more constrained than the median area. For this reason, a median hernia typical exerts a lesser compression on the spinal nerves, determining a less severe clinical scenario [77].

51. **According to Combined Task Force (CTF) classification system, lumbar disc can be classified in which categories among the following?**
    a. Normal disc, focal protrusion, broad-based protrusion or extrusion.
    b. Normal disc, median protrusion, paramedian protrusion, lateral protrusion.
    c. Normal disc, partially expelled disc, totally expelled disc, migrated disc expulsion.
    d. Normal disc, dehydrated disc, partially expelled disc, migrated disc.
    e. Normal disc, herniated disc.

A: In 2001, in the attempt of standardize definitions of lumbar disc pathology, the North American Spine Society collaborated in a joint project with the American Society of Neuroradiology and American Society of Spine Radiology, defining the Combined Task Force (CTF) classification system. According to that system, lumbar disk can be classified as normal when it is fully and normally developed and free of any changes due to diseases, trauma or aging. A herniated disc refers to a localized displacement of nucleus, cartilage, fragments of apophyseal bone or fragments of annular tissue beyond the intervertebral disc space. The herniation is classified as protruded disc, if the greatest plane in any direction between the edges of the herniated disc portion beyond the disc space result to be inferior in relation to the distance of the edges of the base. In cases of protrusion, this may also be discriminated in focal, if the circumference of the protrusion is less than 25% of the circumference of the whole disc, or broad-based, if the circumference is between 25 and 50% of the whole disc perimeter. Finally, in cases where no continuity exists between the disc material beyond the disc space and that within the disc space the hernia is defined as extrusion [80].

52. **Which one among the following is not a classification system for lumbar disc pathology?**
    a. Combined Task Force (CTF) classification system.
    b. Jansen classification system.
    c. MSU classification system.
    d. All the listed.
    e. None of the above.

E: The CTF classification system is the most used system for radiological classification of lumbar disc herniation classification, that describes vertebral discs as normal, focal protrusion, broad-based protrusion and extrusion [80]. The Jansen classification is another classification system with the same meaning of the CTF one, identifying 4 different radiological grades of lumbar disc herniation [81]. MSU classification is a classification system developed for herniated lumbar disc, based on Axial T2 MRI. According to this classification, size and location of the hernia are measured in terms of grade of herniation and location of the hernia [77].

53. **A patient comes to your attention with antalgic gait, relying more on the right then the left leg, which appears a little bit more flexed in the attempt of reducing the pain. At the neurological examination, the patient describes a reduction in tactile, thermic and pain sensibility along the S1 dermatome. Which one among the following sentences regarding lumbar disc herniation radiculopathy pathogenesis is true?**
    a. Radiculopathy is only due to mechanical deformation of the involved nerve caused by the herniated material pressure.
    b. Radiculopathy is only the result of chemical irritation of the nerve due to the direct biochemical effects of nucleolus pulposus components on nerve fiber structure.
    c. Radiculopathy is a consequence of both, mechanical deformation and chemical irritation of the nerve, to the point that it is not possible to have a radiculopathy in the absence of one of this two elements.
    d. Radiculopathy is usually due to both mechanical deformation and chemical irritation of the nerve

acting simultaneously but the presence of one of them alone may induce clinical manifestations.

e. Radiculopathy is the cause of lumbar disc herniation and not the contrary.

D: There is evidence that mechanical deformation of the nerve root as well as its chemical irritation due to lumbar disc herniation are both causes of radiculopathy. However, many studies have demonstrated that root compression alone is capable of causing sciatica [82] by causing impaired blood supply, edema, onset of compression and nerve suffering. On the other hand, also chemical irritation may provoke radiculopathy by itself via a direct biochemical effects of nucleus components on nerve fiber structures and function, inducing microvascular changes and inflammatory reactions in the nerve [83].

54. **In approaching a patient with high lumbar disc herniation, which of the following anatomical aspects should be considered:**
    a. The upper lumbar spine is similar to the L4-L5 and L5-S1 levels.
    b. The upper lumbar spine is characterized by anatomically lager spinal canal.
    c. The upper lumbar spine has the same density of rootlets than the lower lumbar area.
    d. Upper lumbar spine is characterized by narrower laminas and isthmus, compared with those in the lower lumbar area.
    e. There are no anatomical differences between upper and lower lumbar spine.

D: The definition of upper lumbar spine usually comprises the levels from L1 to L4 [84]. This area presents a narrower spinal canal than the lower lumbar area, with a major density of rootlets and narrow laminas and isthmus. These are important anatomical differences between the two segments of the lumbar spine and they should be kept in mind when surgically approaching lumbar spine.

55. **For which reason fully endoscopic transforaminal lumbar discectomy is more suitable for upper lumbar disc herniations than lower lumbar ones?**
    a. Because the higher lumbar space offers a larger interlaminar space
    b. The upper lumbar area has narrow isthmi, providing higher instruments maneuverability.
    c. The spinal canal is larger than in the lower lumbar area, allowing for more room for endoscopic movements.
    d. The upper lumbar area has wide lumbar foramen, offering more possibility for endoscope angulations.
    e. There is no indication for fully endoscopic transforaminal lumbar discectomy in the lower lumbar area.

D: Endoscopic transforaminal lumbar discectomy is particularly indicated for herniation occurring in the upper lumbar area because of the wider foramina diameter. This aspect translates in more available space for endoscopic maneuverability, making the transforaminal endoscopic approach for lumbar disc hernia removal more suitable in this area, especially for upward migrated disc herniations [72]. In upper lumbar area interlaminar space is not large and the spinal canal is narrower than lower lumbar area.

56. **Which one among the following is a percutaneous endoscopic lumbar discectomy (PELD) systems?**
    a. YESS.
    b. TESSYS.
    c. A + b.
    d. MIS-TLIF.
    e. PLIF.

C: YESS stands for Yeung endoscopic spine systems that is one of the most used system for PELD. The technology of this system relies on the Kambin triangle as entry point for the procedure. TESSYS stands for transforaminal endoscopic spine system and is a system for PELD as well. This system, however, refers to a different entry point. In particular, the entry point for this system is the inferior intervertebral foramen. Both the systems are used for transforaminal PELD approaches [85].

57. **What is the role of transforaminal epidural steroid injections for treatment of lumbar disc herniation, according to NASS 2014 lumbar disc herniation guidelines?**
    1. This conservative treatment modality does not carry any benefits for the lumbar disc herniation patients with radicular symptoms.
    2. This conservative treatment modality carries the same benefits of lumbar microdiscectomy.
    3. This conservative treatment is superior to lumbar microdiscectomy in terms of pain relief for the patient.
    4. This conservative treatment modality is recommended by the NASS with the aim to provide short-term (2–4 weeks) pain relief to patients with lumbar disc herniation and radiculopathy.

5. This conservative treatment modality presents a lower efficacy rate in comparison to interlaminar epidural steroid injections, in terms of pain relief.

D: According to NASS, transforaminal epidural steroids injections are recommended to provide short-term (2–4 weeks) pain relief in patients with lumbar disc herniation and radiculopathy. This recommendation presents grade A evidence. Interlaminar epidural steroid injections may be considered, but with a recommendation level C [69].

58. **Which one among the following epidural steroid injection modalities, has the strongest recommendation?**
    a. Interlaminar.
    b. Caudal
    c. Transforaminal.
    d. All the listed has the same level of recommendation.
    e. None of the listed is recommended.

A: According to the 2012 North American Spine Society Guidelines, epidural steroid injections are recommended in non-surgical management of lumbar disc herniation, especially for short-term pain relief [69]. The results of 2 years follow-up of 3 randomized double-blind controlled trials, proved that interlaminar steroids injection are superior to the transforaminal one at 12-months [86].

59. **In a patient with clinical symptoms of radiculopathy due to lumbar disc herniation, when is the optimal timing for surgical intervention?**
    a. Prior to 2 months.
    b. As soon as possible.
    c. Prior to one year.
    d. Prior to 6 months.
    e. Timing does not affect the outcome.

D: According to NASS 2014 guidelines, best surgical intervention timing in lumbar disc herniation patients is within 6 months from the onset of clinical symptoms, with a grade B recommendation. This is associated with a faster recovery and improved in long-term outcomes [69].

60. **Which one among the following localizations of lumbar disc herniation is the most frequent?**
    a. Lateral intraforaminal.
    b. Lateral extraforaminal.
    c. Medio-lateral.
    d. Medial
    e. All the locations have the same prevalence.

C: The majority of lumbar disc herniations present a medio-lateral localization (65%). This aspect has an anatomical explanation due to the fact that the medial fibers of the deep layer of the Posterior Longitudinal Ligament (PLL) are firmly attached to the medial portion of the annulus fibrosus, reinforcing this portion and making medial lumbar disc herniations rare. On the lateral portion of the annulus fibrosus, instead, they attach to the lateral membrane that is a thin and translucent anatomical structure. Therefore, the mediolateral portion of the annulus fibrous, the conjunction point of the PLL and the lateral membrane, is to consider as a point of weakness favoring the formation of medio-lateral herniations [87].

61. **In patients affected by lumbar disc herniation, in order to avoid recurrence:**
    a. It is suggested to always make discectomy along with herniectomy.
    b. Discectomy alone is enough because the freed space is sufficient to obtain decompression, without removing the herniated fragment.
    c. The association of discectomy to the herniectomy has not shown a clear advantage in terms of lumbar disc herniation recurrence, so no clear indications are present.
    d. Discectomy associated with herniectomy has shown to be detrimental, increasing the recurrence rate.
    e. None of the listed sentences is true.

C: Recurrence of lumbar disc herniation is an important issue with a mean prevalence rate ranging between 4 and 21% [88–90]. According to the literature, the re-operation rate do not clearly increase following removal of the herniated material, with contrasting results among different authors [88, 91]. Total removal of disc material leads to reduced intervertebral disc space height, that can cause segmental instability and acceleration of spondylosis, finally causing failed back syndrome. Besides, preservation of intervertebral disc reduces the risk of very life-threating complications like abdominal or retroperitoneal neuro-vascular structures injuries. For these reasons, the opportunity of limiting the surgery to the herniectomy has been evaluated in the literature with encouraging results in terms of relapsing rate. Nevertheless, discectomy has shown slightly better results in terms of low-back pain relief [88].

At this moment, clear indications are lacking, and more high-quality studies are needed with longer follow-up periods.

62. **Which one among the following radiological exams is not useful in lumbar foraminal stenosis diagnosis?**
    a. Myelography.
    b. Lumbar MRI.
    c. Lumbar CT.
    d. Plain radiographic lateral views.
    e. Dynamic flexion and extension lumbar studies.

A: Myelography has a limited use in detecting lumbar foraminal stenosis because is not able in depicting lateral pathology for the reason that the dural sac terminates at the lateral aspect of the midzone. As a consequence, that aspect avoids contrast-filling of the distal nerve root sheaths. Plain radiographs in the lateral views allow to depict the two most important anatomical parameters for lumbar foraminal stenosis diagnosis: posterior disc height (< 4 mm) and foraminal height ($\leq$ 15 mm). Dynamic flexion and extension lumbar studies are also useful in detecting dynamic foraminal changes and stenosis. CT is precious in showing bony encroachment into the foraminal area as well as the presence of bony spurs. MRI is the gold standard providing visualization of the foramen and at the same time a better resolution on non-osseous components, namely intervertebral disc and paucity of perineural fat surrounding the nerve root (in T1-weighted images) [92].

63. **In a patient with foraminal stenosis:**
    a. Conservative treatment is not indicated.
    b. Surgery is indicated also in asymptomatic patients.
    c. Surgery just consists in foramen enlargement, because other treatments are only more invasive but do not impact clinical outcome.
    d. Fusion surgery in always indicated in cases of foraminal decompression.
    e. Fusion surgery is necessary only in cases when direct foraminal decompression does not provide enough enlargement or when preoperative instability is detected.

E: Patients with symptomatic Lumbar Foramen Stenosis (LFS) are primarily treated conservatively. In cases of failure to improve a surgical foraminal enlargement should be performed and, in cases of failure, a fusion surgery can be performed. However, the latter should be conceived as first strategy in cases of significant preoperative instability [93].

64. **Which one among the following sentences regarding the clinical presentation of lumbar spinal stenosis is true?**
    a. Patients do not present with radiculopathy.
    b. Lumbar stenosis is not always symptomatic. Patients can also present without symptoms.
    c. Neurogenic claudication is a rare manifestation of spinal stenosis.
    d. Low back pain is almost always present among lumbar stenosis patients.
    e. All the listed sentences are true.

B: Lumbar stenosis is a chronic degenerative alteration of lumbar spinal canal with spinal cord or nerve compression. Neurogenic claudication is the cardinal symptom of this pathology, while low-back pain is not always present. Pain improves when bending forward and is alleviated by sports like bicycling, since during this sport the trunk is flexed forward [94]. Some patients can also present with a radiculopathy that persists during resting worsening during the night.

65. **A 70 years old patient comes to your attention with a clinical picture of mild low-back pain, worsening in supine position and improving in sitting position. The main complaint referred by the patient is a severe gait fatiguability, making him unable to walk for more than 100 m without resting. After resting, however, he can restart again without leg pain. His walking autonomy is longer in anterior bending position and on uphill. Moreover, the patient refers that bicycling is less a problem for him than walking. On clinical examination, he presented hyporeflexia, without sensibility or strength alterations, with worsening of lumbar pain during back extension maneuvers and Straight Leg Test negativity. Lumbar MRI is showed in the figure. Which is the diagnosis for this patient?**
    a. Lumbar stenosis.
    b. Lumbar disc herniation.
    c. Spondylolisthesis.
    d. Spondylodiscitis
    e. None of the listed hypothesis is true.

A: The clinical scenario and the magnetic resonance imaging is compatible with a diagnosis of lumbar stenosis. The patient does not present signs of radiculopathy or infection. Moreover, the aspects of the pain, that improves with lumbar anterior flexion and worsens with spine extension is typically associated with degenerative lumbar stenosis. Contrariwise, spondylolisthesis presents with pain improving during physical effort. Finally, patients with lumbar stenosis use to better perform bicycling and uphill walking, because both require spine flexion, enlarging intracanal space and reducing spinal cord compression. Magnetic resonance shows an L3-L4 lumbar stenosis, that is also compatible with the neurologic examination [95].

66. **Considering MRI pictures of question number 56, which one among the following classification scales is the most suitable to define its severity?**
    a. MSU classification.
    b. Meyerding system.
    c. Schizas system.
    d. Modic system.
    e. None of the listed system has been improved for this pathology.

C: The patient presented in question number 56 is affected by lumbar stenosis. Schizas classification represents a qualitative grading system based on the morphologic appearance of the dural sac as seen in T2-weighted axial images of the lumbar spine. Many radiological evaluation systems have been developed, most of all concerning almost exclusively about spinal canal diameter measurements, such as the surface measurement methodology or the stenosis ratio system [96]. The Schizas' system is different from these methodologies because it focuses on morphological parameters. This classification systems identifies 4 different grades of stenosis severity, based on CSF morphology: Grade A, describes the condition where CSF is clearly visible but has an inhomogeneous aspect; Grade B consider the case where CSF is slightly present and rootlets occupy the whole dural sac area, but they are still individualized; Grade C is the case where no rootles are recognizable and no CSF signal is detectable, making the dural sac showing an homogeneous gray signal; Grade D patients, on the other hand, present with no rootles recognizable with no epidural fat posteriorly [97].

67. **The clinical history of a patient with spinal stenosis usually consists in:**
    a. An acute onset with intense lumbar pain and sciatica.
    b. An acute onset with only sciatica.
    c. Chronic course of mild low back pain interspaced with critical episodes of lumbar painful blockage, worsening during the bending position and coupled with falling due to hyposthenia.
    d. Chronic course of numbness, weakness and discomfort in the legs while walking or prolonged, usually without a long history of low back pain.
    e. None of the following sentences describes the typical clinical picture of lumbar stenosis.

D: Lumbar spinal stenosis is a chronic condition, typically manifesting with neurogenic claudicatio, with regression of the symptoms during sitting, resting and forward bending. An acute onset is rare and if present the diagnosis should be reconsidered, except in the cases of patients with a congenitally narrow canal that can develop major neurologic deficit in a brief period due to the insurgence of an additional disc protrusion [98].

68. **Which one among the followings sentences is not true regarding the anatomy of lumbar foramina?**
    a. Vertebral pedicles contribute to form the anterior wall of the lumbar foramina.
    b. Superior articular facet composes the posterior wall of the foramina.
    c. Intervertebral discs participate in the composition of the anterior wall of lumbar foramina.
    d. Inferior articular facet composes the anterior wall of the foramina.
    e. Ligamentum flavum participates in the formation of the posterior wall of the foramina.

D: Intervertebral foramina are oval or round anatomic structures, forming between upper and lower vertebra, that contains the emergence of nerve roots. They present anterior and posterior boundaries. The anterior profile is made by adjacent superior-inferior vertebral pedicles, the posteroinferior margin of the superior vertebral body, the intervertebral disc, the postero-superior margin of the inferior vertebral body. Posterior foraminal boundary is made by the ligamentum flavum and the superior and inferior articular facets [93].

69. **Which one among the following radiological aspects of the nerve root is indicative of lumbar foraminal stenosis (LFS) on MRI?**
    a. The paucity of perineural fat surrounding the nerve root.

b. The excessive posterior deviation of the nerve root direction in exiting the foramen, depicting an obtuse angle.
c. The excessive anterior bending of the nerve root in exiting the foramen, depicting a pathologically acute angle.
d. The reduction of the nerve diameter < of 2 mm.
e. None of the listed has a value in determining foraminal stenosis.

A: MRI is an important tool in diagnosis of LFS, mainly because it allows to gain information regarding both foraminal alterations and central canal narrowing, at the same time. Moreover, it allows to define the degeneration of intervertebral discs and vertebral bodies. The most indicative sing of LFS on parasagittal MRI images is the loss of perineural fat surrounding the nerve root [93]. Nerves direction deviations are better visible on MR myelography. Nerve root swelling and increased diameter are more likely associated to LFS than diameter reduction [99].

70. **In evaluating the lumbar foramen on plain radiographs of a patient suspected for lumbar foraminal stenosis (LFS):**
   a. Posterior disc height < 4 mm.
   b. Foraminal height $\leq$ 15 mm.
   c. a + b.
   d. Kyphotic grade of lumbar lordosis < 5°.
   e. None among the listed sentences is true.

C: Plain radiographic lateral views have shown to detect the lowering of posterior disc height (< 4 mm) and the foraminal height (< 15 mm) [100].

71. **A 65-year-old male patient comes to your attention reporting left leg pain and paresthesia in a crural distribution. The symptoms are present during rest, worsen during gait, reaching a peak always after 200 m. Moreover, he refers that pain improves with anteflexion of the trunk and intensifies while lying, especially whit left side decubitus. Clinical evaluation shows weakness in reflex elicitation at the left side, and ante-flexed trunk gaiting. Kemp's sign was present on the left side, reproducing radicular symptoms early. Which one is the most probable pathology affecting this patient?**
   a. Radiculopathy secondary to lumbar disc herniation.
   b. Central canal lumbar stenosis.
   c. Neurogenic claudication with radiculopathy, due to lumbar foraminal stenosis.
   d. Isthmic spondylolisthesis.
   e. None of the listed hypothesis is correct.

B: Lumbar foraminal stenosis (LFS) is a common degenerative alteration of the lumbar spine, causing radicular pain and neurogenic claudication, mainly due to degeneration of the intervertebral disc. This degeneration, indeed, associates to anterior or posterior subluxation of the superior articular process of the inferior vertebra, leading to reduction of the foramen height and thus foramen area. From a clinical point of view, this pathology presents predominantly with radicular leg pain and limited lumbar range of motion, especially in extension. Typically, leg pain often presents a dermatomal distribution with the aspects of an entrapping nerve pathology. In fact, in affected patients, pain is triggered by lumbar extension, in particular on the affected side, by sitting or by supine position, for example during bed lying. Contrariwise, it improves with anterior flexion of the trunk [101]. These aspects explained considering that lumbar foraminal stenosis is the result of both fixed anatomical anomalies and dynamic factors. In particular, cadaveric studies clearly showed that spine extension decreases all foraminal dimensions by an average of 15% while flexion causes a significant average increase of 12% [102]. In cases of lumbar disc herniation, compression causes neural distraction, provoking a pain that worsens during trunk flexion and tension-based sings, warranting Lasègue test positivity [93].

72. **Lumbar MRI of the patient at the question 71 showed an L2-L3 left foraminal stenosis. Which type of foraminal stenosis is the one that affected this patient?**
   a. Transverse foraminal stenosis.
   b. Vertical foraminal stenosis.
   c. Circumferential foraminal stenosis.
   d. Half circumscriptive stenosis.
   e. None of the listed is a possible category of foraminal stenosis.

C: Lumbar foraminal stenosis (LFS) is a common degenerative alteration of the lumbar spine, mainly due to reduction of the foraminal area and height, that is often clinically and radiologically unrecognized. Anatomically, three major types of LFS can be distinguished. *Vertical stenosis*, featured by craniocaudal compression of the exiting nerve, exerted by posterolateral osteophytes and herniated disc at the same time, pushing the root against the superior pedicle. *Transverse stenosis* defines the cases of a subluxation of the superior facet is and associated to a hypertrophic ligamentum flavum and/or bony spurs that simultaneously participate in root compression on a transversal plane.

Finally, the *circumferential stenosis characterized by a* combination of the described compression mechanisms. The distinctive element individuating this category is the absence of intraforaminal fat in both, anterior and posterior portion of the foramen. Therefore, the patient in the clinical case is affected by a circumferential foraminal stenosis [93].

73. **In the management of lumbar foraminal stenosis:**
    a. Electrophysiological preoperative studies are always indicated, independently to the extension and location of the peripheral disorder.
    b. Plain radiographs are not useful anymore because no information's regarding the foramen pathology are provided.
    c. After foraminal decompression, spine fusion is advisable in the majority of cases considering that foraminal decompression leads to spine instability.
    d. In cases of patients affected by both, foraminal and intra-canalar stenosis, intraoperative electrophysiology may be useful.
    e. Lumbar foraminal stenosis has primarily to be surgically treated.

D: In some cases, lumbar foraminal stenosis (LFS) also associates with an immediately higher medial canal stenosis, depicting a clinical pathological situation called "double crash" lesion. In these cases, it can be difficult to understand which one among the two pathological alterations is the main responsible for the symptomatology. In these cases, intraoperative electrophysiology may be helpful in overcoming this problem by measuring the distal latency of the spinal nerve to compare intracanal and extraforaminal lesions [103]. Electrophysiological preoperative studies are useful in clinical management of this pathology. However, they are not always applicable because they can lead to false positive results when Wallerian degeneration does not extend below the knee. Plain radiographs are still useful in foraminal stenosis management setting because they allow to gain precious information regarding posterior disc height and foraminal height that, in cases of pathological reduction, are indicators of potential LFS. After practicing foraminal surgical decompression, spinal fusion is not advised as default but is restricted to the cases when also spinal instability has been detected. Usually, in cases of lumbar foramina stenosis, conservative treatment is the first line treatment of choice, leaving surgical management for the cases where conservative treatment has failed [93].

74. **Speaking of lumbar stenosis, the narrowing:**
    a. Is located into the central spinal canal.
    b. Is located in the central spinal canal and in the neural foramina. Cases of only central spinal canal narrowing are called incomplete lumbar stenosis.
    c. Can be located in the central spinal canal and/or the neural foramina and/or under the facet joint (subarticular stenosis).
    d. Can be located in the central spinal canal and/or the neural foramina and/or under the facet joint (subarticular stenosis), also involving the interlaminar space.
    e. Has to be located just in the foramina.

C: In patients affected by lumbar stenosis, the narrowing may involve the central spinal canal, the neural foramina (foraminal stenosis) but also the area under the facet joint (subarticular stenosis) [104].

75. **In the surgical treatment of lumbar stenosis:**
    a. Decompression alone is more effective than decompression and fusion in relieving pain.
    b. Decompression alone is generally not enough in obtaining pain relief and fusion should always been associated.
    c. There is no advantage in associating fusion to decompression in treating lumbar stenosis.
    d. Decompression and fusion have shown to be more effective in relieving pain in comparison to decompression alone, but only in cases of lumbar stenosis due to spondylolisthesis.
    e. Decompression and fusion are more effective than decompression alone.

D: According to the literature, decompression along with fusion is a more effective strategy than decompression alone in treating pain and in increasing functional status, but only in patients with lumbar stenosis associated to spondylolisthesis [105]. The same benefit has not been achieved in cases of lumbar stenosis without spondylolisthesis [106].

76. **In patients affected by lumbar stenosis, the most typical clinical sign is neurogenic claudication, that improves in lumbar flexion. Which one among the following may be a possible explanation?**
    a. Extension of the spine reduces the cross-sectional area of the central canal as well as of the neural foramina stretching the myelin of the intraformational tract of peripheral spine nerves and slowing nerve conduction.
    b. Flexion of the spine moves forward the center of gravity, moving the body weight from the hips to the ankle, reducing in this way axial and groin pain.

c. Extension of the spine obstacles the liquor pathways to the medulla, causing catabolites accumulation in the spine and lack of anabolites, inducing spinal suffering and pain.
d. Extension of the spine reduces the cross-sectional area of the central canal as well as of the neural foramina, exerting further pressure on the veins surrounding the nerve roots, leading to nerve compression. Spine flexion inverts this process.
e. Extension of the spine reduces the cross-sectional area of the central canal as well as of the neural foramina, exerting further pressure on the arterioles surrounding the nerve roots, leading to nerves suffering. Spine flexion is able to invert this process.

D: Typically, patients affected by lumbar stenosis present with neurogenic claudication that improves with rest and spine flexion. Moreover, these patients usually better tolerate exercises performed during lumbar flexion, such as cycling [104]. Extension of the spine reduces the cross-sectional area of the central canal and of the neural foramina, exerting further pressure on the veins surrounding the nerve roots, leading to nerves engorgement and ischemic suffering. Spine flexion is able to invert this process [107].

77. **In patients with lumbar stenosis surgically treated for decompression:**
    a. Physical therapy is contraindicated in the post-operative management because it results dangerous.
    b. Physical therapy is indicated but it useful only if started at least two months after surgery.
    c. Physical therapy has shown to be useful in the post-operative management, independently to the post-surgical starting time.
    d. Physical therapy has shown to be useful in the post-operative management, when started six weeks to three months after surgery.
    e. Physical therapy is superior to surgical treatment in all cases of degenerative lumbar stenosis.

D: The role of physical therapy in the post-operative period is supported by randomized controlled trials, showing that active rehabilitation started from six weeks to three months after surgery is more effective than standard care in long-term improvement of functionality, low back pain and leg pain [108].

78. **Regarding the preoperative factors to consider in predicting post-surgical outcomes in lumbar spinal stenosis, which one among the following is incorrect:**
    a. Patients' age has a strong impact on the outcomes because older patients have shown worse outcomes in comparison to younger ones.
    b. Depression is associated to worse outcomes.
    c. Smoking impacts post-operative outcomes.
    d. Preoperative leg pain is associated with more evident post-operative improvements
    e. Obese patients have worse post-surgical outcomes.

A: Obesity, smoking habit and preoperative depression are detrimental for post-surgical patient course. Age and gender, however, have proved to have no impact in determining post-operative outcomes [109].

79. **In endoscopic laminectomy for treatment of lumbar stenosis, which one among the following is a possible starting point?**
    a. Kambin triangle in the intervertebral foramen.
    b. Inferior intervertebral foramen.
    c. Superior articular process.
    d. Inferior articular process.
    e. None of the listed.

C: Endoscopic corridors for treating lumbar stenosis requires an higher starting point. Kambin triangle is the entry point for YESS (Yeung endoscopic spine system) and inferior intervertebral foramen is the entry point for TESSYS (Transforaminal endoscopic spine system), which are two PELD (percutaneous endoscopic lumbar discectomy) modalities, that have the common goal of approaching the intervertebral disc. For this reason, their viewing window is not suitable for practicing a laminectomy. The superior articular process is more indicated [110].

80. **Sagittal Balance has shown to be strictly correlated with spinal pathology. In particular, lumbar lordosis (LL) has shown to be strongly correlated with low back pain. How does this parameter change with age and how is it correlated with low back pain?**
    a. This parameter decreases with age. A decreased lumbar lordosis increases the risk of low back pain because the two elements are connected by an inverse correlation.

b. This parameter increases with age and increased lumbar lordosis reduces the risk of low back pain.
c. This parameter decreases with age and the same does the risk of developing low back pain considering that this risk is directly correlated to the grade of lumbar lordosis.
d. This parameter increases with age and the same dose the risk of low back pain because the latter increasing proportionally at the increasing of the former.
e. Lumbar lordosis does not affect the risk of developing low back pain.

A: Loss of the lumbar lordosis is a distinctive finding in the aging spine, leading to an increased prevalence of low back pain (LBP). In fact, patients with LBP tend to have an attenuated lumbar lordosis compared to healthy patients [111].

81. **According to WFNS 2020 guidelines, which among the following radiological parameters is considered as cut-off for central lumbar canal stenosis definition?**
a. Anteroposterior canal diameter < 10–15 mm.
b. Anteroposterior canal diameter < 4–5 mm.
c. Cross-sectional area < 75–145 mm^2.
d. a + c.
e. b + c.

D: According to WFNS 2020 guidelines, an antero-posterior canal inferior than 10–15 mm and/or a cross-sectional area inferior than 75–145 mm^2 should be considered as cut-off values to define central stenosis [112].

82. **Which one among the following is not a suitable surgical approach in treating lumbar stenosis?**
a. Laminectomy.
b. Bilateral laminotomies.
c. \.
d. Laminoplasty.
e. Bilateral decompression through unilateral laminotomy.

C: Laminectomy, bilateral laminotomies, bilateral decompression through unilateral laminotomy and laminoplasty are all surgical techniques indicated in lumbar stenosis according to WFNS 2020 guidelines. YESS is a PELD (percutaneous endoscopic lumbar discectomy) technique that does not allow endoscopic canal decompression [110, 112, 113].

83. **According to the WFNS 2020 guidelines for spinal stenosis, which one among the following is the best surgical management of a patient with lumbar degenerative spinal stenosis, with loss of sagittal balance and related symptoms?**
a. Decompression alone in sufficient.
b. Decompression and associated fusion is necessary.
c. Decompression, fixation and deformity correction are all indicated.
d. There is no difference among the approaches.
e. There is no consensus regarding this issue.

C: According to the WFNS 2020 guidelines, in cases of lumbar degenerative spinal stenosis with concomitant loss of sagittal balance and related symptoms, decompression should be coupled with fixation and deformity correction [112].

84. **Which one among the following spinal decompressing techniques allow preservation of posterior elements?**
a. Standard posterior laminectomy.
b. Bilateral laminotomy.
c. Unilateral laminotomy with bilateral decompression.
d. a + c.
e. b + c.

E: Standard posterior approach with open laminectomy and facet sparing is the only one approach among the listed that contemplate the whole resection of posterior elements (spinous processes and laminas). Bilateral laminotomy allows the preservation of pars of the laminas and the spinous process. In the unilateral laminotomy with bilateral decompression technique, part of the lamina on one side, the whole lamina on the opposite side and the whole spinous process are preserved [114].

85. **According to 2020 WFNS recommendations for lumbar stenosis surgical treatment:**
a. Microscopic techniques are equal to standard laminectomy in achieving adequate spinal canal decompression.

b. Microscopic techniques are more effective than standard laminectomy in achieving adequate spinal canal decompression.
c. Standard laminectomy is more effective than microscopic techniques in achieving adequate spinal canal decompression.
d. There is no consensus regarding the best technique for spinal decompression in lumbar spine degenerative stenosis.
e. WFNS recommendation does not mention about best surgical decompression technique in cases of lumbar stenosis.

D: The WFNS spine committee does not reached a consensus regarding the most indicated decompression technique for lumbar stenosis. For this reason the choose is still left to the surgeons according to their preferences [114].

86. **According to 2016 NASS guidelines, which is the definition of "isthmic spondylolisthesis":**
a. The anterior translation of one lumbar vertebra over the next inferior segment as a result of a lesion of the pars interarticularis.
b. The anterior translation of one lumbar vertebra over the next inferior segment as a result of the rupture of a vertebral hemangioma.
c. The anterior translation of one lumbar vertebra over the next inferior segment as a result of spinal disc degeneration.
d. The anterior translation of one lumbar vertebra over the next inferior segment as a result of a lesion of the facet joints, generating lumbar spinal and/or foraminal stenosis.
e. The anterior translation one lumbar vertebra over the next inferior segment as a result of a lesion of the posterior ligamentous complex, generating lumbar spinal canal and/or foraminal stenosis and a clinical picture of claudicatio and hyporeflexia.

A: According to 2016 NASS guidelines, isthmic spondylolisthesis is the anterior translation of one lumbar vertebra over the next inferior segment as a result of a lesion of the pars interarticularis, regardless to the presence of spinal canal or foraminal stenosis and a compatible clinical picture [115]. Vertebral hemangiomas are well described benign lesions of the spine consisting in a pathological proliferation of normal thin-walled capillary, cavernous or venous vessels within the marrow space and the bony trabeculae of the vertebra [116]. Only rarely they cause isthmic spondylolisthesis [117].

87. **In treating a patient with lumbar degenerative spondylolisthesis, according with 2014 NASS guidelines:**
a. Conservative treatment is not advised.
b. A first try with conservative treatment is suggested, independently from the severity of spondylolisthesis.
c. Conservative treatment is a valid option in patients with low-grade spondylolisthesis and low back pain.
d. Conservative treatment is indicated as a first-line treatment in patients with low-grade spondylolisthesis and low back pain, but only in cases where neurological deficits are absent.
e. The 2014 NASS guidelines do not mention conservative treatment for spondylolisthesis.

D: 2014 NASS guidelines suggest conservative management as first-line therapy only in patients affected by low-grade spondylolisthesis and low back pain, but without neurological deficits [118].

88. **Which ones among the following are main clinical signs of spondylolisthesis?**
a. Back pain worsening during motion and meliorating with rest. The presence of leg pain indicates another diagnosis.
b. Back pain and leg pain worsening during motion and improving with rest.
c. Constant back pain, worsening especially during night. The aspect of pain that improves during rest should move toward another diagnosis.
d. Constant leg pain, worsening with nerve stretching maneuverers.
e. Neurological claudication.

B: The cardinal symptoms of spondylolisthesis are mechanical low back pain, namely a pain that worsens with motion and improves with rest, and leg pain [119]. They are thought to be the result of abnormal distribution of load across the vertebral endplates. Constant back pain worsening especially at night time is more typical of tumoral vertebral lesions, like spinal metastasis [120], while leg pain with crural or sciatic distribution, especially exacerbated by nerve stretching maneuverers like Wasserman or Lasègue, is indicative of nerve root inflammation and compression, usually due to intervertebral disc herniation [69].

89. **Which one among the following is the best clinical test for diagnosis of facet joint pain syndrome?**
    a. Kemp's test.
    b. Quadrant test
    c. Extension-rotation test.
    d. All of the above are different names for the Kemp's test.
    e. None of the listed tests.

The Kemp's test has shown to be a clinical test useful for clinical diagnosis of facet joint syndrome. This test has been described with different names, such as Quadrant test and extension-rotation test [121, 122].

90. **Regarding low back pain in patients affected by spondylolisthesis, which one of the following descriptions of the pain is correct?**
    a. pain is constant and does not change with posture or motion.
    b. pain improves with rest and worsens with motion.
    c. Pain is more intense during the night, improving when patient wakes up starting his/her daily activities.
    d. Pain does not change with changes in position, but it is worse at rest.
    e. None of the sentences are true.

B: One of the main symptoms affecting spondylolisthesis' patients is mechanical low back pain., namely a pain that worsens during motion and changes from sitting to standing position, and improves with rest. It is considered to be due to an abnormal distribution of load across the vertebral endplates following disc degeneration [123].

91. **A thirty-six-years-old patient comes to your attention referring long history of low back pain, worse during physical demanding activities and improving with rest, forcing the patient to rest after walking for less than 200 m. A seven months pharmacological therapy with both steroids and not steroidal drugs has led to poor improvement. Mri of the lumbar spine depicts a grade 1 spondylolisthesis according to Meyerding classification, and lumbar stenosis. Which one among the following treatment strategies may lead to a better clinical outcome?**
    a. Physiotherapy.
    b. Steroids infiltrations.
    c. Surgical management with laminectomy alone.
    d. Surgical management with laminectomy and fusion.
    e. Surgical management with no differences among laminectomy alone and laminectomy and fusion.

D: The Spinal Laminectomy versus instrumented pedicle screw (SLIP) trial showed that laminectomy with the addiction of fusion is superior to laminectomy alone in patients affected by grade 1 spondylolisthesis with lumbar stenosis[124]. When a 3–6 months of conservative treatment does not show results in spondylolisthesis patients, laminectomy and fusion is the most suitable option [118].

92. **In surgical treatment of lumbar degenerative spondylolisthesis, according to the most recent guidelines and clinical trials:**
    a. Instrumentation must always be considered after decompression and fusion, due to the peculiar pathogenetic pattern of the pathology, to prevent recurrences.
    b. After decompression and fusion, instrumentation should be avoided in consideration of the excessively high complication rate.
    c. Instrumentation after decompression and fusion has shown to be effective in improving patients' clinical outcome but not the fusion rates.
    d. Instrumentation after decompression and fusion has shown to be effective in improving fusion rates, but without effects on clinical outcomes.
    e. Instrumentation after decompression and fusion has shown to be effective in improving clinical outcomes, without effects on fusion rates.

D: Studies have shown statistical significant evidence that fixation improves fusion rates without affecting clinical outcomes [124]. Instrumentation is notably associated to longer operations and more blood loss than decompression and fusion alone [125] and according to 2016 NASS guidelines for surgical treatment of lumbar degenerative spondylolisthesis, instrumentation is only indicated to improve fusion rate but not with the aim of obtaining a better surgical outcome [126].

93. **In surgical treatment of lumbar degenerative spondylolisthesis, in comparison to open fusion techniques:**
    a. Minimally invasive surgery (MIS) is not recommended because it has not reached yet a sufficient level of efficacy in terms of clinical outcomes.

b. MIS has shown better results in terms of clinical outcomes but has higher costs. For these reasons it should be considered as the gold standard approach, but only in western countries.
c. MIS has technical limitations that lead to worse clinical outcomes including higher failure rates and with higher costs.
d. MIS is a possible option to consider because has shown similar clinical results, but with lower costs and shorter recovery time.
e. MIS is a possible option to consider because has shown similar clinical results, but it is not very much applied because of its major costs.

D: MIS for surgical management of lumbar degenerative spondylolisthesis has shown same results in terms of clinical outcomes when compared with open fusion techniques. Moreover, this approach is associated with lower costs and shorter recovery time [124]. Its indications are still surgeon's preference although there is data proving lesser tissue injury, reduced blood loss and the limited postoperative pain in cases of 2-level fusion [127, 128].

94. **Which one among the following is the gold standard method in diagnosis of facet joint pain?**
a. MRI of the spine.
b. Spine TC.
c. Intra-articular anesthetic injections and medial branch blocks.
d. Spine SPECT.
e. Spine radiographs.

C: Although MRI allows to define radiologically facet joints changes, the diagnostic strategy recognized as the gold standard for correlating the pain referred from a patient to its origin from vertebral articulations are facet joints (intra-articular) or their never supply (medial nerve blocks) anesthetic injections. Due to the risk of false-positive rates from single blocking, literature suggests to perform double blockings [129].

95. **An important test in evaluating etiology of spinal pain consists in making the patient perform an extension combined with a rotation of the spinal region of interest, in the attempt of exacerbate pain. Which one among the following is the name of this clinical test?**
a. Lasègue.
b. Wasserman.
c. Romberg.
d. Babinski.
e. Kemp.

E: The Kemp's test has shown to be useful for clinical diagnosis of facet joint syndrome. This test has been described with different names, such as Quadrant test and extension-rotation test. It consists in manipulating the patient with the aim of making him to extent and rotate the spinal region of interest, cervical or lumbar as well, affected by the pain. Pain exacerbation defines the test as positive [130].

96. **Which of the following sentences is true about pedicle screws fixation after lumbar fusion?**
a. Pedicle screw fixation has to be avoided because, differently from lumbar traumatic pathology, the gains from the procedure do not justify its use.
b. Pedicle screw fixation is indicated, only with bilateral pedicle screws.
c. Pedicle screw fixation is indicated, only with one unilateral screw.
d. Pedicle screw fixation is indicated mainly with bilateral pedicles even if unilateral technique has shown same clinical results in terms of VAS, JOA, ODI, SF-36, and complication rate.
e. Pedicle screw fixation is indicated mainly with bilateral pedicles even if unilateral technique has shown better clinical results in terms of VAS, JOA, ODI, SF-36, and rate of complications.

D: Lumbar spinal fusion is recognized as an effective surgical procedure. The method that has become the standard is lumbar interbody fusion followed by bilateral pedicle screw fixation. However, a unilateral approach has been also implemented in the attempt of reducing post-operative complications. According to the literature, the latter is less invasive and thus associated with a reduced blood loss and operation time [131]. Nevertheless, this innovative procedure has not improved fusion rates, complications rates, length of hospital stay and post-operative pain [132]. Moreover, unilateral screw fixation is associated with a major rate of cage migration as compared to bilateral pedicle screw fixation [133].

97. **Degenerative sspondylolisthesis:**
a. Is only a degenerative condition.
b. Is located, in the majority of cases, at the cervical level.
c. Presents predominantly in young adults.
d. Is prevalent among females.

   e. In cases of degenerative lumbar subtype, it more often involves the L5-S1 level.

D: Degenerative sspondylolisthesis is a pathological condition featured by the translation of one vertebra over the next inferior one, caused by instability of that specific segment [118]. It involves the lumbar segment in the majority of cases and manifests usually in patients that are 70 or older. Females are considerably more affected than males, with a male-to-female ratio of 1:6 [134]. Moreover, preferential location of the degenerative form of lumbar spondylolistheses is at the L4-L5 level [135], while L5-S1 is the most involved one in cases of spondylolisthesis due to spondylolysis.

98. **Spondylolisthesis indicates a pathological condition:**
   a. Where the soma of a vertebra is split in different parts, mostly due to an excessive axial load applied to the vertebral column.
   b. A pathological condition that relates to the presence of a neoplastic lesion causing disruption of the vertebral soma.
   c. An infection of the vertebra that involves only the posterior vertebral arch structures.
   d. An infection of the vertebra that involves only the articular processes.
   e. A pathological condition that consists in the misplacement of one vertebra on the other.

E: The word spondylolisthesis is derived from the Greek word "olisthanein," which means "to slip" [136]. It consists in the translation of one vertebra over the other, due to instability of that specific spinal segment. Etiologically, it is possible to define six different forms: isthmic, traumatic, degenerative, pathologic, dysplastic, and postsurgical; among these, the most commonly reported is degenerative spondylolisthesis (DS) [118].

99. **In the pathogenesis of degenerative spondylolistheses, the first event that triggers the pathogenetic process is:**
   a. Rupture of the vertebral ring.
   b. Fracture of the pars interarticularis.
   c. A misalignment of the ventral vertebral body of a vertebra when compared to the above and below.
   d. Degeneration with weakening of the anterior and posterior longitudinal ligament.
   e. Vertebral disc degeneration.

E: Degenerative spondylolisthesis is a pathological condition defined as the slippage of one vertebra over the subjacent one, but with an intact vertebral ring. Although in the past it was hypothesized that this phenomenon was due to degenerative arthritis of the lumbar facet joints [137], nowadays is known that degeneration of the intervertebral disc is the first step in the pathogenesis of the degenerative form. This leads to motion segment rigidity and high reduction of the discal space. The result is the generation of micro instability and forward or backward vertebral slipping [123].

100. **The Spinal Deformity Study Group (SDSG) Classification System for spondylolisthesis:**
   a. Is a recent classification system for spondylolisthesis that consists in a modification of the Meyerding classification system, adding a sixth category including the cases of rotational slippage > 50° versus one side or the other.
   b. Is a recent classification system that consists in an attempt at better defining the prognosis of spondylolisthesis coupling the Meyerding classification system to spinal balance.
   c. Is a recent classification system that aims aT better defining the prognosis of spondylolisthesis patients matching the Meyerding classification system to the degree of dysplasia.
   d. Is a recent classification system that refers to patients' Karnofsky score matched to the Marchetti and Bartolozzi classification system as anatomopathological grading system.
   e. Defines 5 different categories, based on the degree of slippage of the involved vertebra over the lower one.

B: Many classification systems for spondylolisthesis have been developed in order to provide an instrument that could be useful for communication among different clinicians and for defining patient's prognosis and best therapeutic management. The most widely used classification system for grading spondylolisthesis is the Meyerding classification. However, although being so precise in defining the grade of slippage, this system is not completely effective in defining the patient's prognosis considering that it lacks the ability to predict the risk of progression. For addressing this shortcoming, the Spinal Deformity Study Group (SDSG) Classification System has been developed, based on the Meyerding Classification System but also considering sacropelvic balance in order to provide a comprehensive classification [138]. Many studies have shown that sacropelvic morphology and spinopelvic alignment have to be taken into account to define the best treatment strategy for spondylolisthesis. SDSG classification systems includes 6 items [139]. Initially also the degree of dysplasia was included but it was subsequently excluded due to low overall inter-observer reliability [140].

101. **Regarding natural progression of degenerative spondylolisthesis:**
    a. It has been widely demonstrated that there is no progression risk of the slippage.
    b. Vertebral slippage progression is present if patient is not adequately treated and the entity of the slippage increases with aging and worsening of the patient clinical state.
    c. Vertebral slippage progression is present if patient is not adequately treated. The slippage entity increases with aging but is not correlated to patient's clinical state.
    d. Vertebral slippage progression is present if patient is not adequately treated but the entity of the slippage decreases with aging, without correlation with patient's clinical state.
    e. Vertebral slippage progression is present if patient is not adequately treated and the entity of the slippage increases with aging leading to a proportional impairment of patient's clinical state.

D: Degenerative spondylolisthesis is a chronic progressive pathology that gets worse with patient's aging. However, slipping progression has shown to decrease with patient's aging. Moreover, the entity of the slippage is not strictly related to the severity of patient's clinical status [141].

102. **In spondylolisthesis, vertebral slippage:**
    a. Is always sagittal, considering the particular anatomy of the spine.
    b. Can be sagittal, rotational or latero-lateral, depending on the type of discal degeneration affecting that patient.
    c. Is mainly on the sagittal plain but less frequently it can be a rotational slippage, depending on the subluxation type of the facet joints.
    d. Is only on the rotational plane, depending on the entity of the degeneration of anterior and posterior longitudinal ligaments.
    e. None of the listed sentences is true.

C: Degenerative spondylolisthesis is a pathological condition defined as the slippage of one vertebra over the subjacent one, with an intact vertebral ring. However, the direction of the slippage can be on both, a sagittal or a coronal plane. Although intervertebral disc degeneration is the premium movens of the pathological process, the main aspects that determines the type of slippage are the symmetry of the facet joints degeneration and the distribution of weight-bearing forces. In cases of symmetric facet joint subluxation, the resultant vertebral slippage will be mainly sagittal. On the other hand, in cases of asymmetric facet joint subluxation, the slippage will be mainly rotational [118].

103. **In conservative treatment of lumbar degenerative spondylolisthesis (DS), with regard to physical rehabilitation, which one among the followings methodologies has shown the best results?**
    a. Extension exercises.
    b. Flexion exercises.
    c. Rehabilitation exercises have shown to be dangerous in not surgically treated spondylolistheses patients.
    d. There are no differences in terms of clinical outcomes between flexion or extension exercises.
    e. None of the listed sentences is correct.

B: Conservative treatment is contemplated in cases of degenerative spondylolisthesis patients [142]. It should be carried out with the same modalities as in degenerative lumbar stenosis, according to the NASS 2014 guidelines for diagnosis and treatment of lumbar DS. These include activities restrictions, anti-inflammatory medications, epidural steroids injections and physical rehabilitation [126]. Among the latter, many strategies are available, namely bracing, exercise, ultrasound and activities modifications. Regarding exercise modalities, the flexion ones have shown the best results in terms of pain relief and functional improvement [118, 143].

104. **Which of the following are the most appropriate for surgical treatment of lumbar degenerative spondylolisthesis?**
    a. Low grade of the spondylolisthesis.
    b. Moderate to severe spondylolisthesis, regardless of the clinical symptoms.
    c. Moderate to severe spondylolisthesis, associated to a severe clinical picture.
    d. Low grade spondylolisthesis, associated to clinical symptoms, but only after conservative treatment failure.
    e. In every case of low grade spondylolisthesis associated to clinical symptoms as first line treatment.

D: Conservative treatment is contemplated in cases of degenerative spondylolisthesis [126, 142]. Conservative treatment is considered to have failed in cases of symptoms persistence after 3–6 months [144]. The type of clinical manifestation should also be considered. The clinical symptoms for which a surgical approach is more suitable are radicular pain and/or neurogenic claudication while, in cases of cauda equina syndrome, urgent surgical intervention is advised [145].

105. **Spondylolysis**
   a. Is a congenital pathology, manifesting in the elderly.
   b. Is an acquired pathological condition due to sedentary lifestyle
   c. Is a pathological condition characterized by vertebral body degeneration, in the presence of neural arch integrity.
   d. Is a pathological degenerative condition that, due to its peculiar pathogenesis, is always associated with back pain.
   e. Involves mostly L5.

E: Spondylolysis is a pathological degenerative alteration of the vertebra, featured by an isolated defect in the neural arch of the vertebra. In the majority of the cases, the pars interarticularis of the L5 vertebra is involved [146]. This pathology can also be asymptomatic and found incidentally. When symptomatic, it presents mainly with low back pain. It is considered as an acquired pathology and not a congenital one, even if biological factors can participate to its development. In particular, the main etiological factor that has been identified consists in repetitive, mechanical stress and for this reason, this anomaly has never been detected in non-ambulatory patients [147].

106. **The Meyerding classification system is the most widely used grading system for spondylolisthesis. Which one among the following sentences is true?**
   a. It is a radiological grading system based on evaluation of T2 sequences of spinal column.
   b. It defines 6 different categories, based on slipped vertebra inclination and the angle that its axis with the lower vertebra.
   c. Grade II consists in a 75% of slippage.
   d. Spondyloptosis corresponds to the Grade I.
   e. It is based on the entity of slippage of the involved vertebra in relation to the vertebral plate of the vertebra below.

E: The Meyerding classification system defines five different degrees of spondylolisthesis. It takes into account the relationship between the involved vertebra and the one below. More specifically, this system individuates the 5 different grades of the slippage by drawing a line in correspondence of the posterior wall of the involved vertebral body and the one of the vertebra below, successively measuring the distance between the two lines. Grade I consists in a distance that corresponds to 0 or 25% of the length of the lower vertebral body; Grade II corresponds to 25–50%; Grade III the 50–75% and Grade IV, also called spondyloptosis, corresponds to 100% of slippage [148].

107. **Associate the correct median age of affected patients to each pathology:**
   a. Lumbar disc herniation: 40 years old; degenerative spondylolisthesis: 50 years old; lumbar stenosis: 70 years old.
   b. Lumbar disc herniation 70 years old; degenerative spondylolisthesis 50 years old; lumbar stenosis 40 years old.
   c. Lumbar disc herniation: 50 years old; degenerative spondylolisthesis: 40 years old; lumbar stenosis: 70 years old.
   d. Lumbar disc herniation: 40 years old; degenerative spondylolisthesis: 70 years old; lumbar stenosis: 50 years old.

A: Lumbar disc herniation has its higher incidence during the fourth decade of life and male patients are affected more than twice than females. L5-S1 is the most frequently affected level [149]. Degenerative spondylolisthesis presents mainly in patients in their 50 s, affecting females much more than males (female: male ratio 6:1), mainly involving the L4-L5 level [135]. Degenerative lumbar stenosis is prevalent among elderly patients being found among individuals older than 64 years in 90–100% of cases [150]. Median age at diagnosis is 70 years old [151].

108. **Which one among the following condition is an absolute indication for surgery among spondylolisthesis patients?**
   a. Presence of radicular symptoms of stenosis.
   b. Presence of mechanical low-back pain, non-responsive to conservative treatment.
   c. The presence of Phalen-Dixon sign.
   d. High-grade spondylolistheses in adults.
   e. All of the above.

Phanel-Dixon sign indicates the presence of sciatic crisis, caused by compression of the cauda equina, leading to spasm of the ischiocrural muscle group. The clinical picture is composed of sciatic pain, due to L5 and S1 roots irritation, vertical sacrum and pelvis, lumbosacral kyphosis, tight hamstrings and unusual pelvic waddling gait. In cases when radicular symptoms of stenosis are prevalent or when mechanical low-back pain is predominant, surgical management is indicated but it is not mandatory, as conservative treatments can also be effective [126]. The isolated radiological finding of spondylolisthesis, even in high grade cases, is not enough to warrant urgent surgery [152].

109. **Buck's fusion technique:**
   a. Is only indicated in symptomatic cases of a very slight slippage and verified recent pars defect.
   b. Is an osteosynthesis technique using Morscher's screws and hooks.
   c. Is an indirect repair technique.
   d. Is a modified variant of Scott's technique.
   e. All the listed sentences are correct.

A: surgical repair of the spondylolysis is a strategy to consider in case of symptomatic patients with a very slight slippage and verified recent pars defect [153]. Many different strategies are possible. Buck's fusion techniques consists in a direct repair of the lysis by screw fixation, without hooks or wires [154]. Morscher's screws and hooks technique consists in a different surgical strategies that includes screws application to the pedicles and hooks under the laminas [155, 156]. Finally, the Scott's technique is a different approach with application of wires.

110. **In surgical treatment of spondylolisthesis:**
   a. Slip reduction is always recommended.
   b. Slip reduction has shown clearly clinical results only in pediatric spondylolisthesis.
   c. Slip reduction has shown clearly clinical results only in adult degenerative spondylolisthesis.
   d. No clear indications are present regarding slippage reduction in degenerative spondylolisthesis, while in situ fixation with or without decompression is an effective surgical method in adult high-grade spondylolisthesis.
   e. Slip reduction has shown clearly clinical results only in high grades of slippage.

D: According to NASS 2016 guidelines on lumbar adult degenerative spondylolisthesis, no clear indications are available regarding slip reduction [126]. In situ fixation with or without decompression, however, has proven to be an effective surgical methods, especially when intervertebral body space has markedly diminished. Associating decompression to fixation depends on patient symptoms [157].

111. **In pedicle screw fixation by a percutaneous technique:**
   a. In order to be safe, general anesthesia is indicated.
   b. If virtual fluoroscopy guidance is used, first step is to apply a dynamic reference array.
   c. Conventional fluoroscopy provides the advantage of visualizing two different planes of view at the same time.
   d. Virtual fluoroscopy carries many advantages compared to conventional fluoroscopy, but at the cost of a major radiation exposure.
   e. All the listed sentences are correct.

B: Percutaneous pedicle screw fixation is a well-described and a very common surgical strategy for spinal stabilization [158]. Although being practiced more often under general anesthesia, it offers the possibility to be performed even under epidural anesthesia [159]. Considering that the spine is not exposed, a radiological guidance is mandatory. Conventional fluoroscopy represents a valid tool, and it is widely used worldwide [160]. However, it has some shortcomings like the inability to visualize more than one plane of view at the time as well as the ergonomic difficulties that derive from working around a C-arm and the radiation exposure [161]. Virtual fluoroscopy is a different modality that allows to overcome some limits of convectional fluoroscopy, combining an image-guideance surgical computer to C-arm fluoroscopy or intraoperative CT. It allows the visualization of different planes of view, with a multiplanar guidance strategy, providing the opportunity of quantifying radiographic information and minor radiation exposure for the surgeons [161]. Placing a dynamic reference array is the first step. In particular, it must be placed with a small incision over the spinous process, one level above the segment designed for the spinal fusion. Then, a percutaneous refence array is attached to the spinous process.

112. **In patients affected by degenerative spondylolisthesis with spinal stenosis, after decompression and fusion, instrumentation by screw fixation can also be made by a percutaneous technique. Which one among the following is true?**
   a. According to 2016 NASS guidelines for adult lumbar degenerative spondylolisthesis treatment, percutaneous approach can achieve better clinical results and is recommended in selected cases (grade "B" recommendation).
   b. Although associated with better clinical results in terms of low back pain reduction, percutaneous approaches are associated with major blood loss.
   c. Percutaneous technique has shown better functional outcomes and a faster reduction in post-operative low back pain, even if more studies with a wider population are required.
   d. Although associated with reduction in blood loss and better clinical outcome in term of low back pain

reduction, percutaneous approaches lead to slower clinical improvements than open techniques.

C: percutaneous screw fixation has been applied in degenerative lumbar spondylolisthesis with spinal stenosis, after decompression and fusion. Compared to the open techniques, it is associated with lesser blood loss, in both intraoperatively and during 1st post-operative day, better results in terms of post-operative functionality [162], and a more rapid post-operative pain reduction [163]. These advantages in comparison to open techniques seem to be due to very restricted skin and fascia incisions and reduced paravertebral muscles damage [164]. Nevertheless, there are no studies that have clearly demonstrated its superiority in terms of clinical outcomes in comparison to the open approaches [126].

113. **Scoliosis consists in:**
 a. A fixed pathological anterior flexion of the spine and the thorax, without altering the profile of the spine on the coronal plane.
 b. A lateral curvature and torsion of the spine, without alterations on the sagittal plane.
 c. A lateral curvature and torsion of the spine and chest, altering the profile of the spine on coronal and axial plane that also affects the sagittal balance.
 d. A lateral curvature and torsion of the spine and chest, altering the profile of the spine on the coronal and axial plane, but not on the sagittal one.
 e. A pathological lateral curvature of the spine without torsion.

C: Scoliosis is a consequence of the deformation of spine elements, resulting in abnormal rotation of the spine assuming a non-physiological conformation on the axial, coronal and sagittal planes. Chest is also affected by the rotational deformation [165].

114. **In treating a patient affected by scoliosis, a conservative approach is also an option, including physical therapy. Which one among the following methods should be avoided?**
 a. Methode Lyonaise.
 b. Side-shift method.
 c. Dobosiewicz method.
 d. Schroth method.
 e. Muscle activation technique.

E: In cases of degenerative scoliosis, surgery is an option to consider only when the non-surgical measures failed. In the spectrum of conservative options, physical therapy is one of the most interesting. An important aspect to keep in mind is that general exercises are not useful and that manipulation and physical activation, like Mézierès method, should be avoided because they can increase the pain [165, 166]. Patients should get involved in a low-impact muscle-strengthening endurance program [167].

115. **In a patient affected by adult degenerative scoliosis, which one among the following is not a possible etiological cause to consider?**
 a. Asymmetric disc degeneration.
 b. Osteoporosis.
 c. Vertebral body compression fractures.
 d. Progression of an infantile or adolescent idiopathic scoliosis.
 e. None of the sentences is a possible cause of adult degenerative scoliosis.

D: idiopathic scoliosis is a lateral deviation of the spine in an otherwise healthy person, without an identifiable cause. Although an adult scoliosis can result from the progression of an infant and adolescent idiopathic scoliosis, in order to define it as *degenerative* (also called *de novo*) adult scoliosis, evidence of congenital idiopathic scoliosis should be excluded. In fact, possible causes of adult degenerative scoliosis are degenerative pathological processes of the spine like asymmetric disc degeneration, osteoporosis and vertebral body compression fractures [166].

116. **In defining the best surgical approach for treating adult degenerative scoliosis, defining the coronal balance is mandatory. The central sacral line is very important parameter in defining coronal balance. How is this line drawn?**
 a. It is a line bisecting another line passing through both iliac crests and ascending perpendicularly.
 b. It is a line passing connecting the middle point of the sacral plate to a point at the center of the femoral head.
 c. It is a line perpendicular to the floor passing through the center of the C7 vertebral body.
 d. It is a line connecting the center point of the sacral plate (on a coronal view) to the center of the C7 vertebral body (on a coronal view as well).
 e. None of the previous definitions describes the central coronal line.

A: The central sacral line is used to assess the coronal balance of a patient. It bisects the line passing through both iliac crests and ascending perpendicularly. The vertebras that are bisected more closely by this line are called *stable vertebras* [166].

117. **In a patient affected by degenerative scoliosis, which one among the following radiological parameters is the most important predictor of outcome of surgery?**
   a. Positive global sagittal balance.
   b. Curve magnitude.
   c. Curve location.
   d. Coronal imbalance.
   e. All the listed elements have the same impact.

A: Several studies showed that positive sagittal balance is the radiological parameter that mainly correlates with outcomes [168].

118. **It is known that positive global sagittal balance is a radiological parameter that affects the incidence of adverse health status outcomes. How is it correlated to the outcomes?**
   a. Severity of symptoms increases in a linear fashion with progressive positive sagittal balance.
   b. The presence of positive balance is enough to determine worse outcomes, but the correlation between the entity of the two elements hasn't been described yet.
   c. The presence of positive balance is enough to determine worse outcomes, but there is no accordance in the literature regarding the correlation between the two elements.
   d. The presence of positive balance is enough to determine worse outcomes, but the lesser is the entity of the positivity, the higher is the probability of having a worse outcome.
   e. The entity of positive balance is directly correlated to the risk of a worse outcome in a linear fashion.

E: Wide population studies have shown that although even mildly positive sagittal balance is somewhat detrimental, severity of symptoms increases in a linear fashion with progressive sagittal imbalance [169].

119. **Positive global sagittal balance is a radiological parameter that has been recognized as a bad prognostic factor in predicting post-operative results in scoliosis patients. How is this parameter defined?**
   a. Anterior deviation of the C7 plumb line.
   b. Positive value of the pelvic incidence.
   c. A value of the sacral slope that is more the one and half times the value of the pelvic tilt.
   d. Negative value of the pelvic incidence.

A: Positive sagittal balance is a pathological misalignment of the spine on the sagittal plane that negatively correlates with scoliosis progression in both treated and untreated patients. It is defined as the anterior deviation of the C7 plumb line measurement [169].

120. **Which one among the following is the most used method to define the curve magnitude in scoliosis patients?**
   a. Meyerding system.
   b. Modic system.
   c. Cobb angle method.
   d. MSU system.
   e. Schizas system.

C: The Cobb angle method is the most used system to define the magnitude of the scoliosis curves. This method has been designed by the Scoliosis Research Society as the system of choice for scoliosis severity evaluation. It consists in individuating the superior surface of the proximal end vertebra and the inferior surface of the distal end vertebra as first step. Subsequently, two intersecting lines, drawn perpendicular to each one vertebral plate lines, are individuated. The angle created by their intersection is the Cobb Angle [170].

121. **Which one among the following is a grading system for evaluation of vertebra's rotation on an axial plane?**
   a. The Pedirolle technique.
   b. The Cobb method.
   c. The Nash and Moe.
   d. The Raimondi Regolo method.
   e. All the listed.

E: Spinal degenerative scoliosis is a pathology that involves the spine in a 3D fashion, due to vertebral rotation. For this reason, it is important not only evaluate the severity of the scoliosis curve on the coronal plane, with a bidimensional approach, but it is also fundamental to evaluate the grade of vertebral rotation on the axial plane. With this aim, many different classifications have been implemented among the years [171].

The Pedirolle technique is based on the measurement of the amount of vertebral rotation by considering vertebral pedicle shadow offset and the edge of the vertebral bodies and measure them with the torsion meter [172]. Likewise, the Nash and Moe method is a grading system developed for studying vertebral rotation. It indirectly deduces the vertebral rotation by considering the pedicle projection on frontal radiographs [173]. However, it has not been widely used due to the complexity of the steps that have to be made in applying this method.

The Regolo Raimondi is another evaluation process similar to the Pedirolle technique. It uses a metric ruler measuring the vertebral pedicle shadow offset in millimeters [171].

Even Cobb, in 1948, provided a vertebral rotation grading system, based on the dislocation of the spinous process tip in comparison to the lower vertebra's one, on X-ray frontal plane [171].

122. **Pedicle subtraction osteotomy (PSO) is a valid technique in surgically correcting spinal degenerative scoliosis. Which one among the following sentences is false?**
    a. PSO is particularly indicated in treating cases of degenerative scoliosis with alterations in the sagittal balance.
    b. It possible to perform PSO in both, dorsal and lumbar spine.
    c. PSO is useful in cases of spinal scoliosis with sharp, angular kyphosis.
    d. PSO in not indicated in cases of circumferential fusion along multiple segments.
    e. PSO is particularly important in cases where anterior and/or posterior release is not sufficient to correct the scoliosis.

D: PSO is widely indicated in treating patients affected by degenerative scoliosis, especially in cases of sagittal imbalance superior to 10–12 cm and/or with sharp angular kyphosis. PSO is also indicated in cases of circumferential fusion along multiple segments, precluding performing other osteotomy techniques like Smith-Petersen Osteotomy (SPO) [174].

123. **The osteotomy technique that consists in a V-shaped resection trough the posterior elements, pedicles and vertebral body in order to gain more lordosis is called:**
    a. Smith-Petersen osteotomy (SPO).
    b. Pedicle Subtraction Osteotomy (PSO).
    c. Chevron osteotomy.
    d. None of the listed described the procedure.
    e. All the listed are different names for the same procedure.

B: PSO is a widely used technique in degenerative scoliosis correction, especially in cases with important sagittal unbalance and sharp angular kyphosis. It consists in a V-shaped resection through the posterior vertebral elements, pedicles and vertebral body in order to gain more lordosis [174].

124. **Scoliosis can be divided in two types: structural and nonstructural. Which one among the following sentences is false?**
    a. Hysterical scoliosis is a type of nonstructural scoliosis.
    b. Neuromuscular scoliosis a type of structural scoliosis.
    c. Nonstructural scoliosis can become structural.
    d. In nonstructural scoliosis, the key difference is that curve has no rotatory component.
    e. Traumatic scoliosis is a type of nonstructural scoliosis.

E: From an etiological, pathological and clinical point of view, it is possible to define two different subgroups of scoliosis: nonstructural and structural scoliosis. Non-structural scoliosis include postural, hysterical, sciatic, inflammatory and compensatory. Structural scoliosis can be congenital, neuromuscular, idiopathic, de novo, traumatic or iatrogenic. The main difference among the two groups is mainly the absence of rotatory component of the curve in the nonstructural type. However, it is possible that a nonstructural type of scoliosis turns in a structural one over time [167].

125. **A sixty-years-old male patient comes to your attention referring inability to walk more than 200 m due to leg fatigue, which developed over a period of two years. A chronic mild lumbar pain is also reported. Neurological examination shows mild bilateral leg muscular hypotrophy, mild (4/5) legs hyposthenia with normal reflexes. He also relates that he can benefit from rest, but that assuming a flexed position does not improve his condition unless supporting his trunk with the arms. Which one among the following spinal degenerative disorders do you expect to find on imaging?**
    a. Lumbar stenosis.
    b. Adult Degenerative Scoliosis.
    c. Cervical disc herniation.
    d. Lumbar disc foraminal hernia.
    e. None of the listed sentences is correct.

B: Adult degenerative scoliosis usually presents in the 6th decade, mostly with symptoms of spinal stenosis. However, an important difference between degenerative stenosis and degenerative scoliosis consists in the fact that in the patient affected by scoliosis, claudication symptoms do not relieve with forward posture except when patient supports his trunk with his arms. This is of utmost importance considering that prognosis and treatment of degenerative scoliosis is widely different from the ones of lumbar stenosis [167].

126. **Nonoperative treatment is not contraindicated in cases of:**
    a. Scoliosis without significant stenotic or radicular symptoms.
    b. Scoliosis with curves < 30°.
    c. Presence of anterior osteophytes.
    d. Scoliosis with < 2 mm subluxation.
    e. Scoliosis with reasonable sagittal and coronal balance.
    f. All of the above

E: Even in degenerative scoliosis, nonsurgical treatment is a recognized treatment option, aimed to just alleviate the symptoms without blocking scoliosis progression. However, a careful patient selection must be made to obtain the best outcomes. It is indicated in patients without significant stenotic or radicular symptoms, with a scoliosis curve that is < 30° and a subluxation < 2 mm, with a reasonable sagittal and coronal balance. Presence of anterior osteophytes does not represent a contraindication to nonoperative treatment [175].

127. **In patients affected by adult degenerative scoliosis:**
    a. Bracing is not an option as it causes a worsening of the clinical picture.
    b. Bracing is an option for conservative treatment by virtue of its well know therapeutic efficacy on correcting the deformity.
    c. Bracing is an option for nonsurgical management. However, although it confers some benefits in terms of short-term pain relief. Indications regarding its application are not well defined.
    d. Bracing is an option for conservative treatment by virtue of its well know therapeutic efficacy on correcting the deformity, but only in tailored well-selected cases.
    e. none of the listed are true.

C: Although conservative care may be useful in degenerative scoliosis management, more evidence are needed before posing clear indications. More concrete indications are only available regarding anti-inflammatory medications and activity modifications. The most used bracing system in adult scoliosis is the one made according to the Veniset's method, that has shown some effects in reducing degenerative scoliosis progression, even if high quality studies are lacking [176]. This aspect may be due to a supposed effect in improving muscle strength as reported for other pathologies like low back pain or vertebral fractures [177]. Actually, only level IV evidence are available supporting bracing or casting in scoliosis. Additional studies should be carried out evaluating custom or general "off the shell" thoracic scoliosis [175, 176, 178].

128. **A sixty-years-old male patient comes to your attention referring inability to walk more than 200 m that he developed over a period of two years. A chronic mild lumbar pain is also reported, irradiated to the right leg. Neurological examination presents right leg upper muscular hypotrophy, mild (4/5) right leg hyposthenia with hyporeflexia and pain irradiation. Full-length standing anteroposterior and lateral radiographs show a left side scoliosis (curve < 30° grades), with L3-L4 rotary subluxation and with an acceptable sagittal balance, without anterior osteophytes. Spine MRI shows a spinal stenosis from L3 to L5. Which one of the following surgical approaches should be chosen, according to the "Lenke-Silva Six Levels of Operative Treatment system"?**
    a. Level I, Decompression alone.
    b. Level II, Decompression and limited instrumented posterior spinal fusion.
    c. Both approaches are suitable with no differences.
    d. Level VI, inclusion of osteotomies.
    e. None of the listed is indicated for this case.

B: According to "Lenke-Silva Six Levels of Operative Treatment System", in a patient with neurological deficits and mild or not back pain and without anterior osteophytes, but necessitating of an extensive decompression, level II operative strategy is to prefer (decompression and posterior spinal fusion) [167].

129. **Which surgical approach is not affected by the presence of anterior osteophytes in the operative region, according to Lenke-Silva Six Levels of Operative Treatment System?**
    a. Level I.
    b. Level II.
    c. Level III.
    d. Level IV.
    e. Level V.

A: According to Lenke-Silva Six Levels of Operative Treatment System, Level I approach (decompression alone) is the one to prefer in cases of anterior osteophytes in the operative region. Anterior osteophytes represents a contraindication to all the other five levels surgical options [167].

130. **Which one among the following is not a method to evaluate in an objective manner the grade of scoliosis of a patient?**
 a. The Cobb method.
 b. The Ferguson's method.
 c. The Pedirolle method.
 d. The Mergel method.
 e. All the listed are methods developed for scoliosis radiological evaluation.

D: The Cobb method is the most used methodology developed for scoliosis measurement, which has been designed by the Scoliosis Research Society as the method of choice [170]. The Ferguson method is a more direct measurement approach, considering that it does not depend on the inclination of the vertebral plates of the end vertebras. However, it is also considered slightly more difficult to use, especially with curves greater than 50–60° [179]. The Pedirolle method is the most used technique for radiological evaluation of vertebral coronal rotation, that is an important pathological aspect in scoliosis patients [171].

131. **For the surgical approach to a thoracic disc herniation (TDH):**
 a. The anterior approach is not possible, because of the presence of the lungs.
 b. The lateral approach is the only one allowed, considering the peculiar anatomy aspects of the dorsal tract.
 c. The posterolateral approach is not allowed for the presence of the ribs in the surgical trajectory.
 d. The posterior approach has been abandoned.
 e. All the previous sentences are right.

D: TDH is an infrequent condition for which surgical management is challenging because is technically difficult and caries a high risk of complications. Different surgical corridors are available, that can be grouped in anterior, lateral and posterolateral [180]. However, posterior approaches to the dorsal disc herniation, such as laminectomy and thoracic discectomy, have been forsaken due to high rate of post-operative neurological deficits [181].

132. **Which one among the following hereditary diseases is known for inducing an increased risk of developing thoracic disc herniation?**
 a. Charcot-Marie-Tooth disease.
 b. Multiple Sclerosis.
 c. Scheuermann's disease.
 d. Turner's syndrome.
 e. Rheumatoid arthritis.

C: Thoracic spine is the less frequent location of disc herniation, accounting for the 0,1–3% of all spinal disc herniation [182]. However, patient affected by Scheuermann's disease present a higher risk of developing disc herniation at the thoracic level, since the classical form of this disease presents with an excessive dorsal kyphosis, leading to a more probable dorsal degenerative disease [183].

133. **The Transient Anterior Spinal Artery Syndrome is a possible clinical manifestation described mainly in cases of:**
 a. Spondylolisthesis.
 b. Thoracic disc herniation
 c. Lumbar disc herniation.
 d. Cervical disc herniation surgery.
 e. Lumbar spine stenosis.

B: Although being rare, Transient Anterior Spinal Artery Syndrome is described as a possible complication of thoracic disc herniation, due to occlusion of Adamkiewicz' artery, also called Arteria Radicularis Magna, compressed by an herniated dorsal disc. This artery is one of the anterior segmental medullary vessels that arises from lateral aspect of the aorta and supplies the anterior spinal artery. In particular, the artery of Adamkiewicz is the biggest anterior segmental medullary vessel. It arises from the posterior branch of the radiculomedullary artery, that is a posterior terminal branch of the intercostal arteries, from T9 to T12 levels. Importantly, these are also the levels more often involved by thoracic disc herniation [184].

The possibility that this artery can be compressed by a thoracic disc is due to the fact that the former enters the spinal canal through the intervertebral foramen and adjacent to the exiting nerve root and the anteriorly placed intervertebral disc [185].

Despite this anatomical proximity this complication is described as rare mainly because the anterior spinal cord blood supply presents a high grade of anastomosis from different arteries. For this reason, cases of anterior cord syndrome, also called anterior spinal artery syndrome, due to thoracic disc herniation are mostly associated to vascular anatomy anomalies [186].

134. **Regarding thoracic disc herniation, which one among the following sentences is correct?**
    a. A dorsal disc herniation can cause sensitivity disturbances only in a distribution territory that is inferior respect to the herniated disc.
    b. Even when it is a lateral intraforaminal disc herniation, it is still able to cause anterior spinal deficit symptoms.
    c. An angiography is not indicated in studying a patient with paraplegia and dorsal disc herniation because it is not able to apport any information regarding the pathology.
    d. In cases of suspected thoracic disc herniation presenting with paraplegia, only a central herniation is expectable.
    e. None of the listed sentences is true.

B: Although being an infrequent occurrence, Transient Anterior Spinal Artery Syndrome has been described as a possible complication of thoracic disc herniation, due to the compression of the Adamkiewicz artery, also called Arteria Radicularis Magna, by an herniated dorsal disc. This syndrome presents with both motor and sensitive disturbances consisting in bilateral loss of temperature and pain sensation, in some cases also distributed slightly above the level of disc herniation (differently from the "simple" thoracic disc herniation). Moreover, another typical aspect of patients affected by thoracic disc herniation is the presence of bilateral spastic paresis, even if the herniated disc is lateral, affecting only one side. Finally, in order to better define the etiology of a clinical picture of anterior spinal cord syndrome in a patient affected by lateral thoracic disc herniation and most importantly to define the best therapeutic approach, an angiography should be carried out [184].

135. **The thoracic spinal cord presents some peculiar aspects that expose it to a particular vulnerability in cases of disc herniation. Which one among the following sentences is not true:**
    a. Thoracic spinal cord is exposed to the opportunity of an intradural extension of the disc herniation, with cord compression.
    b. The presence of a kyphosis in the thoracic tract, moves the cord against the disc, making it more vulnerable to an eventual compression.
    c. The presence of the dentate ligament contributes to determine less mobility of the thoracic spinal cord, making it more prone to suffer from compression.
    d. The spinal cord presents smaller diameter in relation to the spinal canal, allowing the thoracic herniated disc to move between the neural tissue and the osseous structures, causing myelopathy.
    e. All the sentences are true.

D: The spinal cord in its dorsal tract presents a diameter (6.5 × 8 mm) with the diameter of the spinal canal (16.8 mm × 17.2 mm). This represents an important anatomical aspect inducing an higher risk of spinal cord damage in cases of disc herniation [180].

136. **Which one among the following is not a prognostic factor for poor surgical outcomes in patients with thoracic myelopathy?**
    a. Longer pre-operative duration of the symptoms.
    b. Worse pre-operative symptoms.
    c. Ossification of the posterior ligament or flavum ligament.
    d. Large operative blood loss.
    e. Maximum ossification of the thoracic posterior longitudinal ligament located at the upper thoracic spine.

E: Thoracic surgery is challenging also for expert spine surgeons because of both anatomical aspects of the thoracic spine and patient's features. Long pre-operative duration of the symptoms, severe pre-operative symptoms, ossification of the posterior longitudinal ligament or flavum ligament are all known as poor prognostic factors. Ligament ossification, in particular, determines obstruction to venous drainage, increasing epidural blood pressure and so leading to a major intraoperative blood loss (which is another prognostic factor of poor outcome). A multi-institutional study of patients treated for thoracic OPLL found that the presence of maximum ossification located at the upper thoracic spine is an aspect that significantly associates with favorable surgical outcomes [49].

137. **Which one among the following levels is the most frequently affected by thoracic disc herniation?**
    a. C7-T1.
    b. T2-T3.
    c. T5-T6.
    d. T11-T12.
    e. There is not a level more affected than the others.

D: Thoracic dorsal herniation is a rare pathology, affecting men more than women at the mean age of 50 years old. It occurs mainly at the T11-T12 level. Not much is known about the pathological mechanisms that underlie this pathology, however some Authors think that this preferred location is due to a relative weakness of the posterior longitudinal ligament at this level, coupled to the higher mobility of the lower thoracic spine [181, 187, 188].

138. **Which one among the followings sentences is not true?**
   a. Treatment of thoracic disc herniation is technically challenging because of the delicate anatomy of the dorsal column.
   b. The transthoracic approach has shown better results compared to the others in the treatment of central and paracentral disc herniations.
   c. The transthoracic approach is associated with very few contraindications.
   d. Thoracic disc herniation is more frequent in male patients.
   e. All the sentences are false.

C: The transthoracic approach is a very effective approach that has shown good results especially in treating central and paracentral disc herniations. However, it is a very invasive procedure with difficult recovery, making this approach not suitable for patients with significant comorbidities such as cardiac or pulmonary disease. During this approach, lungs, heart and great vessels are at risk. During the post-operative period chest tube placement, intensive monitoring and increased risk of deep venous thrombosis, atelectasis and pneumonia should be considered [181, 189].

139. **Which one among the following approaches to thoracic disc herniation has shown the best surgical outcomes in cases of central thoracic disc herniation?**
   a. Conventional laminectomy.
   b. Transthoracic approach.
   c. Posterolateral approach.
   d. Lateral extracavitary approach.
   e. All the listed approaches showed the same efficacy.

B: Thoracic disc herniation is a technical demanding pathology. Historically, gold standard surgical treatment was the standard posterior approach featured by laminectomy and discectomy. However, due to high post-operative complication rates, this approach has been subsequently abandoned in favor to other less invasive surgical strategies, namely posterolateral or lateral extracavitary variants. Anterior approaches, like the transthoracic approach have shown better clinical outcomes compared to the others, especially in treating central or paracentral thoracic disc herniations [181, 190].

140. **Regarding endoscopic approach to thoracic disc herniation:**
   a. It is possible only by an anterior transthoracic route.
   b. It is also possible by a posterior approach, making the endoscope to pass between the laminas in a bone sparing fashion, using a straight 0 grades lens endoscope.
   c. It is also possible by a posterior approach, the route for the endoscope is gained by practicing a partial facetectomy and pedicle removal.
   d. Only a 0 grades lens endoscope is necessary in order to practice this approach.
   e. None of the listed is correct.

C: Anterior endoscopic approaches are associated with thoracic invasiveness and the need of different thoracic skin incisions and many transthoracic drainage tubes. For these reasons, posterior endoscopic approaches have been implemented over the years. The classical well-described posterior endoscopic technique includes, after a transverse paramedian skin incision of 2 cm, the introduction of an operative 0° endoscope, in order to locate and remove the medial portion of the facet and of the pedicle. After this phase, it is possible to visualize the protrude disc. Successively, a 4-mm rigid endoscope with a 70° lens is introduced to complete the herniectomy and ventral spine surgical decompression, by also using customized 90° instruments [191].

141. **When a thoracic disc herniation has to be defined giant?**
   a. Giant thoracic disc herniation is not a clinical described condition.
   b. A thoracic disc herniation occupying more than the 40% of the diameter of the spinal canal.
   c. A thoracic disc herniation occupying more than the 70% of the diameter of the spinal canal, associated to a clinical picture of myelopathy.
   d. A thoracic disc herniation protruding inside the spinal canal, associated to a clinical picture of myelopathy.
   e. A thoracic disc herniation invading the intradural space.

B: According to Hott et al., a thoracic disc herniation is defined giant when it occupies more than 40% of the spinal canal on CT myelography or MRI imaging. There are no correlation to clinical manifestations, the presence or not of myelopathy or dural involvement [192].

142. **In giant thoracic disc herniations:**
   a. Posterior approach is usually the approach of choice, because their removal by an anterior root can put thoracic organs at risk.
   b. Herniated disc is usually soft, as a consequence of their capacity of causing an immediate catastrophic clinical picture, leading to an early diagnosis.

c. Thoracotomy and anterior approaches are preferred to endoscopic ones, in consideration of the technical demanding nature of the pathology.
d. Patient's neurological condition are more unlikely to worsen as majority of the disc herniates right away with less nucleus polposus available to herniate.
e. None of the listed sentences is true.

D: Thoracic disc hernias are defined giant when occupying more of the 40% of the spinal canal space. These pathological entities present some unique clinical, pathological and surgical aspects. From a clinical point of view, affected patients more easily tend to become symptomatic with severe progressive neurological deficit and myelopathy. Nevertheless, patients' neurological condition is more refractory to worsening, considering that almost all the disc herniates at the first phase and no more disc prone to herniation is available. Giant thoracic disc herniation are associated with dural involvement with dural erosion or dura mater incorporation in the ossified mass. In fact, these herniations usually are calcified manifesting more like osseous masses than calcified disc herniations making them very hard to remove. From the surgical point of view, posterior approaches have been banned in their treatment, expect except in selected cases of laterally located hernias. Endoscopic anterior approaches are not only allowed but also preferred by some authors, considering that in these patients, spinal dura mater is often already damaged. In this sense, open approaches offer the opportunity of having a more solid control of the pathology and of eventual complication, making gentle dissection of the ossified material from the dura and eventual dura reconstruction both feasible [192].

143. **Regarding surgical treatment of thoracic disc herniation (TDH) by a trans-facet pedicle sparing technique, which one among the following sentences is not true?**
   a. This technique offers the advantage of a smaller skin incision, with a longer surgical time.
   b. This technique offers the advantage of a shorter surgical time, with a bigger skin incision.
   c. This technique offers the advantage of a shorter surgical time, with a smaller skin incision but it is more difficult to remove the centrally located herniated discs.
   d. This technique offers the advantage of a smaller skin incision, with a shorter surgical time especially in cases of centrally located herniated discs.
   e. All the listed sentences are not true.

C: The first described approach for removing TDHs was a posterior standard laminectomy. Due to the poor clinical outcomes the posterior standard laminectomy approaches have been abandoned in favor of more recent anterior, lateral and posterolateral approaches. Anterior approaches have become the gold standard, but they are technically demanding and really invasive for the patient. Among the posterolateral approaches, the trans-facet pedicle sparing approach is an effective and safe approach, providing some advantages, namely a smaller skin incision and shorter surgical time. However, this approach is not suitable for all types of thoracic disc herniations, considering that is not possible to easily remove central disc herniations, especially without dedicated instruments [193].

144. **Transpedicular approach for thoracic disc herniation:**
   a. Belongs to the lateral approaches to the thoracic spine.
   b. Is indicated also as a prophylactic approach, due to its really low morbidity.
   c. Although being an effective approach, it has shown slightly worse neurological outcomes than anterior and lateral approaches.
   d. It is indicated for both soft and calcified thoracic disc herniations (TDHs).
   e. It is indicated for medial, lateral or medio-lateral TDHs.

D: Transpedicular approach for TDH is an effective approach for removal of TDHs, that is counted among the posterolateral approaches to the thoracic spine since the patient is put in prone position and approached from the back. Nevertheless, it provides the most lateral of the posterior routes to the disc. For this reason, this approach is indicated in cases of both, soft and calcified consistency TDHs, but it is not the best choice for central disc herniation, because of the excessive dislocation and manipulation of the spinal cord required. However, it is not completely discouraged for calcified central TDHs [194]. Prophylactic surgery is never indicated for disc herniations, especially, in consideration of their low rate of clinical manifestation [195].

145. **In posterior endoscopic approach to dorsal disc herniation:**
   a. Patient is placed in prone position.
   b. Evoked sensory potentials usage is not recommended.
   c. After the exposure has been completed, nerve root appears to be usually rostral to the herniated disc.

d. Partial pedicle and facet removal are done without any magnification technique.
e. None of the listed is correct.

C: Posterior endoscopic approach is a well-described minimally-invasive approach to dorsal spinal column useful in thoracic disc herniation removal. This approach comprises different phases that, at the end, allow the visualization of the nerve root that usually is located rostral to the involved vertebral disc (even if rarely is also possible to visualize it above the resected portion of the pedicle). Patient is not placed in a prone position but in a lateral decubitus that puts the lesion side upward with also a 60° forward inclination. Due to the extreme proximity of the procedure to the spinal cord, somatosensory evoked potentials are usually monitored during the entire procedure, even if no clear guidelines are present in this regard. Medial portion of the facet, lateral portion of the lamina and rostral one-third portion of the pedicle are exposed with a 1.5 cm diameter tubular retractor and removed by a 0° grade lens endoscope or using the microscope [191].

146. **In vertebral interbody fusion approaches:**
a. Anterior approaches require smaller graft due to the higher risk of spinal cord damage.
b. Posterior fusion approaches are associated with a major risk to vital structures.
c. Combined approaches are associated with a higher rate of fusion better clinical outcomes than anterior or posterior only approaches.
d. In cases of reduction for spondylolisthesis, fusion is not recommended.
e. Anterior approaches provide the advantage of allowing for an easier discectomy.

E: Considering that spondylolisthesis is to consider as a spinal instability, fusion surgery is of particular importance, especially in cases of reduction [196]. Anterior surgical approaches offer the double advantage of allowing for discectomy and also of giving the opportunity of placing a bigger structural graft because there is a lower risk of damaging dural sac or nerve roots as compared with posterior approaches. Nevertheless, in order to gain access to the anterior column, a retroperitoneal approach is required. Thus, these approaches carry a major risk of complication due proximity of vascular structures, sympathetic plexus and retro and intraperitoneal structures. Circumferential approaches for fusion have shown bigger fusion rates, without leading to better clinical outcomes [197].

147. **A 46 years old woman affected by a rare form of Charcot-Marie-Tooth syndrome, comes to your attention with a long history of leg hyposthenia, hyporeflexia and sphincters deficiency, compatible with the underlying neurodegenerative pathology, and multiple vertebral fracture due to iatrogenic severe osteoporosis. Clinical picture has recently changed with a two months history of painful leg cramps and rapid worsening of leg hyposthenia. At clinical evaluation, the patient showed spastic paraparesis and hyperreflexia at the lower limbs. The cervico-dorsal MRI is showed in the picture. Which one among the followings is the least invasive surgical approach to the pathology in this patient?**
a. Open transthoracic approach.
b. Thoracoscopic approach.
c. Constotransversectomy.
d. Transpedicular approach.
e. All the listed approaches have the same value.

The patient under discussion is affected by a thoracic disc herniation, with a clinical background of a severe neurodegenerative pathology [198]. Regardless of their underlying disease, surgical treatment should be considered, due to the acute manifestation of new-onset pathological pyramidal signs. Anterior and lateral approaches are very invasive, with potential for long post-operative curse with the possibility of developing cardiothoracic complications including atelectasis, lung contusion, intercostal neuralgia, pneumothorax, and hemothorax Considering the chronic degenerating neurological condition of the patient, a posterolateral approach is advisable.

References

1. Le Huec JC, Demezon H, Aunoble S. Sagittal parameters of global cervical balance using EOS imaging: normative values from a prospective cohort of asymptomatic volunteers. Eur Spine J. 2015;24(1):63–71. https://doi.org/10.1007/s00586-014-3632-0.
2. Le Huec JC, Thompson W, Mohsinaly Y, Barrey C, Faundez A. Sagittal balance of the spine. Eur Spine J. 2019;28(9):1889–905. https://doi.org/10.1007/s00586-019-06083-1.
3. Fehlings MG, Tetreault LA, Riew KD, Middleton JW, Wang JC. A clinical practice guideline for the management of degenerative cervical myelopathy: introduction, rationale, and scope. Global Spine J. 2017;7(3 Suppl):21S-S27. https://doi.org/10.1177/2192568217703088.
4. Cahueque Lemus MA, Cobar Bustamante AE, Ortiz Muciño A, Caldera HG. Clinical outcome of anterior vs posterior approach for cervical spondylotic myelopathy. J Orthop. 2016;13(3):123–6. https://doi.org/10.1016/j.jor.2016.03.006.
5. Deora H, Kim SH, Behari S, Rudrappa S, Rajshekhar V, Zileli M, et al. Anterior surgical techniques for cervical spondylotic myelopathy: WFNS Spine Committee recommendations. Neurospine. 2019;16(3):408–20. https://doi.org/10.14245/ns.1938250.125.

6. Zhu B, Xu Y, Liu X, Liu Z, Dang G. Anterior approach versus posterior approach for the treatment of multilevel cervical spondylotic myelopathy: a systemic review and meta-analysis. Eur Spine J. 2013;22(7):1583–93. https://doi.org/10.1007/s00586-013-2817-2.
7. Ranawat CS, O'Leary P, Pellicci P, Tsairis P, Marchisello P, Dorr L. Cervical spine fusion in rheumatoid arthritis. J Bone Joint Surg Am. 1979;61(7):1003–10.
8. Ferrante A, Ciccia F, Giammalva GR, Iacopino DG, Visocchi M, Macaluso F, et al. The craniovertebral junction in rheumatoid arthritis: state of the art. Acta Neurochir Suppl. 2019;125:79–86. https://doi.org/10.1007/978-3-319-62515-7_12.
9. Baker JF. Evaluation and treatment of tandem spinal stenosis. J Am Acad Orthop Surg. 2020;28(6):229–39. https://doi.org/10.5435/JAAOS-D-18-00726.
10. Steinmetz MPBEC. Benzel's spine surgery: techniques, complication avoidance, and management. 2017.
11. Sakaura H, Hosono N, Mukai Y, Ishii T, Iwasaki M, Yoshikawa H. Long-term outcome of laminoplasty for cervical myelopathy due to disc herniation: a comparative study of laminoplasty and anterior spinal fusion. Spine (Phila Pa 1976). 2005;30(7):756–9. https://doi.org/10.1097/01.brs.0000157415.79713.7e
12. Baba H, Uchida K, Maezawa Y, Furusawa N, Azuchi M, Imura S. Lordotic alignment and posterior migration of the spinal cord following en bloc open-door laminoplasty for cervical myelopathy: a magnetic resonance imaging study. J Neurol. 1996;243(9):626–32. https://doi.org/10.1007/BF00878657.
13. Cuccia A, Caradonna C. The relationship between the stomatognathic system and body posture. Clinics (Sao Paulo). 2009;64(1):61–6. https://doi.org/10.1590/s1807-59322009000100011.
14. Nagata K, Ohashi T, Abe J, Morita M, Inoue A. Cervical myelopathy in elderly patients: clinical results and MRI findings before and after decompression surgery. Spinal Cord. 1996;34(4):220–6. https://doi.org/10.1038/sc.1996.41.
15. Dickman KV. Surgical anatomy and techniques to the spine, 2nd ed. Elsevier Saunders; 2013.
16. Hejrati N, Moghaddamjou A, Marathe N, Fehlings MG. Degenerative cervical myelopathy: towards a personalized approach. Can J Neurol Sci. 2021:1–12. https://doi.org/10.1017/cjn.2021.214.
17. Rhee J, Tetreault LA, Chapman JR, Wilson JR, Smith JS, Martin AR, et al. Nonoperative versus operative management for the treatment degenerative cervical myelopathy: an updated systematic review. Global Spine J. 2017;7(3 Suppl):35S-41S. https://doi.org/10.1177/2192568217703083.
18. Eck JC, Humphreys SC, Hodges SD, Levi P. A comparison of outcomes of anterior cervical discectomy and fusion in patients with and without radicular symptoms. J Surg Orthop Adv. 2006;15(1):24–6.
19. Saunders RL, Bernini PM, Shirreffs TG, Reeves AG. Central corpectomy for cervical spondylotic myelopathy: a consecutive series with long-term follow-up evaluation. J Neurosurg. 1991;74(2):163–70. https://doi.org/10.3171/jns.1991.74.2.0163.
20. Somma T, de Rosa A, Mastantuoni C, Esposito F, Meglio V, Romano F, et al. Multidisciplinary management of osteoporotic vertebral fractures. An overview. Minerva Endocrinol (Torino). 2021. https://doi.org/10.23736/S2724-6507.21.03515-6.
21. Fernyhough JC, White JI, LaRocca H. Fusion rates in multilevel cervical spondylosis comparing allograft fibula with autograft fibula in 126 patients. Spine (Phila Pa 1976). 1991;16(10 Suppl):S561–4. https://doi.org/10.1097/00007632-199110001-00022.
22. Hwang SL, Lee KS, Su YF, Kuo TH, Lieu AS, Lin CL, et al. Anterior corpectomy with iliac bone fusion or discectomy with interbody titanium cage fusion for multilevel cervical degenerated disc disease. J Spinal Disord Tech. 2007;20(8):565–70. https://doi.org/10.1097/BSD.0b013e318036b463.
23. Eck KR, Bridwell KH, Ungacta FF, Lapp MA, Lenke LG, Riew KD. Analysis of titanium mesh cages in adults with minimum two-year follow-up. Spine (Phila Pa 1976). 2000;25(18):2407–15. https://doi.org/10.1097/00007632-200009150-00023.
24. Lee GP, Ahir B, Chaudhry N, Engelhard HH. Cervical spondylotic myelopathy: an updated review. Neurosurg Cases Rev. 2021;4:056. https://doi.org/10.23937/2643-4474/1710056.
25. Omerovic S. Chvostek Sign. StatPearls. Treasure Island (FL): StatPearls Publishing; 2022.
26. Tan LA, Riew KD, Traynelis VC. Cervical spine deformity-Part 2: management algorithm and anterior techniques. Neurosurgery. 2017;81(4):561–7. https://doi.org/10.1093/neuros/nyx388.
27. Vaccaro AR, Falatyn SP, Scuderi GJ, Eismont FJ, McGuire RA, Singh K, et al. Early failure of long segment anterior cervical plate fixation. J Spinal Disord. 1998;11(5):410–5.
28. Sasso RC, Ruggiero RA, Reilly TM, Hall PV. Early reconstruction failures after multilevel cervical corpectomy. Spine (Phila Pa 1976). 2003;28(2):140–2. https://doi.org/10.1097/00007632-200301150-00009.
29. Fehlings MG, Smith JS, Kopjar B, Arnold PM, Yoon ST, Vaccaro AR, et al. Perioperative and delayed complications associated with the surgical treatment of cervical spondylotic myelopathy based on 302 patients from the AOSpine North America cervical spondylotic myelopathy study. J Neurosurg Spine. 2012;16(5):425–32. https://doi.org/10.3171/2012.1.SPINE11467.
30. Smith JS, Ramchandran S, Lafage V, Shaffrey CI, Ailon T, Klineberg E, et al. Prospective multicenter assessment of early complication rates associated with adult cervical deformity surgery in 78 patients. Neurosurgery. 2016;79(3):378–88. https://doi.org/10.1227/NEU.0000000000001129.
31. Taniyama T, Hirai T, Yamada T, Yuasa M, Enomoto M, Yoshii T, et al. Modified K-line in magnetic resonance imaging predicts insufficient decompression of cervical laminoplasty. Spine (Phila Pa 1976). 2013;38(6):496–501. https://doi.org/10.1097/BRS.0b013e318273a4f7.
32. Taniyama T, Hirai T, Yoshii T, Yamada T, Yasuda H, Saito M, et al. Modified K-line in magnetic resonance imaging predicts clinical outcome in patients with nonlordotic alignment after laminoplasty for cervical spondylotic myelopathy. Spine (Phila Pa 1976). 2014;39(21):E1261–8. https://doi.org/10.1097/BRS.0000000000000531.
33. Madhavan K, Chieng LO, Foong H, Wang MY. Surgical outcomes of elderly patients with cervical spondylotic myelopathy: a meta-analysis of studies reporting on 2868 patients. Neurosurg Focus. 2016;40(6):E13. https://doi.org/10.3171/2016.3.FOCUS1657.
34. Gillis CC, Kaszuba MC, Traynelis VC. Cervical radiographic parameters in 1- and 2-level anterior cervical discectomy and fusion. J Neurosurg Spine. 2016;25(4):421–9. https://doi.org/10.3171/2016.2.spine151056.
35. Acharya AB, Fowler JB. Chaddock Reflex. StatPearls. Treasure Island (FL): StatPearls Publishing LLC.; 2022.
36. Morrow JM, Reilly MM. The Babinski sign. Br J Hosp Med (Lond). 2011;72(10):M157–9. https://doi.org/10.12968/hmed.2011.72.sup10.m157.
37. Miczak K, Padova J. Muscle overactivity in the upper motor neuron syndrome: assessment and problem solving for complex cases: the role of physical and occupational therapy. Phys Med Rehabil Clin N Am. 2018;29(3):529–36. https://doi.org/10.1016/j.pmr.2018.03.006.

38. Barman B. Clinical Sign Revisited: Hoffman's sign. Indian J Med Specialities. 2010;1:44–5. https://doi.org/10.7713/ijms.2010.0012.
39. Bono CM, Ghiselli G, Gilbert TJ, Kreiner DS, Reitman C, Summers JT, et al. An evidence-based clinical guideline for the diagnosis and treatment of cervical radiculopathy from degenerative disorders. Spine J. 2011;11(1):64–72. https://doi.org/10.1016/j.spinee.2010.10.023.
40. Xie JC, Hurlbert RJ. Discectomy versus discectomy with fusion versus discectomy with fusion and instrumentation: a prospective randomized study. Neurosurgery. 2007;61(1):107–16; discussion 16–7. https://doi.org/10.1227/01.neu.0000279730.44016.da.
41. Epstein NE. A review of complication rates for anterior cervical diskectomy and fusion (ACDF). Surg Neurol Int. 2019;10:100. https://doi.org/10.25259/SNI-191-2019.
42. Leven D, Cho SK. Pseudarthrosis of the cervical spine: risk factors, diagnosis and management. Asian Spine J. 2016;10(4):776–86. https://doi.org/10.4184/asj.2016.10.4.776.
43. Karadimas SK, Erwin WM, Ely CG, Dettori JR, Fehlings MG. Pathophysiology and natural history of cervical spondylotic myelopathy. Spine (Phila Pa 1976). 2013;38(22 Suppl 1):S21–36. https://doi.org/10.1097/BRS.0b013e3182a7f2c3.
44. Tetreault LA, Nouri A, Singh A, Fawcett M, Fehlings MG. Predictors of outcome in patients with cervical spondylotic myelopathy undergoing surgical treatment: a survey of members from AOSpine International. World Neurosurg. 2014;81(3–4):623–33. https://doi.org/10.1016/j.wneu.2013.09.023.
45. Tetreault L, Wilson JR, Kotter MRN, Côté P, Nouri A, Kopjar B, et al. Is preoperative duration of symptoms a significant predictor of functional outcomes in patients undergoing surgery for the treatment of degenerative cervical myelopathy? Neurosurgery. 2019;85(5):642–7. https://doi.org/10.1093/neuros/nyy474.
46. Spurling RGSW. Lateral rupture of the cervical intervertebral discs: a common cause of shoulder and arm pain. Surg Gynecol Obstet. 1944;78:350–8.
47. Shah KC, Rajshekhar V. Reliability of diagnosis of soft cervical disc prolapse using Spurling's test. Br J Neurosurg. 2004;18(5):480–3. https://doi.org/10.1080/02688690400012350.
48. Kato S, Chikuda H, Seichi A, Ohtsu H, Kimura A, Toyama Y. Radiographical risk factors for major intraoperative blood loss during laminoplasty in patients with ossification of the posterior longitudinal ligament. Spine (Phila Pa 1976). 2012;37(25):E1588–93. https://doi.org/10.1097/BRS.0b013e3182712b74.
49. Onishi E, Yasuda T, Yamamoto H, Iwaki K, Ota S. Outcomes of surgical treatment for thoracic myelopathy: a single-institutional study of 73 patients. Spine (Phila Pa 1976). 2016;41(22):E1356–63. https://doi.org/10.1097/BRS.0000000000001622.
50. Joaquim A, Riew K. Axis screw fixation—a step-by-step review of the surgical techniques. Arquivos Brasileiros de Neurocirurgia: Braz Neurosurg. 2017;36. https://doi.org/10.1055/s-0037-1601455.
51. Joaquim AF, Tan L, Riew KD. Posterior screw fixation in the subaxial cervical spine: a technique and literature review. J Spine Surg. 2020;6(1):252–61. https://doi.org/10.21037/jss.2019.09.28.
52. Cho W, Maeda T, Park Y, Buchowski JM, Nabb CE, Riew D. The incidence of bifid c7 spinous processes. Global Spine J. 2012;2(2):99–104. https://doi.org/10.1055/s-0032-1319776.
53. Klekamp JW, Ugbo JL, Heller JG, Hutton WC. Cervical transfacet versus lateral mass screws: a biomechanical comparison. J Spinal Disord. 2000;13(6):515–8. https://doi.org/10.1097/00002517-200012000-00009.
54. Roy-Camille R, Salient G, Mazel C. Internal fixation of the unstable cervical spine by a posterior osteosynthesis with plates and screws. In: Sherk HH, Dunn EJ, Eismont FJ, et al., editors. The cervical spine. 2nd ed. Philadelphia, PA: JB Lippincott; 1989. p. 390–403.
55. An HS, Coppes MA. Posterior cervical fixation for fracture and degenerative disc disease. Clin Orthop Relat Res. 1997;335:101–11.
56. Nazarian SM, Louis RP. Posterior internal fixation with screw plates in traumatic lesions of the cervical spine. Spine (Phila Pa 1976). 1991;16(3 Suppl):S64–71. https://doi.org/10.1097/00007632-199103001-00011.
57. Jeanneret B, Magerl F, Ward EH, Ward JC. Posterior stabilization of the cervical spine with hook plates. Spine (Phila Pa 1976). 1991;16(3 Suppl):S56–63. https://doi.org/10.1097/00007632-199103001-00010.
58. Anderson PA, Henley MB, Grady MS, Montesano PX, Winn HR. Posterior cervical arthrodesis with AO reconstruction plates and bone graft. Spine (Phila Pa 1976). 1991;16(3 Suppl):S72–9. https://doi.org/10.1097/00007632-199103001-00012.
59. Joaquim AF, Ghizoni E, Rubino PA, Anderle DV, Tedeschi H, Rhoton AL Jr, et al. Lateral mass screw fixation of the atlas: surgical technique and anatomy. World Neurosurg. 2010;74(2–3):359–62. https://doi.org/10.1016/j.wneu.2010.05.010.
60. Bogduk N, Mercer S. Biomechanics of the cervical spine. I: Normal kinematics. Clin Biomech (Bristol, Avon). 2000;15(9):633–48. https://doi.org/10.1016/s0268-0033(00)00034-6.
61. Daniels AH, Hart RA, Hilibrand AS, Fish DE, Wang JC, Lord EL, et al. Iatrogenic spinal cord injury resulting from cervical spine surgery. Global Spine J. 2017;7(1 Suppl):84S-90S. https://doi.org/10.1177/2192568216688188.
62. Radhakrishnan K, Litchy WJ, O'Fallon WM, Kurland LT. Epidemiology of cervical radiculopathy. A population-based study from Rochester, Minnesota, 1976 through 1990. Brain. 1994;117(Pt 2):325–35. https://doi.org/10.1093/brain/117.2.325.
63. Joaquim AF, Makhni MC, Riew KD. Post-operative nerve injuries after cervical spine surgery. Int Orthop. 2019;43(4):791–5. https://doi.org/10.1007/s00264-018-4257-4.
64. Liu G, Reyes MR, Riew KD. Why does C5 palsy occur after prophylactic bilateral C4–5 foraminotomy in open-door cervical laminoplasty? A risk factor analysis. Global Spine J. 2017;7(7):696–702. https://doi.org/10.1177/2192568217699191.
65. Than KD, Mummaneni PV, Smith ZA, Hsu WK, Arnold PM, Fehlings MG, et al. Brachial plexopathy after cervical spine surgery. Global Spine J. 2017;7(1 Suppl):17S-20S. https://doi.org/10.1177/2192568216687297.
66. Stoker GE, Kim HJ, Riew KD. Differentiating c8–t1 radiculopathy from ulnar neuropathy: a survey of 24 spine surgeons. Global Spine J. 2014;4(1):1–6. https://doi.org/10.1055/s-0033-1354254.
67. Ebraheim NA, Lu J, Yang H, Heck BE, Yeasting RA. Vulnerability of the sympathetic trunk during the anterior approach to the lower cervical spine. Spine (Phila Pa 1976). 2000;25(13):1603–6. https://doi.org/10.1097/00007632-200007010-00002.
68. Abumi K, Kaneda K. Pedicle screw fixation for nontraumatic lesions of the cervical spine. Spine (Phila Pa 1976). 1997;22(16):1853–63. https://doi.org/10.1097/00007632-199708150-00010.
69. Kreiner DS, Hwang SW, Easa JE, Resnick DK, Baisden JL, Bess S, et al. An evidence-based clinical guideline for the diagnosis and treatment of lumbar disc herniation with radiculopathy. Spine J. 2014;14(1):180–91. https://doi.org/10.1016/j.spinee.2013.08.003.
70. Jensen OH. The level-diagnosis of a lower lumbar disc herniation: the value of sensibility and motor testing. Clin Rheumatol. 1987;6(4):564–9. https://doi.org/10.1007/BF02330594.
71. Pape E, Eldevik P, Vandvik B. Diagnostic validity of somatosensory evoked potentials in subgroups of patients with sciatica. Eur

Spine J. 2002;11(1):38–46. https://doi.org/10.1007/s005860100322.
72. Heo DH, Lee DK, Lee DC, Kim HS, Park CK. Fully endoscopic transforaminal lumbar discectomy for upward migration of upper lumbar disc herniation: clinical and radiological outcomes and technical considerations. Brain Sci. 2020;10(6). https://doi.org/10.3390/brainsci10060363.
73. Ahn Y. Endoscopic spine discectomy: indications and outcomes. Int Orthop. 2019;43(4):909–16. https://doi.org/10.1007/s00264-018-04283-w.
74. Huang W, Qian Y, Zheng K, Yu L, Yu X. Is smoking a risk factor for lumbar disc herniation? Eur Spine J. 2016;25(1):168–76. https://doi.org/10.1007/s00586-015-4103-y.
75. Seidler A, Bergmann A, Jäger M, Ellegast R, Ditchen D, Elsner G, et al. Cumulative occupational lumbar load and lumbar disc disease–results of a German multi-center case-control study (EPILIFT). BMC Musculoskelet Disord. 2009;10:48. https://doi.org/10.1186/1471-2474-10-48.
76. Ravichandran D, Pillai J, Krishnamurthy K. Genetics of intervertebral disc disease: a review. Clin Anat. 2022;35(1):116–20. https://doi.org/10.1002/ca.23803.
77. Mysliwiec LW, Cholewicki J, Winkelpleck MD, Eis GP. MSU classification for herniated lumbar discs on MRI: toward developing objective criteria for surgical selection. Eur Spine J. 2010;19(7):1087–93. https://doi.org/10.1007/s00586-009-1274-4.
78. Vader JP, Porchet F, Larequi-Lauber T, Dubois RW, Burnand B. Appropriateness of surgery for sciatica: reliability of guidelines from expert panels. Spine (Phila Pa 1976). 2000;25(14):1831–6. https://doi.org/10.1097/00007632-200007150-00015.
79. McCulloch JA. Focus issue on lumbar disc herniation: macro- and microdiscectomy. Spine (Phila Pa 1976). 1996;21(24 Suppl):45S–56S. https://doi.org/10.1097/00007632-199612151-00005.
80. Appel B. Nomenclature and classification of lumbar disc pathology. Neuroradiology. 2001;43(12):1124–5.
81. Li Y, Fredrickson V, Resnick DK. How should we grade lumbar disc herniation and nerve root compression? A systematic review. Clin Orthop Relat Res. 2015;473(6):1896–902. https://doi.org/10.1007/s11999-014-3674-y.
82. Smyth MJ, Wright V. Sciatica and the intervertebral disc; an experimental study. J Bone Joint Surg Am. 1958;40-A(6):1401–18.
83. Olmarker K, Rydevik B, Nordborg C. Autologous nucleus pulposus induces neurophysiologic and histologic changes in porcine cauda equina nerve roots. Spine (Phila Pa 1976). 1993;18(11):1425–32.
84. Albert TJ, Balderston RA, Heller JG, Herkowitz HN, Garfin SR, Tomany K, et al. Upper lumbar disc herniations. J Spinal Disord. 1993;6(4):351–9. https://doi.org/10.1097/00002517-199306040-00009.
85. Xin G, Shi-Sheng H, Hai-Long Z. Morphometric analysis of the YESS and TESSYS techniques of percutaneous transforaminal endoscopic lumbar discectomy. Clin Anat. 2013;26(6):728–34. https://doi.org/10.1002/ca.22286.
86. Manchikanti L, Singh V, Pampati V, Falco FJ, Hirsch JA. Comparison of the efficacy of caudal, interlaminar, and transforaminal epidural injections in managing lumbar disc herniation: is one method superior to the other? Korean J Pain. 2015;28(1):11–21. https://doi.org/10.3344/kjp.2015.28.1.11.
87. Ebeling U, Reulen HJ. Are there typical localisations of lumbar disc herniations? A prospective study. Acta Neurochir (Wien). 1992;117(3–4):143–8. https://doi.org/10.1007/BF01400611.
88. Park JS, Choi SE, Cho TK, Kim SH, Rhee W, Kim WJ, et al. Recurrence rate after herniotomy only versus discectomy in lumbar disc herniation. Korean J Spine. 2013;10(4):227–31. https://doi.org/10.14245/kjs.2013.10.4.227.
89. Rogers LA. Experience with limited versus extensive disc removal in patients undergoing microsurgical operations for ruptured lumbar discs. Neurosurgery. 1988;22(1 Pt 1):82–5. https://doi.org/10.1227/00006123-198801010-00013.
90. Williams RW. Microlumbar discectomy: a conservative surgical approach to the virgin herniated lumbar disc. Spine (Phila Pa 1976). 1978;3(2):175–82.
91. Wenger M, Mariani L, Kalbarczyk A, Gröger U. Long-term outcome of 104 patients after lumbar sequestrectomy according to Williams. Neurosurgery. 2001;49(2):329–34; discussion 34–5. https://doi.org/10.1097/00006123-200108000-00013.
92. Waguespack A, Schofferman J, Slosar P, Reynolds J. Etiology of long-term failures of lumbar spine surgery. Pain Med. 2002;3(1):18–22. https://doi.org/10.1046/j.1526-4637.2002.02007.x.
93. Orita S, Inage K, Eguchi Y, Kubota G, Aoki Y, Nakamura J, et al. Lumbar foraminal stenosis, the hidden stenosis including at L5/S1. Eur J Orthop Surg Traumatol. 2016;26(7):685–93. https://doi.org/10.1007/s00590-016-1806-7.
94. Dyck P, Doyle JB. Bicycle test" of van Gelderen in diagnosis of intermittent cauda equina compression syndrome. Case report. J Neurosurg. 1977;46(5):667–70. https://doi.org/10.3171/jns.1977.46.5.0667.
95. Porter RW. Spinal stenosis and neurogenic claudication. Spine (Phila Pa 1976). 1996;21(17):2046–52. https://doi.org/10.1097/00007632-199609010-00024.
96. Laurencin CT, Lipson SJ, Senatus P, Botchwey E, Jones TR, Koris M, et al. The stenosis ratio: a new tool for the diagnosis of degenerative spinal stenosis. Int J Surg Investig. 1999;1(2):127–31.
97. Schizas C, Theumann N, Burn A, Tansey R, Wardlaw D, Smith FW, et al. Qualitative grading of severity of lumbar spinal stenosis based on the morphology of the dural sac on magnetic resonance images. Spine (Phila Pa 1976). 2010;35(21):1919–24. https://doi.org/10.1097/BRS.0b013e3181d359bd.
98. Amundsen T, Weber H, Lilleås F, Nordal HJ, Abdelnoor M, Magnaes B. Lumbar spinal stenosis. Clinical and radiologic features. Spine (Phila Pa 1976). 1995;20(10):1178–86. https://doi.org/10.1097/00007632-199505150-00013.
99. Aota Y, Niwa T, Yoshikawa K, Fujiwara A, Asada T, Saito T. Magnetic resonance imaging and magnetic resonance myelography in the presurgical diagnosis of lumbar foraminal stenosis. Spine (Phila Pa 1976). 2007;32(8):896–903. https://doi.org/10.1097/01.brs.0000259809.75760.d5.
100. Hasegawa T, An HS, Haughton VM. Imaging anatomy of the lateral lumbar spinal canal. Semin Ultrasound CT MR. 1993;14(6):404–13. https://doi.org/10.1016/s0887-2171(05)80034-4.
101. Yamada K, Aota Y, Higashi T, Ishida K, Nimura T, Konno T, et al. Lumbar foraminal stenosis causes leg pain at rest. Eur Spine J. 2014;23(3):504–7. https://doi.org/10.1007/s00586-013-3055-3.
102. Inufusa A, An HS, Lim TH, Hasegawa T, Haughton VM, Nowicki BH. Anatomic changes of the spinal canal and intervertebral foramen associated with flexion-extension movement. Spine (Phila Pa 1976). 1996;21(21):2412–20. https://doi.org/10.1097/00007632-199611010-00002.
103. Iwasaki H, Yoshida M, Yamada H, Hashizume H, Minamide A, Nakagawa Y, et al. A new electrophysiological method for the diagnosis of extraforaminal stenosis at L5–s1. Asian Spine J. 2014;8(2):145–9. https://doi.org/10.4184/asj.2014.8.2.145.
104. Katz JN, Harris MB. Clinical practice. Lumbar spinal stenosis. N Engl J Med. 2008;358(8):818–25. https://doi.org/10.1056/NEJMcp0708097.

105. Kornblum MB, Fischgrund JS, Herkowitz HN, Abraham DA, Berkower DL, Ditkoff JS. Degenerative lumbar spondylolisthesis with spinal stenosis: a prospective long-term study comparing fusion and pseudarthrosis. Spine (Phila Pa 1976). 2004;29 (7):726–33; discussion 33–4. https://doi.org/10.1097/01.brs.0000119398.22620.92.
106. Grob D, Humke T, Dvorak J. Significance of simultaneous fusion and surgical decompression in lumbar spinal stenosis. Orthopade. 1993;22(4):243–9.
107. Sekiguchi M, Kikuchi S. Experimental studies of lumbar spinal stenosis. Clin Calcium. 2005;15(3):51–6.
108. McGregor AH, Probyn K, Cro S, Doré CJ, Burton AK, Balagué F, et al. Rehabilitation following surgery for lumbar spinal stenosis. A Cochrane review. Spine (Phila Pa 1976). 2014;39 (13):1044–54. https://doi.org/10.1097/BRS.0000000000000355.
109. Bagley C, MacAllister M, Dosselman L, Moreno J, Aoun SG, El Ahmadieh TY. Current concepts and recent advances in understanding and managing lumbar spine stenosis. F1000Research. 2019;8:F1000 Faculty Rev-137. https://doi.org/10.12688/f1000research.16082.1.
110. Sun F, Liang Q, Yan M, Wang H, Liu Z, Li F, et al. Unilateral laminectomy by endoscopy in central lumbar canal spinal stenosis: technical note and early outcomes. Spine (Phila Pa 1976). 2020;45(14):E871–E7. https://doi.org/10.1097/BRS.0000000000003478.
111. Chun SW, Lim CY, Kim K, Hwang J, Chung SG. The relationships between low back pain and lumbar lordosis: a systematic review and meta-analysis. Spine J. 2017;17(8):1180–91. https://doi.org/10.1016/j.spinee.2017.04.034.
112. Sharif S, Shaikh Y, Bajamal AH, Costa F, Zileli M. Fusion surgery for lumbar spinal stenosis: WFNS Spine Committee recommendations. World Neurosurg X. 2020;7: 100077. https://doi.org/10.1016/j.wnsx.2020.100077.
113. Lurie J, Tomkins-Lane C. Management of lumbar spinal stenosis. BMJ (Clin Res Ed). 2016;352: h6234. https://doi.org/10.1136/bmj.h6234.
114. Costa F, Alves OL, Anania CD, Zileli M, Fornari M. Decompressive Surgery for Lumbar Spinal Stenosis: WFNS Spine Committee recommendations. World Neurosurg X. 2020;7: 100076. https://doi.org/10.1016/j.wnsx.2020.100076.
115. Kreiner DS, Baisden J, Mazanec DJ, Patel RD, Bess RS, Burton D, et al. Guideline summary review: an evidence-based clinical guideline for the diagnosis and treatment of adult isthmic spondylolisthesis. Spine J. 2016;16(12):1478–85. https://doi.org/10.1016/j.spinee.2016.08.034.
116. Mariniello G, Pagano S, Meglio V, Barbato M, Russo C, Pontillo G, et al. Multiple vertebral hemangiomas of the thoracic spine with atypical radiological features and aggressive behavior causing myelopathy: a case report. Interdiscipl Neurosurg. 2021;23: 100954. https://doi.org/10.1016/j.inat.2020.100954.
117. Butt S, Saifuddin A. The imaging of lumbar spondylolisthesis. Clin Radiol. 2005;60(5):533–46. https://doi.org/10.1016/j.crad.2004.07.013.
118. Bydon M, Alvi MA, Goyal A. Degenerative lumbar spondylolisthesis: definition, natural history, conservative management, and surgical treatment. Neurosurg Clin N Am. 2019;30(3):299–304. https://doi.org/10.1016/j.nec.2019.02.003.
119. Möller H, Sundin A, Hedlund R. Symptoms, signs, and functional disability in adult spondylolisthesis. Spine (Phila Pa 1976). 2000;25(6):683–9; discussion 90. https://doi.org/10.1097/00007632-200003150-00006.
120. Aielli F, Ponzetti M, Rucci N. Bone metastasis pain, from the bench to the bedside. Int J Mol Sci. 2019;20(2). https://doi.org/10.3390/ijms20020280.
121. Schneider GM, Jull G, Thomas K, Smith A, Emery C, Faris P, et al. Intrarater and interrater reliability of select clinical tests in patients referred for diagnostic facet joint blocks in the cervical spine. Arch Phys Med Rehabil. 2013;94(8):1628–34. https://doi.org/10.1016/j.apmr.2013.02.015.
122. Stuber K, Lerede C, Kristmanson K, Sajko S, Bruno P. The diagnostic accuracy of the Kemp's test: a systematic review. J Can Chiropr Assoc. 2014;58(3):258–67.
123. Herkowitz HN. Spine update. Degenerative lumbar spondylolisthesis. Spine (Phila Pa 1976). 1995;20(9):1084–90. https://doi.org/10.1097/00007632-199505000-00018.
124. Chan AK, Sharma V, Robinson LC, Mummaneni PV. Summary of guidelines for the treatment of lumbar spondylolisthesis. Neurosurg Clin N Am. 2019;30(3):353–64. https://doi.org/10.1016/j.nec.2019.02.009.
125. Thomsen K, Christensen FB, Eiskjaer SP, Hansen ES, Fruensgaard S, Bünger CE. 1997 Volvo Award winner in clinical studies. The effect of pedicle screw instrumentation on functional outcome and fusion rates in posterolateral lumbar spinal fusion: a prospective, randomized clinical study. Spine (Phila Pa 1976). 1997;22(24):2813–22. https://doi.org/10.1097/00007632-199712150-00004.
126. Matz PG, Meagher RJ, Lamer T, Tontz WL, Annaswamy TM, Cassidy RC, et al. Guideline summary review: An evidence-based clinical guideline for the diagnosis and treatment of degenerative lumbar spondylolisthesis. Spine J. 2016;16 (3):439–48. https://doi.org/10.1016/j.spinee.2015.11.055.
127. Mummaneni PV, Bisson EF, Kerezoudis P, Glassman S, Foley K, Slotkin JR, et al. Minimally invasive versus open fusion for Grade I degenerative lumbar spondylolisthesis: analysis of the quality outcomes database. Neurosurg Focus. 2017;43(2):E11. https://doi.org/10.3171/2017.5.FOCUS17188.
128. Minimally invasive vs. open spine surgery: 6 key points.
129. Cohen SP, Raja SN. Pathogenesis, diagnosis, and treatment of lumbar zygapophysial (facet) joint pain. Anesthesiology. 2007;106(3):591–614. https://doi.org/10.1097/00000542-200703000-00024.
130. Marks MC, Stanford CF, Mahar AT, Newton PO. Standing lateral radiographic positioning does not represent customary standing balance. Spine (Phila Pa 1976). 2003;28(11):1176–82. https://doi.org/10.1097/01.brs.0000067271.00258.51.
131. Dickman CA, Yahiro MA, Lu HT, Melkerson MN. Surgical treatment alternatives for fixation of unstable fractures of the thoracic and lumbar spine. A meta-analysis. Spine (Phila Pa 1976). 1994;19(20 Suppl):2266S–73S. https://doi.org/10.1097/00007632-199410151-00003.
132. Lu P, Pan T, Dai T, Chen G, Shi KQ. Is unilateral pedicle screw fixation superior than bilateral pedicle screw fixation for lumbar degenerative diseases: a meta-analysis. J Orthop Surg Res. 2018;13(1):296. https://doi.org/10.1186/s13018-018-1004-x.
133. Duncan JW, Bailey RA. An analysis of fusion cage migration in unilateral and bilateral fixation with transforaminal lumbar interbody fusion. Eur Spine J. 2013;22(2):439–45. https://doi.org/10.1007/s00586-012-2458-x.
134. Jacobsen S, Sonne-Holm S, Rovsing H, Monrad H, Gebuhr P. Degenerative lumbar spondylolisthesis: an epidemiological perspective: the Copenhagen Osteoarthritis study. Spine (Phila Pa 1976). 2007;32(1):120–5. https://doi.org/10.1097/01.brs.0000250979.12398.96.
135. Matsunaga S, Sakou T, Morizono Y, Masuda A, Demirtas AM. Natural history of degenerative spondylolisthesis. Pathogenesis and natural course of the slippage. Spine (Phila Pa 1976). 1990;15(11):1204–10. https://doi.org/10.1097/00007632-199011010-00021.

136. Golder W. Spondyl-olisthesis more than a problem of etymology (author's transl). Rontgenblatter. 1982;35(3):111.
137. Newman PH, Stone KH. The etiology of spondylolisthesis. J Bone Joint Surg Br. 1963;45-B(1):39–59. https://doi.org/10.1302/0301-620X.45B1.39.
138. Mac-Thiong JM, Duong L, Parent S, Hresko MT, Dimar JR, Weidenbaum M, et al. Reliability of the Spinal Deformity Study Group classification of lumbosacral spondylolisthesis. Spine (Phila Pa 1976). 2012;37(2):E95–102. https://doi.org/10.1097/BRS.0b013e3182233969.
139. Mac-Thiong JM, Wang Z, de Guise JA, Labelle H. Postural model of sagittal spino-pelvic alignment and its relevance for lumbosacral developmental spondylolisthesis. Spine (Phila Pa 1976). 2008;33(21):2316–25. https://doi.org/10.1097/BRS.0b013e318186b236.
140. Mac-Thiong JM, Labelle H, Parent S, Hresko MT, Deviren V, Weidenbaum M, et al. Reliability and development of a new classification of lumbosacral spondylolisthesis. Scoliosis. 2008;3:19. https://doi.org/10.1186/1748-7161-3-19.
141. Fredrickson BE, Baker D, McHolick WJ, Yuan HA, Lubicky JP. The natural history of spondylolysis and spondylolisthesis. J Bone Joint Surg Am. 1984;66(5):699–707.
142. Samuel AM, Moore HG, Cunningham ME. Treatment for degenerative lumbar spondylolisthesis: current concepts and new evidence. Curr Rev Musculoskelet Med. 2017;10(4):521–9. https://doi.org/10.1007/s12178-017-9442-3.
143. Gramse RR, Sinaki M, Ilstrup DM. Lumbar spondylolisthesis: a rational approach to conservative treatment. Mayo Clin Proc. 1980;55(11):681–6.
144. Faldini C, Pagkrati S, Acri F, Miscione MT, Francesconi D, Giannini S. Surgical treatment of symptomatic degenerative lumbar spondylolisthesis by decompression and instrumented fusion. J Orthop Traumatol. 2007;8(3):128–33. https://doi.org/10.1007/s10195-007-0079-7.
145. Eismont FJ, Norton RP, Hirsch BP. Surgical management of lumbar degenerative spondylolisthesis. J Am Acad Orthop Surg. 2014;22(4):203–13. https://doi.org/10.5435/JAAOS-22-04-203.
146. Lovell WWWR, Morrissy RT, et al. Lovell and Winter's pediatric orthopaedics. Philadelphia: Lippincott Williams & Wilkins; 2006.
147. Berger RG, Doyle SM. Spondylolysis 2019 update. Curr Opin Pediatr. 2019;31(1):61–8. https://doi.org/10.1097/mop.0000000000000706.
148. Meyerding HW. Low backache and sciatic pain associated with spondylolisthesis and protruded intervertebral disc: Incidence, significance, and treatment. JBJS 1941;23(2):461–70.
149. Spangfort EV. The lumbar disc herniation: a computer-aided analysis of 2,504 operations. Acta Orthop Scand. 1972;43(sup142):1–99. https://doi.org/10.3109/ort.1972.43.suppl-142.01.
150. Larsen JL, Smith D. Size of the subarachnoid space in stenosis of the lumbar canal. Acta Radiol Diagn (Stockh). 1980;21(5):627–32. https://doi.org/10.1177/028418518002100509.
151. Sasaki K. Magnetic resonance imaging findings of the lumbar root pathway in patients over 50 years old. Eur Spine J. 1995;4(2):71–6. https://doi.org/10.1007/BF00278915.
152. Möller H, Hedlund R. Instrumented and noninstrumented posterolateral fusion in adult spondylolisthesis–a prospective randomized study: part 2. Spine (Phila Pa 1976). 2000;25(13):1716–21. https://doi.org/10.1097/00007632-200007010-00017.
153. Disorders S. Fundamentals of diagnosis and treatment. Am J Neuroradiol. 2009;30(3): e44. https://doi.org/10.3174/ajnr.A1299.
154. Beckers L. Buck's operation for treatment of spondylolysis and spondylolisthesis. Acta Orthop Belg. 1986;52(6):819–23.
155. Hefti F, Seelig W, Morscher E. Repair of lumbar spondylolysis with a hook-screw. Int Orthop. 1992;16(1):81–5. https://doi.org/10.1007/BF00182992.
156. Scott JC. Spinal fusion. J Bone Joint Surg Br. 1953;35-B(2):169–71. https://doi.org/10.1302/0301-620X.35B2.169-a.
157. DeWald CJ, Vartabedian JE, Rodts MF, Hammerberg KW. Evaluation and management of high-grade spondylolisthesis in adults. Spine (Phila Pa 1976). 2005;30(6 Suppl):S49–59. https://doi.org/10.1097/01.brs.0000155573.34179.7e.
158. Gaines RW. The use of pedicle-screw internal fixation for the operative treatment of spinal disorders. J Bone Joint Surg Am. 2000;82(10):1458–76. https://doi.org/10.2106/00004623-200010000-00013.
159. Foley KT, Gupta SK. Percutaneous pedicle screw fixation of the lumbar spine: preliminary clinical results. J Neurosurg. 2002;97(1 Suppl):7–12. https://doi.org/10.3171/spi.2002.97.1.0007.
160. Lowery GL, Kulkarni SS. Posterior percutaneous spine instrumentation. Eur Spine J. 2000;9(Suppl 1):S126–30. https://doi.org/10.1007/pl00008318.
161. Rampersaud YR, Foley KT, Shen AC, Williams S, Solomito M. Radiation exposure to the spine surgeon during fluoroscopically assisted pedicle screw insertion. Spine (Phila Pa 1976). 2000;25(20):2637–45. https://doi.org/10.1097/00007632-200010150-00016.
162. Schizas C, Tzinieris N, Tsiridis E, Kosmopoulos V. Minimally invasive versus open transforaminal lumbar interbody fusion: evaluating initial experience. Int Orthop. 2009;33(6):1683–8. https://doi.org/10.1007/s00264-008-0687-8.
163. Kotani Y, Abumi K, Ito M, Sudo H, Abe Y, Minami A. Mid-term clinical results of minimally invasive decompression and posterolateral fusion with percutaneous pedicle screws versus conventional approach for degenerative spondylolisthesis with spinal stenosis. Eur Spine J. 2012;21(6):1171–7. https://doi.org/10.1007/s00586-011-2114-x.
164. Fan S, Hu Z, Zhao F, Zhao X, Huang Y, Fang X. Multifidus muscle changes and clinical effects of one-level posterior lumbar interbody fusion: minimally invasive procedure versus conventional open approach. Eur Spine J. 2010;19(2):316–24. https://doi.org/10.1007/s00586-009-1191-6.
165. Weiss HR, Negrini S, Rigo M, Kotwicki T, Hawes MC, Grivas TB, et al. Indications for conservative management of scoliosis (SOSORT guidelines). Stud Health Technol Inform. 2008;135:164–70.
166. Birknes JK, White AP, Albert TJ, Shaffrey CI, Harrop JS. Adult degenerative scoliosis: a review. Neurosurgery. 2008;63(3 Suppl):94–103. https://doi.org/10.1227/01.neu.0000325485.49323.b2.
167. Silva FE, Lenke LG. Adult degenerative scoliosis: evaluation and management. Neurosurg Focus. 2010;28(3):E1. https://doi.org/10.3171/2010.1.FOCUS09271.
168. Glassman SD, Berven S, Bridwell K, Horton W, Dimar JR. Correlation of radiographic parameters and clinical symptoms in adult scoliosis. Spine (Phila Pa 1976). 2005;30(6):682–8. https://doi.org/10.1097/01.brs.0000155425.04536.f7.
169. Glassman SD, Bridwell K, Dimar JR, Horton W, Berven S, Schwab F. The impact of positive sagittal balance in adult spinal deformity. Spine (Phila Pa 1976). 2005;30(18):2024–9. https://doi.org/10.1097/01.brs.0000179086.30449.96.
170. Scholten PJ, Veldhuizen AG. Analysis of Cobb angle measurements in scoliosis. Clin Biomech (Bristol, Avon). 1987;2(1):7–13. https://doi.org/10.1016/0268-0033(87)90039-8.
171. Weiss HR. Measurement of vertebral rotation: Perdriolle versus Raimondi. Eur Spine J. 1995;4(1):34–8. https://doi.org/10.1007/bf00298416.
172. Richards BS. Measurement error in assessment of vertebral rotation using the Perdriolle torsionmeter. Spine (Phila Pa 1976).

1992;17(5):513–7. https://doi.org/10.1097/00007632-199205000-00008.
173. Nash CL Jr, Moe JH. A study of vertebral rotation. J Bone Joint Surg Am. 1969;51(2):223–9.
174. Bridwell KH. Decision making regarding Smith-Petersen vs. pedicle subtraction osteotomy vs. vertebral column resection for spinal deformity. Spine (Phila Pa 1976). 2006;31(19 Suppl): S171–8. https://doi.org/10.1097/01.brs.0000231963.72810.38.
175. Everett CR, Patel RK. A systematic literature review of nonsurgical treatment in adult scoliosis. Spine (Phila Pa 1976). 2007;32(19 Suppl):S130–4. https://doi.org/10.1097/BRS.0b013e318134ea88.
176. Palazzo C, Montigny JP, Barbot F, Bussel B, Vaugier I, Fort D, et al. Effects of bracing in adult with scoliosis: a retrospective study. Arch Phys Med Rehabil. 2017;98(1):187–90. https://doi.org/10.1016/j.apmr.2016.05.019.
177. Wang G, Hu J, Liu X, Cao Y. Surgical treatments for degenerative lumbar scoliosis: a meta analysis. Eur Spine J. 2015;24(8):1792–9. https://doi.org/10.1007/s00586-015-3942-x.
178. van Dam BE. Nonoperative treatment of adult scoliosis. Orthop Clin North Am. 1988;19(2):347–51.
179. George K, Rippstein J. A comparative study of the two popular methods of measuring scoliotic deformity of the spine. JBJS. 1961;43(6).
180. Bouthors C, Benzakour A, Court C. Surgical treatment of thoracic disc herniation: an overview. Int Orthop. 2019;43(4):807–16. https://doi.org/10.1007/s00264-018-4224-0.
181. Carr DA, Volkov AA, Rhoiney DL, Setty P, Barrett RJ, Claybrooks R, et al. Management of thoracic disc herniations via posterior unilateral modified transfacet pedicle-sparing decompression with segmental instrumentation and interbody fusion. Global Spine J. 2017;7(6):506–13. https://doi.org/10.1177/2192568217694140.
182. Quint U, Bordon G, Preissl I, Sanner C, Rosenthal D. Thoracoscopic treatment for single level symptomatic thoracic disc herniation: a prospective followed cohort study in a group of 167 consecutive cases. Eur Spine J. 2012;21(4):637–45. https://doi.org/10.1007/s00586-011-2103-0.
183. Palazzo C, Sailhan F, Revel M. Scheuermann's disease: an update. Joint Bone Spine. 2014;81(3):209–14. https://doi.org/10.1016/j.jbspin.2013.11.012.
184. Guest JD, Griesdale DE, Marotta T. Thoracic disc herniation presenting with transient anterior spinal artery syndrome. A case report. Interv Neuroradiol. 2000;6(4):327–31. https://doi.org/10.1177/159101990000600408.
185. Lindeire S, Hauser JM. Anatomy, back, artery of Adamkiewicz. StatPearls. Treasure Island (FL): StatPearls Publishing LLC.; 2022.
186. Fried LC, Di Chiro G, Doppman JL. Ligation of major thoraco-lumbar spinal cord arteries in monkeys. J Neurosurg. 1969;31(6):608–14. https://doi.org/10.3171/jns.1969.31.6.0608.
187. Dickman CA, Rosenthal D, Regan JJ. Reoperation for herniated thoracic discs. J Neurosurg. 1999;91(2 Suppl):157–62. https://doi.org/10.3171/spi.1999.91.2.0157.
188. Melissano G, Bertoglio L, Civelli V, Amato AC, Coppi G, Civilini E, et al. Demonstration of the Adamkiewicz artery by multidetector computed tomography angiography analysed with the open-source software OsiriX. Eur J Vasc Endovasc Surg. 2009;37(4):395–400. https://doi.org/10.1016/j.ejvs.2008.12.022.
189. Charles YP, Barbe B, Beaujeux R, Boujan F, Steib JP. Relevance of the anatomical location of the Adamkiewicz artery in spine surgery. Surg Radiol Anat. 2011;33(1):3–9. https://doi.org/10.1007/s00276-010-0654-0.
190. Bohlman HH, Zdeblick TA. Anterior excision of herniated thoracic discs. J Bone Joint Surg Am. 1988;70(7):1038–47.
191. Jho HD. Endoscopic transpedicular thoracic discectomy. Neurosurg Focus. 2000;9(4): e4. https://doi.org/10.3171/foc.2000.9.4.5.
192. Hott JS, Feiz-Erfan I, Kenny K, Dickman CA. Surgical management of giant herniated thoracic discs: analysis of 20 cases. J Neurosurg Spine. 2005;3(3):191–7. https://doi.org/10.3171/spi.2005.3.3.0191.
193. Arnold PM, Johnson PL, Anderson KK. Surgical management of multiple thoracic disc herniations via a transfacet approach: a report of 15 cases. J Neurosurg Spine. 2011;15(1):76–81. https://doi.org/10.3171/2011.3.SPINE10642.
194. Bilsky MH. Transpedicular approach for thoracic disc herniations. Neurosurg Focus. 2000;9(4): e3. https://doi.org/10.3171/foc.2000.9.4.4.
195. Williams MP, Cherryman GR, Husband JE. Significance of thoracic disc herniation demonstrated by MR imaging. J Comput Assist Tomogr. 1989;13(2):211–4. https://doi.org/10.1097/00004728-198903000-00004.
196. Boos N, Marchesi D, Zuber K, Aebi M. Treatment of severe spondylolisthesis by reduction and pedicular fixation. A 4–6-year follow-up study. Spine (Phila Pa 1976). 1993;18(12):1655–61. https://doi.org/10.1097/00007632-199309000-00014.
197. Kwon BK, Albert TJ. Adult low-grade acquired spondylolytic spondylolisthesis: evaluation and management. Spine (Phila Pa 1976). 2005;30(6 Suppl):S35–41. https://doi.org/10.1097/01.brs.0000155561.70727.20.
198. Pareyson D, Marchesi C. Diagnosis, natural history, and management of Charcot-Marie-Tooth disease. Lancet Neurol. 2009;8(7):654–67. https://doi.org/10.1016/s1474-4422(09)70110-3.

Pediatric Spine

8

Christopher Sy, Alexander Villahermosa, Jonathan Fisher, Molly Farrell, Ryan McDermott, and Daniel Smerin

Question 1

A 6-month-old male child is referred to your clinic with a dimple that the mother noticed on his lower back. There is no obvious tract or drainage. It lies below the gluteal fold and overlies the coccyx. On examination, the patient has no other lesions and appears to have a grossly intact neurological exam for his age. The mother reports that he has been meeting usual milestones. What is the next best step?

a. MRI
b. Ultrasound
c. CT
d. Observation

Preferred answer: (d) Observation [1]

Question 2

You were consulted on an 11-year-old female who was found to have an intramedullary lesion at the level of T2. The decision was made to undergo surgical biopsy/resection while utilizing intra-operative neuromonitoring including MEPs and SSEPs. As soon as you make a midline myelotomy, the SSEPs bilaterally completely disappear. There are no changes with MEPs. What is the next best step?

a. Abort the procedure and close the patient. Get a prompt neurological exam and MRI.
b. Check positioning and vital signs. Ask anesthesia to increase the patient's mean arterial pressure.
c. Proceed with surgery as planned.
d. Perform additional laminectomies above the level of the lesion due to concern for stenosis/compression.

Preferred answer: (c) Proceed with surgery as planned [2].

Question 3

The following radiographic findings in pediatric patients can be considered normal variants EXCEPT for:

a. 3-year-old female. Anterior wedging of the vertebral bodies.
b. 4-year-old male. C1 lateral masses displaced up to 6mm with respect to dens on open mouth x-ray.
c. 9-year-old female. Atlanto-dens interval up to 10mm on lateral x-ray.
d. 6-year-old male. About 1mm anterior displacement of C2 on C3 on lateral x-ray.

Preferred answer: (c) 9-year-old female. Atlanto-dens interval up to 10mm on lateral x-ray [3].

Question 4

A 10-year-old male presents to the ED with severe, worsening low back pain and a grossly intact neurological exam. CT scan demonstrates an expansile, radiolucent lesion involving the left pedicle and vertebral body of L1. MRI demonstrates fluid levels. What is the most likely diagnosis and best course of treatment?

A. Villahermosa · J. Fisher · M. Farrell · R. McDermott · D. Smerin
Department of Neurosurgery, University of Texas Health Science Center at San Antonio, San Antonio, TX, USA
e-mail: villahermosa@uthscsa.edu

J. Fisher
e-mail: fisherj1@uthscsa.edu

M. Farrell
e-mail: farrelm1@uthscsa.edu

R. McDermott
e-mail: McDermottRA@uthscsa.edu

D. Smerin
e-mail: smerin@uthscsa.edu

C. Sy (✉)
Department of Neurosurgery, Houston Methodist Sugar Land Hospital, Sugar Land, TX, USA
e-mail: casy@houstonmethodist.org

C. Gragnaniello et al. (eds.), *MCQs in Spine Surgery*,
https://doi.org/10.1007/978-3-031-69332-8_8

a. Osteoid Osteoma: conservative management and observation.
b. Aneurysmal Bone Cyst: curettage, high-speed burr, electrocautery, phenolization.
c. Hemangioma: surgical excision.
d. Osteoblastoma: surgical excision and instrumented fusion.

Preferred answer: (b) Aneurysmal Bone Cyst: curettage, high-speed burr, electrocautery, phenolization [4].

Question 5

A 4-year-old female presents to your clinic with a diagnosis of tethered cord syndrome based on a recent MRI ordered by her pediatrician. She is here for evaluation and to establish multidisciplinary care. All of the following additional consults are commonly needed for these patients EXCEPT:

a. Neurology: due to weakness and spasticity.
b. Urology: due to urinary dysfunction and fecal incontinence.
c. Ophthalmology: due to papilledema.
d. Orthopedics: due to leg asymmetry and valgus deformity.

Preferred answer: (c) Ophthalmology: due to papilledema [5].

Question 6

There is a 15-year-old male with a history of cerebral palsy at birth and known coronal and sagittal deformity that you have been following with serial exams and imaging. He is non-ambulatory at baseline and uses a wheelchair. What is a commonly accepted indication for surgical intervention in regard to this patient's deformity?

a. Curvature progressing beyond 10 degrees
b. Curvature change of more than 5 degrees per year
c. Recurrent urinary tract infections
d. Inability to maintain upright posture and a comfortable sitting position

Preferred answer: (d) Inability to maintain upright posture and a comfortable sitting position [6].

Question 7

Myelomeningoceles are often associated with all of the following EXCEPT:

a. Chiari I
b. Chiari II
c. Hydrocephalus
d. Paraplegia

Preferred answer: (a) Chiari I [7].

Question 8

The suboccipital triangle is made up of the obliquus capitis superior, the rectus capitis posterior major, and the obliquus capitis inferior. What important structure can be found within it?

a. Cranial nerve XI
b. Vertebral artery
c. Occipital artery
d. C2 nerve root

Preferred answer: (b) Vertebral artery [8]

Question 9

The MOMS Trial (2011) demonstrated that there may be potential benefits to prenatal treatment of myelomeningoceles. Which of the following was the significant finding?

a. Safer delivery with lower chance of complications
b. Reduction in rate of shunt insertion for hydrocephalus
c. Lower likelihood of developing a Chiari malformation
d. Preserved urinary/bowel function

Preferred answer: (b) Reduction in rate of shunt insertion for hydrocephalus [9]

Question 10

All of the following radiographic findings are suggestive of atlanto-occipital dislocation (AOD) EXCEPT?

a. Basion-dens interval (BDI) > 15mm on lateral x-ray
b. Powers ratio > 1.0 on lateral x-ray
c. Condyle-C1 interval (CCI) > 4mm on CT
d. Atlanto-dens interval (ADI) > 1mm on CT

Preferred answer: (d) Atlanto-dens interval (ADI) > 1mm on CT [10]

Question 11

A patient who had a baclofen pump for spasticity placed years ago presents to the ED with worsening spasticity, tachycardia, hyperthermia, and seizures. What is likely happening and what is the best course of treatment?

a. Baclofen overdose - > turn off pump, CSF aspiration, ICU admission
b. Pump infection - > pan-cultures and broad-spectrum antibiotics
c. Pump infection - > emergent OR for pump explantation
d. Baclofen withdrawal - > intrathecal administration of baclofen

Preferred answer: (d) Baclofen withdrawal - > intrathecal administration of baclofen [11]

Question 12

Pediatric patients with achondroplasia are more likely to develop each of the following EXCEPT?

a. Spinal stenosis
b. Hydrocephalus
c. Foramen magnum stenosis
d. Recurrent spine fractures

Preferred answer: (d) Recurrent spine fractures [12]

Question 13

A 10-year-old female presents to the ED with worsening arm weakness and inability to walk. She was found to have an intramedullary spinal cord lesion at C4-C5. What is the most likely diagnosis?

a. Meningioma
b. Neurofibroma
c. Astrocytoma
d. Myxopapillary ependymoma

Preferred answer: (c) Astrocytoma [13]

Question 14

An 8-year-old male with bilateral lower extremity weakness was found to have a type 2 split cord malformation. What is the primary goal of surgery in cases of progressive neurological deficit?

a. Repositioning both hemicords within the same dural sleeve
b. Resection of the midline septum
c. Decompression via laminectomies or laminoplasties
d. Release of intradural arachnoid adhesions

Preferred answer: (b) Resection of the midline septum [14]

Question 15

Selective dorsal rhizotomy is a technique that is most effective at which of the following:

a. Decreasing neuropathic type pain in the lower extremities after trauma
b. Decrease in frequency of seizures in epilepsy patients
c. Decrease in spasticity in cerebral palsy patients
d. Decrease in urinary frequency in tethered cord patients

Preferred answer: (c) Decrease in spasticity in cerebral palsy patients [15]

Question 16

A 2-year old child who was developing normally has recently regressed and has only very weak movement in his legs. He was found to have a spinal cord lipoma on MRI. What is the primary goal of surgery for spinal cord lipomas in patients with neurologic deficit?

a. Untethering of the spinal cord
b. Decompression and debulking of the lipoma only
c. Gross total resection of lipoma
d. Biopsy for diagnosis followed by adjuvant therapies

Preferred answer: (a) Untethering of the spinal cord [16]

Question 17

A child with cerebral palsy and severe spastic quadriparesis presents to your clinic for evaluation and he is deemed a good candidate for intrathecal baclofen pump placement. What is the appropriate level shown to have the best efficacy?

a. C1-C2
b. C5-T2
c. T10-T12
d. L3-L4

Preferred answer: (b) C5-T2 [17]

Question 18

Primary neurulation, or the enfolding of the lateral edges of the neural plate to form the neural tube, happens approximately at what time?

a. Days 14–18, forming the most caudal part of the neural tube

b. Days 18–28, forming the most rostral part of the neural tube
c. Days 25–35, forming the most rostral part of the neural tube
d. Days 10–15, forming the most caudal part of the neural tube

Preferred answer: (b) Days 18–28, forming the most rostral part of the neural tube [18]

Question 19

The pediatrics team calls you for an inpatient consult on a newborn patient with a large cystic sac on the lumbar spine, noticeable lower extremity weakness, and clubfeet. Of note, the mother's alpha fetoprotein was significantly elevated during pregnancy. This is an example of what sort of spinal dysraphism?

a. Primary neurulation
b. Secondary neurulation
c. Gastrulation
d. Resegmentation

Preferred answer: (a) Primary neurulation [19]

Question 20

A 4-year-old male is referred to your office after falling from standing, with initial concern of a type 3 odontoid fracture. The patient denies any neck pain and does not seem to be acting abnormally. He has normal alignment on upright imaging, and no evidence of instability of flexion/extension x-rays. What would you recommend as management?

a. Observation. This is a normal anatomical finding of a non-ossified dentocentral synchondrosis
b. Repeat Xrays in 6 weeks
c. MRI of the cervical spine
d. Posterior cervical fixation

Preferred answer: (a) Observation. This is a normal anatomical finding of a non-ossified dentocentral synchondrosis [20]

Question 21

The os terminale of the odontoid fuses by what age approximately?

a. 3 years
b. 5 years
c. 9 years
d. 13 years

Preferred answer: (d) 13 years [20]

Question 22

A pediatric patient is referred to you with concern for difficulty swallowing and paresis of tongue movement. On exam, the patient has a noticeably short neck, low hairline, and decreased range of neck motion. Imaging demonstrates basilar invagination and compression of the mesencephalon. What is the likely diagnosis?

a. McArdle's syndrome
b. Odontoid insufficiency
c. Down Syndrome
d. Klippel-Feil Syndrome

Preferred answer: (d) Klippel-Feil Syndrome [21]

Question 23

A 15 years old female presents for evaluation of her scoliosis. She states her grandmother also had scoliosis. On exam, she has a rightward thoracic curve with mild cosmetic deformity. She has noticed a worsening of her pain over the last few years, however she describes the pain as mild. She denies breathing issues. What is the first form of treatment you would recommend?

a. Surgical fusion
b. Conservative observation and repeat imaging
c. Pain management with no further follow up
d. Bracing

Preferred answer: (b) Conservative observation and repeat imaging [22]

Question 24

A 7-year-old male presents with progressive back pain over a few months and frequent urinary tract infections to the ER. On X-ray imaging, he is noted to have a major left thoracic curve with a kyphotic component. What is your recommendation for management?

a. Pain management
b. MRI imaging with gadolinium to evaluate for intraspinal neoplasm or Chiari malformation
c. CT imaging for evaluation of fractures

d. Ultrasound of bladder to assess for urinary outlet obstruction

Preferred answer: (b) MRI imaging with gadolinium to evaluate for intraspinal neoplasm or Chiari malformation [23]

Question 25

The rostral neuropore closes around what day?

a. Day 14–16
b. Day 18–21
c. Day 23–25
d. Day 25 to 27

Preferred answer: (c) Day 23–25 [24]

Question 26

A 2-year-old patient is brought to the trauma bay after a low impact car accident where the patient was restrained, complaining of neck pain. On CT imaging, the trauma surgeon notices three discontinuities in the arch of C1- one anteriorly, and two posteriorly, adjacent bilaterally to the lateral masses. What is your recommendation?

a. Cervical MRI to evaluate for disc herniation
b. Upright AP/Lateral/Open mouth odontoid view x-ray imaging and follow up in 6 weeks with repeat imaging for cervical fractures of C1
c. Treatment in cervical collar for neck sprain only, as CT imaging consistent with normal ossification centers of C1

Preferred answer: (c) Treatment in cervical collar for neck sprain only, as CT imaging consistent with normal ossification centers of C1 [25]

Question 27

A 15-year-old female presents with the primary complaint of months of headache. These headaches are often exacerbated by laughing, coughing or straining on the toilet. She recently was taken to the hospital after she had a syncopal episode following a coughing episode. Given this clinical scenario, what is the most likely finding on imaging studies?

a. Supratentorial brain mass causing cerebral mass effect
b. Cervical stenosis with spinal cord compression
c. Cerebellar ectopia with syrinx formation
d. Basilar invagination

Preferred answer: (c) Cerebellar ectopia with syrinx formation [26]

Question 28

A patient with neurofibromatosis type 1 presents with known optic glioma and cerebellar gliomas for evaluation of worsening bilateral hand weakness, numbness, and worsening gait imbalance. MRI imaging demonstrates stable intracranial gliomas, however of note there appear to be dilations of the neural foramen of the cervical spine with spinal cord compression in the spinal canal. What is your diagnosis and management?

a. Decompression alone, with or without laminoplasty for plexiform neurofibromas
b. Decompression and resection of plexiform neurofibromas
c. Conservative management with observation
d. Refer patient to physical and occupational therapy

Preferred answer: (a) Decompression alone, with or without laminoplasty for plexiform neurofibromas [27]

Question 29

How long is it safe to postpone surgical closure of a newborn with myelomeningocele while having its cardiopulmonary and genitourinary systems investigated?

a. 24 h
b. 48 h
c. 72 h
d. 96 h

Preferred answer: (c) 72 h [28]

Question 30

During closure of a myelomeningocele, special attention to separation of the fused neural placode to surrounding tissue at the junctional zone is made circumferentially in order to obtain a primary closure of the underlying dura. Why is it important also to remove any residual epidermal or dermal elements from the periphery of the neural placode?

a. Assists with water-tight closure to prevent CSF leak
b. Prevents CNS infection
c. Prevents future development of dermoids or lipomas
d. This step is not necessary during myelomeningocele repair

Preferred answer: (c) Prevents future development of dermoids or lipomas [29]

Question 31

During intraoperative debulking of a lipomeningocele, the neuromonitoring tech alerts you to a decrease in pudendal sensory evoked potentials. What does this information indicate?

a. Over-stretch or damage of the lumbar plexus
b. Over-stretch or damage to S2-4 segments
c. Nothing, this is unrelated to your surgery
d. Motor damage to the iliopsoas

Preferred answer: (b) Over-stretch or damage to S2-4 segments [30]

Question 32

What is the best way to prevent post laminectomy kyphosis following suboccipital decompression for Chiari 1 syndrome in a child?

a. Decompressing C1 until you see the lateral dural edges only
b. Decompressing further than the lateral dural edges
c. Leaving the paraspinal musculature and bone of C2 intact
d. Preventing excessive force on the C1 arch that could cause breakdown of the anterior synchondrosis

Preferred answer: (c) Leaving the paraspinal musculature and bone of C2 intact [31]

Question 33

A patient is referred for evaluation of dermal sinus tract. On physical exam, his lower back area appears normal, with no signs of hemangiomas, subcutaneous lipomas or focal hirsutism. The tract appears to be a dimple located deep in the gluteal cleft, overlying the coccyx, has a downward incline, and almost disappears when the skin is spread. What is the most likely diagnosis?

a. Lipomeningocele
b. Dermal sinus tract
c. Benign sacrococcygeal dimple
d. Myelomeningocele

Preferred answer: (c) Benign sacrococcygeal dimple [32]

Question 34

A 7-year-old boy presents to the trauma bay following a car accident and presents with significant paresis of their upper and lower extremities. A stat MRI is done, demonstrating a rupture of the anterior longitudinal ligament without mass lesion or increased spinal cord signal, and a CTA performed is normal. The child is diagnosed with Spinal Cord Injury Without Radiographic Abnormality. What can you determine prognostically in terms of this child's neurological exam?

a. No improvement after 6 months
b. Permanent neurological decline following injury
c. Significant improvement in neurological condition after 6 months

Preferred answer: (c) Significant improvement in neurological condition after 6 months [33]

Question 35

What is generally considered the most reliable diagnostic criteria for atlanto-occipital dislocation (AOD) for pediatric patients?

a. Dens-Basion (DB) distance > 12.5 mm
b. Basion-Axial Interval (BAI) > 12 mm
c. Powers Ratio of > 1
d. Condyle-C1 interval (CCI) > 4.0 mm

Preferred answer: (d) Condyle-C1 interval (CCI) > 4.0 mm [34]

Question 36

A 3-year-old female with no past medical history, meeting developmental milestones presents after being involved in a motor vehicle accident. Patient's neurological exam is non focal except for some neck pain. Radiology report returns with a reading concerning for a type II odontoid fracture. This radiology finding is less likely due to the fact that dentocentral synchondrosis occurs during the ages:

a. 1–2 years of age
b. 2–3 years of agec
c. 4–8 years of age
d. 11–14 years of age

Preferred answer: (c) 4–8 years of age [20]

Question 37

A 12-year-old female with dextroscoliosis that is followed closely by her PCP was noted to have progressive abnormality and worsening back pain. Patient also notes that she had one episode of bladder incontinence. On exam, she is noted to have weakness in her left lower extremity. On MRI, the patient is found to have a tumor with a "meniscus sign" at T12. What kind of tumor do you expect with this radiological finding?

a. Intradural, intramedullary
b. Intradural, extramedullary
c. Extradural

Preferred answer: (b) Intradural, extramedullary [35]

Question 38

Which of the following tumors listed below would you anticipate this patient to have?

a. Neuroblastoma
b. Astrocytoma
c. Dermoid
d. Sarcoma
e. Teratoma
f. Ependymoma

Preferred answer: (c) Dermoid [36]

Question 39

After surgical resection of this patient's spinal tumor which included posterior approach with laminectomies, what postoperative complication should be considered especially in the pediatric population?

a. Increased infection rates
b. Delayed spinal deformity
c. Development of cerebrospinal fluid fistulas
d. Aseptic meningitis

Preferred answer: (b) Delayed spinal deformity [37]

Question 40

After removal of a dermoid spinal tumor, what type of post-operative care should this patient have in particular?

a. Chemotherapy
b. Radiation therapy
c. Proton beam therapy
d. Serial MRI to monitor for recurrence

Preferred answer: (d) Serial MRI to monitor for recurrence [38]

Question 41

A 5-year-old male patient presented to the ER with acute back pain. Patient was found to have a pathologic fracture of T3 on XR. On further imaging, a mass is visualized within the bone and noted to have a fluid level with a thin "eggshell" rim surrounding it. What is this patient's likely diagnosis?

a. Osteochondroma
b. Osteosarcoma
c. Aneurysmal Bone Cyst
d. Eosinophilic Granuloma

Preferred answer: (c) Aneurysmal Bone Cyst [39]

Question 42

The patient with an aneurysmal bone cyst (ABC) should follow up closely with their physician because other conditions are often associated with his diagnosis. What are those other conditions?

a. Osteoblastoma or giant cell tumor
b. Neuroblastoma
c. NF1 or NF2
d. Chordoma

Preferred answer: (a) Osteoblastoma or giant cell tumor [40]

Question 43

An incidental, single, dumbbell shaped tumor through the neural foramina is found in an 8-year-old patient. An MRI shows that the lesion is hypointense to the spinal cord on T1 weighted imaging, hyperintense on T2 weighted imaging, and with homogenous enhancement on postcontrast studies. The patient has no neurological deficits but does have a significant cardiac and pulmonary history. A biopsy is completed and shows a high-grade malignant lesion consistent with neuroblastoma. What treatment should be offered to this patient?

a. Surgical resection of a malignant tumor
b. Chemotherapy
c. Radiation

d. Surgical resection followed by chemotherapy
e. Surgical resection followed by radiation

Preferred answer: (b) Chemotherapy [38]

Question 44

What is the oncologic stage of this tumor according to Enneking system?

a. Stage IA G1, T1, M0
b. Stage IB G1, T2, M0
c. Stage IIA G2, T1, M0
d. Stage IIB G2, T2, M0
e. Stage III G1/2, T1/2, M1

Preferred answer: (c) Stage IIA G2, T1, M0 [41]

Question 45

Maternal serum testing for detecting open neural tube defects is associated with the following:

a. Elevated alpha fetoprotein
b. Low alpha fetoprotein, low inhibin A, low human chorionic gonadotropin, low estriol
c. Low alpha fetoprotein, elevated inhibin A, elevated human chorionic gonadotropin, low estriol

Preferred answer: (a) Elevated alpha fetoprotein [42]

Question 46

A 7-year-old male with past medical history of myelomeningocele who is status post-surgical repair and ventriculoperitoneal shunt placement presents with progressive difficulties with walking and multiple urinary tract infections. The patient denies any headaches, nausea, vomiting, or visual changes. The patient's head CT ventricle size appears stable, and his shunt is on the correct setting and appears intact. What is the patient's most likely diagnosis?

a. Tethered spinal cord
b. Ruptured spinal arteriovenous malformation
c. Large, herniated disc in the lower lumbar region

Preferred answer: (a) Tethered spinal cord [43]

Question 47

Which of the following is true regarding epidermoids, dermoids, and teratomas of the spine?

a. Dermoid tumors consist of only desquamated cells
b. Epidermoid tumors have germ layers that include elements such as skin, hair, sweat, and sebaceous glands
c. Teratomas are made of one germ layer
d. Dermoid tumors are made up of two germ layers

Preferred answer: (d) Dermoid tumors are made up of two germ layers [44]

Question 48

Newborn infant on exam was discovered to have a tuft of hair and cutaneous midline changes at the lumbosacral junction and a small opening. The etiology of this patient's particular diagnosis is due to incomplete separation of neural ectoderm from epithelial ectoderm. This description is consistent with,

a. Dermal sinus
b. Terminal syrinx
c. Meningocele Manque
d. Diastematomyelia

Preferred answer: (a) Dermal sinus [44]

Question 49

Widening of the atlantodental interval (ADI) is consistent with injury to what structure?

a. Alar ligament
b. Transverse ligament
c. Deep accessory tectorial membrane
d. Anterior atlantoaxial ligament

Preferred answer: (b) Transverse ligament [45]

Question 50

A 5-year-old male with no significant past medical history is involved in a motor vehicle accident. The patient reports that his neck hurts and his hands are tingling. On a neurological exam, the patient's hands are decreased in strength but otherwise he is neurologically intact. Work-up and imaging for the patient are all normal. What is true of spinal cord injury without radiographic abnormality (SCIWORA)?

a. Suggested etiology due to the increased malleability of the spinal column leading to less protection of the spinal cord
b. Patients < 8 years old experience this injury most commonly in the lower cervical region

c. It is a functional phenomenon that is commonly seen in children after a traumatic event
d. The rate of occurrence is similar for pediatric patients compared with adult patients

Preferred answer: (a) Suggested etiology due to the increased malleability of the spinal column leading to less protection of the spinal cord [46]

Question 51

Many biomechanical factors contribute to the hypermobility of the pediatric cervical spine, which makes this portion of the spine particularly vulnerable to injury. While the adult fulcrum for maximal flexion–extension is located at C5-C6, an infant's fulcrum is located at:

a. C6-C7
b. C4-C5
c. C3-C4
d. C2-C3
e. C1-C2

Preferred answer: (d) C2-C3 [47]

Question 52

During a transoral approach to the cervical spine in a pediatric patient, lateral exposure beyond 15 mm to the right of midline in the posterior pharyngeal mucosa will most likely lead to which post-operative complication?

a. Tongue deviation to the right
b. Tongue deviation to the left
c. Apnea
d. Bradycardia

Preferred answer: (a) Tongue deviation to the right [48]

Question 53

During subperiosteal dissection as part of the posterior approach to the pediatric cervical spine, excessive pressure on which spinous structure is most likely to cause a fracture and leave the underlying cord vulnerable to injury?

a. C1 lateral mass
b. C2 lamina
c. C1 posterior tubercle
d. C2 transverse foramen

Preferred answer: (c) C1 posterior tubercle [49]

Question 54

Meticulous dissection and avoidance of unintended periosteal exposure is particularly important in pediatric spine surgery due to the pediatric patient's greater propensity for what physiologic response?

a. Hematoma formation
b. Callus formation
c. Abscess formation
d. Seroma formation

Preferred answer: (b) Callus formation (causing bystander fusion) [50]

Question 55

Incompetence of the cruciate ligament such as in pediatric patients with Down syndrome or os odontoideum can lead to pathologic predental space widening primarily due to load placement on which structure(s)?

a. Apical and alar ligaments
b. Tectorial membrane
c. Atlanto-occipital joint
d. Atlanto-axial joint

Preferred answer: (a) Apical and alar ligaments [51]

Question 56

Which of the following structural aspects of the pediatric cranio-vertebral junction is not a cause of increased mobility at the junction relatively to adults?

a. Head to neck ratio
b. Horizontal orientation of cervical facets
c. Lack of uncovertebral joints
d. Strength of paracervical musculature

Preferred answer: (d) Strength of paracervical musculature [51]

Question 57

Which imaging modality is most important to order prior to posterior fossa decompression of a suspected Chiari 0 malformation?

a. XR lumbar spine
b. CT thoraco-lumbar spine
c. MRI neuro-axis

d. CTA head and neck

Preferred answer: (c) MRI neuro-axis

Question 58

A twelve-year-old female is found to have a standing lateral curvature of 12 degrees on plain radiograph. Which accompanying structural abnormality will most likely be found on ensuing MRI evaluation?

a. Cerebellar tonsillar herniation 6 mm below the foramen magnum and syrinx
b. Spina bifida occulta and herniation of cerebellar vermis
c. Parietal bone hypoplasia
d. Dysgenesis of the corpus callosum

Preferred answer: (a) Cerebellar tonsillar herniation 6 mm below the foramen magnum and syrinx [53]

Question 59

Which of the following is least likely to complicate a pediatric Chiari II decompression?

a. Extension of cerebellar tissue into the lower cervical spine
b. Adherence of cerebellar tissue to the medulla
c. High-riding torcula
d. Pre-operative illness due to medullary dysfunction

Preferred answer: (c) High-riding torcula [54]

Question 60

Astrocytomas and ependymomas constitute 80% of pediatric intramedullary tumors. All of the following are radiographic differences that can help distinguish between astrocytoma and ependymoma except:

a. Ependymomas tend to be centrally located within the spinal cord while astrocytomas are more likely eccentrically located
b. Ependymomas have distinct margins while astrocytomas have indistinct margins
c. Ependymomas demonstrate variable enhancement while astrocytomas have uniform enhancement
d. Ependymomas are more likely to have calcification and hemorrhage compared to astrocytomas

Preferred answer: (c) Ependymomas demonstrate variable enhancement while astrocytomas have uniform enhancement [55]

Question 61

Following repair of a myelomeningocele in a 24-week-old patient, post-operative MRI demonstrates an intramedullary lesion at T12. Which of the following radiographic findings will help determine whether this lesion is more likely an epidermoid cyst or arachnoid cyst?

a. Perifocal edema
b. Peripheral enhancement
c. Intensity on T1/T2 MRI
d. Diffusion restriction

Preferred answer: (d) Diffusion restriction [56]

Question 62

Which of the following pediatric neoplasms does not have a well-defined surgical plane and therefore is usually not amenable to gross total resection?

a. Lipoma
b. Juvenile pilocytic astrocytomas
c. Ependymoma
d. Epidermoid cyst

Preferred answer: (a) Lipoma [57]

Question 63

A 7-year-old patient is found to have primary intramedullary oligodendroglioma. Which symptoms are most likely an indication for additional imaging and radiation with adjuvant chemotherapy?

a. Focal weakness
b. Focal sensory loss
c. Bowel incontinence
d. Nausea and blurry vision

Preferred answer: (d) Nausea and blurry vision (Oligodendrogliomatosis-induced hydrocephalus) [58]

Question 64

A 12-month-old patient is found to have a rapidly growing myofibroma of the trunk without visceral involvement or compression of the spinal cord. Which of the following is the appropriate next step in management?

a. Gross total resection
b. Radiation

c. Radiation and chemotherapy
d. Observation

Preferred answer: (d) Observation [59]

Question 65

Which of the following is not a characteristic MRI finding for pediatric intramedullary hemangioblastoma?

a. Isointense on T1-weighted MRI and hyperintense on T2 if tumor is less than 10 mm
b. Presence of flow void
c. Deep location of intramedullary tumor
d. Large size of associated syrinx compared to intramedullary portion of tumor

Preferred answer: (c) Deep location of intramedullary tumor [60]

Question 66

Following removal of a thoracic cavernous malformation in a 14-year-old patient, there is persistent venous bleeding from the surgical bed despite application of gentle pressure with cotton pledges. This bleeding is most likely indicative of which intraoperative complication?

a. Iatrogenic fistula
b. Incomplete resection of cavernous malformation
c. Damage to vertebral venous plexus
d. Damage to perilesional gliotic layer

Preferred answer: (b) Incomplete resection of cavernous malformation [61]

Question 67

A 12-year-old patient with a history of retinoblastoma presents with new-onset lumbar back pain and peri-lumbar soft tissue swelling. Where is this patient most likely to have metastatic lesions?

a. Lung
b. Brain
c. Liver
d. Adrenal gland

Preferred answer: (a) Lung [62]

Question 68

When is surgical stabilization of scoliotic deformity commonly performed in children with Duchenne Muscular Dystrophy (DMD)?

a. When vital capacity falls below 1 L
b. When a child transitions from ambulating to wheelchair use
c. Before 5 years of age
d. Surgery is not indicated; bracing alone is adequate

Preferred answer: (b) When a child transitions from ambulating to wheelchair use [63]

Question 69

In the surgical management of pediatric scoliotic deformity, consideration of which of the following should be considered for the prevention of postoperative incision dehiscence?

a. Nutrition assessment and metabolic demand
b. Presence of spasticity and limb contractures
c. Availability of sufficient subcutaneous tissue
d. All of the above

Preferred answer: (d) All of the above [64]

Question 70

Spasticity is primarily mediated by which of the following fibers?

a. Ia fibers
b. Ib fibers
c. II fibers
d. Alpha-motor fibers
e. Gamma-motor fibers

Preferred answer: (a) Ia fibers [65]

Question 71

When should selective dorsal rhizotomy be considered in the management of cerebral palsy?

a. When hypertonia is present
b. For spasticity implicated in functional impairment
c. Significant motor weakness with standing
d. When dyskinesia is present

Preferred answer: (b) For spasticity implicated in functional impairment [66]

Question 72

A pediatric trauma patient presenting with subarachnoid hemorrhage at the craniocervical junction, prevertebral soft tissue edema, and lower cranial nerve deficits is most concerning for which of the following?

a. Traumatic aneurysm rupture
b. Grade 3 diffuse axonal injury
c. Basilar skull fracture
d. Atlanto-occipital dissociation

Preferred answer: (d) Atlanto-occipital dissociation [67]

Question 73

Neural arches typically fuse to form a solid posterior ring at C1 by the age of:

a. 32 weeks gestational age
b. 1 month
c. 1 year
d. 3 years

Preferred answer: (d) 3 years [68]

Question 74

The atlanto-dental interval is used to assess the integrity of which of the following ligaments?

a. Tectorial membrane
b. Transverse ligament
c. Alar ligaments
d. Apical odontoid ligament

Preferred answer: (b) Transverse ligament [69]

Question 75

When should myelomeningocele repair be undertaken?

a. 20 weeks gestational age
b. Within 72 h of birth
c. Not before 1 week
d. Not before 1 month

Preferred answer: (b) Within 72 h of birth [70]

Question 76

The goals of myelomeningocele repair include all of the following except:

a. Improved urodynamics
b. Reducing risk of meningitis
c. Minimize CSF loss
d. Protect the functional spinal cord tissue

Preferred answer: (a) Improved urodynamics [71]

Question 77

Which occipital sclerotome differentiates into the apical ligament and apex of the dens?

a. 1st
b. 2nd
c. 3rd
d. 4th

Preferred answer: (c) 3rd [72]

Question 78

Inflammatory, spontaneous subluxation of the atlantoaxial joint following parapharyngeal infection is also known as:

a. Grisel syndrome
b. Apert syndrome
c. Scheuermann's disease
d. Pfeiffer syndrome

Preferred answer: (a) Grisel syndrome [73]

Question 79

Symptomatic incidence of atlantoaxial instability in Down syndrome is estimated to be:

a. Less than 1%
b. 14–24%
c. 50%
d. Atlantoaxial instability is not associated with Down syndrome

Preferred answer: (a) Less than 1% [74]

Question 80

The NF2 suppressor gene on 22q12.2 is found in 50% of which pediatric spinal cord tumors?

a. Astrocytoma
b. Ganglioglioma
c. Ependymoma
d. Hemangioblastoma

Preferred answer: (c) Ependymoma [75]

Question 81

The most important oncogene associated with neuroblastoma:

a. MYCN
b. RAS
c. EGFR
d. NF1

Preferred answer: (a) MYCN [76]

Question 82

In the evaluation of a pediatric patient presenting with axial back pain and finding of "vertebra plana" (pancaked vertebral body) on imaging studies, the most likely diagnosis is:

a. Osteochondroma
b. Aneurysmal bone cyst
c. Chordoma
d. Langerhans cell histiocytosis

Preferred answer: (d) Langerhans cell histiocytosis [77]

Question 83

In the pediatric population, chordoma should be suspected with lesions found in the:

a. Craniocervical junction
b. Thoracic spine
c. Lumbar spine
d. Sacrococcygeal region
e. Both A and D
f. Chordoma is found only in the adult population

Preferred answer: (e) Both A and D [77]

Question 84

The presence of C3-C4 anterolisthesis and smooth spinolaminar lines on dynamic imaging is most consistent with:

a. Pseudosubluxation
b. Posterior longitudinal ligament instability
c. Down syndrome
d. Incomplete endochondral ossification

Preferred answer: (a) Pseudosubluxation [78]

Question 85

A 12-year-old male patient with von Hippel-Lindau disease presents with frequent falls and difficulty ambulating. He is found to have an intramedullary spinal cord lesion. On MRI thoracic spine, the mass has a cystic component, enhances with gadolinium, and there is significant spinal cord edema at T8. What is the most appropriate management for this patient's most likely diagnosis?

a. Spinal angiogram with embolization of the draining vein
b. Total surgical resection, followed by chemotherapy and radiation
c. Radiation alone
d. Total surgical resection followed by observation
e. Observation

Preferred answer: (d) Total surgical resection followed by observation [52]

Question 86

Which of the following is true regarding intrauterine repair of myelomeningocele?

a. Decreased rate of post-natal shunt placement
b. Improved motor function at 30 months
c. Decreased rate of tonsillar herniation on imaging studies
d. A and C
e. All of the above

Preferred answer: (e) All of the above [79]

Question 87

An 8-year-old female with Down syndrome presents to the ER complaining of neck pain. Her mother states that she has been having increased difficulty with activities of daily living. On exam, the patient has generalized weakness in all extremities, 3 + hyperreflexia throughout, and an upgoing plantar reflex bilaterally. Lateral x-rays reveal an atlanto-dental interval of 6 mm. Which of the following is the most appropriate management for this patient?

a. Occiput to C2 fusion and C1-2 laminectomy
b. C1 laminectomy and posterior C1-C2 fusion
c. Rigid cervical orthosis
d. Halo placement
e. Cervical laminectomy alone

Preferred answer: (b) C1 laminectomy and posterior C1-C2 fusion [52]

Question 88

A patient presents with progressive scoliosis, at what degree does a patient typically begin to experience respiratory compromise:

a. 45 degrees
b. 60 degrees
c. 90 degrees
d. 100 degrees
e. 120 degrees

Preferred answer: (c) 90 degrees [52]

Question 89

A 9-year-old patient with cerebral palsy undergoes selective dorsal rhizotomy. The patient returns to a four-week post op check and the patient's spasticity is the same as pre-operatively. The patient is complaining of mild lower back pain in the region of the surgery. Which of the following is the most appropriate management?

a. Observation and follow-up in 1–2 months
b. Repeat surgery and possible further root sectioning
c. MRI lumbar spine to assess for infection
d. Intrathecal baclofen administration for possible intrathecal baclofen pump placement
e. Flexion–extension x-rays of L spine to assess for instability

Preferred answer: (a) Observation and follow-up in 1–2 months [80]

Question 90

An infant is found to have a fatty filum terminale. At what stage did this patient have failure of embryological development?

a. Primary neuralation
b. Secondary neuralation
c. Gastrulation
d. Cranial neuropore closure
e. Caudal neuropore closure

Preferred answer: (b) Secondary neuralation[52]

Question 91

A 3-year-old male presents to the ER with fatigue, mild back pain and failure to thrive. MRI of the spine does not reveal any spinal cord compression. The patient is found to have a ventral T10-11 paravertebral mass. Urine testing reveals elevated urine catecholamines. Radionucleotide MiBG testing shows uptake at the same location. What is the best treatment for this patient?

a. Observation
b. Chemotherapy
c. Radiation and Chemotherapy
d. Surgical excision followed by observation
e. Surgical excision followed by chemotherapy

Preferred answer: (b) Chemotherapy. The patient has neuroblastoma. Chemotherapy is first line treatment, especially in absence of neurological deficit or cord compression [81]

Question 92

Approximately what percentage of spinal myelomeningoceles occur outside of the lumbosacral spine?

a. 1%
b. 5%
c. 15%
d. 35%
e. 50%

Preferred answer: (c) 15% [52]

Question 93

A 14-year-old female with history of spinal cord lipoma resection presents to establish care with a screening MRI of the lumbar spine. On the MRI, the conus medullaris terminates at L3. The patient has no back pain, has stable motor exam, and has not had any change in bowel or bladder habits. What is the most appropriate management for this patient?

a. Redo surgery for release of retethering
b. Follow up in MRI in 6 months
c. CT myelogram
d. Urodynamicse. Flexion–extension x-rays

Preferred answer: (b) Follow up in MRI in 6 months [52]

Question 94

A 15-year-old patient sustains a C5 burst fracture with associated spinal cord injury. The patient undergoes surgical decompression stabilization. At the patient's 3 month follow up visit, upright cervical x-rays show bony fusion and stable alignment. However, the patient is reporting radiating pain from the neck into both hands. The pain is worsened during defecation. The patient also reports that his baclofen dose has been increasing due to worsening spasticity. What is the next step in management for the patient's most likely condition?

a. Flexion–extension X-rays of Cervical spine
b. CT scan of the cervical spine
c. MRI Cervical spine without contrast
d. Observation and follow up in 6 weeks
e. Occupational therapy for worsening spasticity

Preferred answer: (c) MRI Cervical spine without contrast to assess for the presence of a syrinx [82]

Question 95

After an MVC, a 6-year-old male patient is found to have a fracture through the C2 synchondrosis. The patient is neurologically intact. MRI shows no spinal canal stenosis or spinal cord injury. Based on 2013 CNS guidelines, how should this fracture be managed?

a. C1-2 posterior spinal fusion
b. Odontoid screw fixation
c. Miami J collar at all times
d. Closed reduction and halo immobilization
e. Occiput to C3 fusion

Preferred answer: (d) Closed reduction and halo immobilization [83]

Question 96

What is the incidence of scoliosis in patients who sustained a spinal cord injury at < 10 years of age?

a. < 10%
b. 10–25%
c. 25–50%
d. 50–75%
e. > 90%

Preferred answer: (e) > 90% [84]

Question 97

Which of the following is true regarding surgery on myelomeningoceles?

a. Preserves all neural elements
b. Complete removal of all skin from the neural elements
c. Cauterization and sectioning of large vessels passing near the placode
d. All of the above
e. A and B

Preferred answer: (e) A and B [52]

Question 98

An 11-year-old patient presents with an intramedullary lipoma. The patient is having progressive weakness and the patient is taken to the OR for resection. Which of the following is important regarding perioperative management?

a. Total resection is needed to prevent recurrence
b. Subtotal resection to decompress the spinal cord is adequate
c. Post-operative adjuvant radiotherapy
d. Bony decompression alone is adequate

Preferred answer: (b) Subtotal resection to decompress the spinal cord is adequate [52]

Question 99

A 12-year-old patient is undergoing a 2nd intramedullary neoplasm resection. After dural opening and prior to myelotomy, SSEP signals are lost. There is no suspicion for blunt injury to the spinal cord. The patient has been hemodynamically stable throughout the case. EEG monitoring is normal. What is the most likely cause?

a. Acute spinal hemorrhage
b. Cerebral infarct
c. Spinal cord infarct
d. Ventral arachnoid cyst
e. Spinal cord hypoperfusion

Preferred answer: (d) Ventral arachnoid cyst [85]

Question 100

A 15-year-old patient presents with acute back pain and quadriparesis with diminished reflexes. MRI with contrast reveals a contrast enhancing non expansile lesion in the thoracic spinal cord. What is the next best step in management?

a. CSF analysis
b. IR biopsy
c. Laminectomy and biopsy
d. Laminectomy and gross total resection
e. Observation

Preferred answer: (a) CSF analysis with high suspicion for transverse myelitis [86]

Question 101

A newborn male is found to have a tethered cord on screening imaging, otherwise spinal imaging is normal. Additionally, the child has tetralogy of Fallot, syndactyly, tracheoesophageal fistula and one kidney. What is the most likely diagnosis?

a. CHARGE SYNDROME
b. VACTERL syndrome
c. 22q11 deletion syndrome
d. Down syndrome
e. Klippel-Feil Syndrome

Preferred answer: (b) VACTERL syndrome [87]

Question 102

When exposing the spinous processes during a posterior approach to the pediatric cervical spine, it is important to stay within which structure to avoid excessive blood loss and post-operative pain?

a. Ligamentum nuchae
b. Prevertebral fascia
c. Alar fascia
d. Trapezius muscle

Preferred answer: (a) Ligamentum nuchae [88]

References

1. Surgery of the Pediatric Spine. Kim. 2008. p. 52–53.
2. Surgery of the Pediatric Spine. Kim. 2008. p. 72–74.
3. Surgery of the Pediatric Spine. Kim. 2008. p. 482–483.
4. Surgery of the Pediatric Spine. Kim. 2008. p. 310–318.
5. Surgery of the Pediatric Spine. Kim. 2008. p. 207–211.
6. Surgery of the Pediatric Spine. Kim. 2008. p. 443–447.
7. Handbook of Pediatric Neurosurgery. Jallo. 2018. p. 321–322.
8. Handbook of Pediatric Neurosurgery. Jallo. 2018. p. 314–316.
9. Handbook of Pediatric Neurosurgery. Jallo. 2018. p. 329–330.
10. Handbook of Pediatric Neurosurgery. Jallo. 2018. p. 391–392.
11. Handbook of Pediatric Neurosurgery. Jallo. 2018. p. 375–376.
12. Handbook of Pediatric Neurosurgery. Jallo. 2018. p. 342–344.
13. Surgery of the Pediatric Spine. Kim. 2008. p. 259–288.
14. Surgery of the Pediatric Spine. Kim. 2008. p. 200–206.
15. Handbook of Pediatric Neurosurgery. Jallo. 2018. p. 372–373.
16. Surgery of the Pediatric Spine. Kim. 2008. p 177–187.
17. Handbook of Pediatric Neurosurgery. Jallo. 2018. p. 373.
18. Carlson B. Human embryology and developmental biology. 3rd ed. St. Louis: CV. Mosby; 2004.
19. Frim et al. Pediatric Surgery. 2006:145–147.
20. Surgery of the Pediatric Spine. Kim. 1st ed. p. 8–9.
21. Surgery of the Pediatric Spine. Kim. 1st ed. p. 28.
22. Surgery of the Pediatric Spine. Kim. 1st ed. p. 32.
23. Surgery of the Pediatric Spine. Kim. 1st ed. p. 33.
24. Surgery of the Pediatric Spine. Kim. 1st ed. p. 83.
25. Surgery of the Pediatric Spine. Kim. 1st ed. p. 97.
26. Surgery of the Pediatric Spine. Kim. 1st ed. p. 153.
27. Youmans, p. 2130.
28. Youmans, p. 2205.
29. Youmans, Page 2205; Surgery of the Pediatric Spine. Kim. 1st ed. p. 174.
30. Youmans, p. 2216.
31. Surgery of the Pediatric Spine. Kim. 1st ed. p. 165.
32. Surgery of the Pediatric Spine. Kim. 1st ed. p. 192.
33. Surgery of the Pediatric Spine. Kim. 1st ed. p. 497.
34. Handbook of Pediatric Neurosurgery. Jallo, p. 392; Principles and Practice of Pediatric Neurosurgery, p. 794–796.
35. Principles and Practice of Pediatric Neurosurgery, p. 599.
36. Principles of Pediatric Neurosurgery, p. 594.
37. Principles of Pediatric Neurosurgery, p. 602.
38. Principles of Pediatric Neurosurgery, p. 600.
39. Principles of Pediatric Neurosurgery, p. 618.
40. Principles of Pediatric Neurosurgery, p. 619.
41. Principles and Practice of Pediatric Neurosurgery, p. 615.
42. Principles and Practice of Pediatric Neurosurgery, p. 295.
43. Principles and Practice of Pediatric Neurosurgery, p. 302.
44. Principles and Practice of Pediatric Neurosurgery, p. 310.
45. Principles and Practice of Pediatric Neurosurgery, p. 797.
46. Principles of Pediatric Neurosurgery, p. 791.
47. Principles of Pediatric Neurosurgery, p. 792.
48. Kim SY, Naqvi IA. Neuroanatomy, Cranial Nerve 12 (Hypoglossal) [Updated 14 Nov 2021]. In: StatPearls [Internet]. Treasure

Island (FL): StatPearls Publishing; 2022 Jan. Available from: https://www.ncbi.nlm.nih.gov/books/NBK532869/
49. Surgery of the Pediatric Spine, p. 100.
50. Surgery of the Pediatric Spine, p. 102.
51. Surgery of the Pediatric Spine, p. 137.
52. None.
53. Surgery of the Pediatric Spine, p. 167.
54. Surgery of the Pediatric Spine. Kim. 1st ed. p. 164.
55. Surgery of the Pediatric Spine. Kim. 1st ed. p. 261.
56. Surgery of the Pediatric Spine. Kim. 1st ed. p. 264.
57. Surgery of the Pediatric Spine. Kim. 1st ed. p. 26.
58. Surgery of the Pediatric Spine. Kim. 1st ed. p. 266.
59. Surgery of the Pediatric Spine. Kim. 1st ed. p. 267.
60. Surgery of the Pediatric Spine. Kim. 1st ed. p. 268.
61. Surgery of the Pediatric Spine. Kim. 1st ed. p. 353.
62. Surgery of the Pediatric Spine. Kim. 1st ed. p. 326.
63. Surgery of the Pediatric Spine. Kim. 1st ed. p. 455.
64. Surgery of the Pediatric Spine. Kim. 1st ed. p. 458.
65. Surgery of the Pediatric Spine. Kim. 1st ed. p. 467.
66. Surgery of the Pediatric Spine. Kim. 1st ed. p. 470.
67. Surgery of the Pediatric Spine. Kim. 1st ed. p. 552.
68. Surgery of the Pediatric Spine. Kim. 1st ed. p. 563.
69. Surgery of the Pediatric Spine. Kim. 1st ed. p. 564.
70. Youmans and Winn, 8th ed., p. 1918.
71. Youmans and Winn, 8th ed., p. 1919.
72. Youmans and Winn, 8th ed., p. 1957.
73. Youmans and Winn, 8th ed., p. 1962.
74. Youmans and Winn, 8th ed., p. 1963.
75. Youmans and Winn, 8th ed., p. 1996.
76. Youmans and Winn, 8th ed., p. 1997.
77. Youmans and Winn, 8th ed., p. 2004.
78. Youmans and Winn, 8th ed., p. 2038.
79. Handbook of Pediatric Neurosurgery, p. 327.
80. Greenberg Handbook of Neurosurgery, p 5440.
81. Handbook of Pediatric Neurosurgery, p. 194.
82. Surgery of the Pediatric Spine. Kim. 1st ed. p. 487.
83. 2013 CNS Management of Pediatric Cervical Spine and Spinal Cord Injuries.
84. ASIA, Surgery of the Pediatric Spine. Kim. 1st ed. p. 399.
85. Surgery of the Pediatric Spine. Kim. 1st ed. p. 269.
86. Absoud M, Greenberg BM, Lim M, Lotze T, Thomas T, Deiva K. Pediatric transverse myelitis Neurology. 2016;87(9 Supplement 2): S46-S52. https://doi.org/10.1212/WNL.0000000000002820
87. Kuo M, Tsai Y, Hsu W, Chen R, Tu Y, Wang H. Tethered spinal cord and VACTERL association. J Neurosurgery: Pediatrics PED. 2007;106(3):201–204. Retrieved 27 May 2022, from https://thejns.org/pediatrics/view/journals/j-neurosurg-pediatr/106/3/article-p201.xml
88. Surgery of the Pediatric Spine. Kim. 1st ed. p. 98.

9 Tumors, Infections, Inflammatory and Vascular Lesions of the Spine

Ravi Nunna, Michael Torres, Wesley Chen, and Sasidhar Karuparti

1. Which of the following most commonly presents with nocturnal back pain in children and adolescents?

   a. Chondrosarcoma
   b. Osteoid osteoma
   c. Hemangioma
   d. Chordoma

Answer: B, osteoid osteoma are non-malignant tumors that often present in the 1st two decades of life, usually involving the posterior elements. They can cause significant pain and sometimes muscle spasms but are not malignant tumors.

2. A patient with intractable neck pain is found to have a vertebra plana at C5. Which of the following lesions is most likely responsible in a patient with no oncological history?
   a. Osteoid osteoma
   b. Prostate cancer
   c. Eosinophilic granuloma
   d. Osteoblastoma

Answer: C, Eosinophilic granuloma of the spine often presents with vertebra plana

3. Which lesion is depicted in the picture (see Fig. 9.1)?

   a. Osteoid osteoma
   b. Chrondrosarcoma
   c. Osteoblastoma
   d. Hemangioma

Answer: D, hemangioma often appears as a spongy appearing vertebral body lesion on CT scan.

4. Which lesion is depicted in the picture below (see Fig. 9.2)?

   a. Chordoma
   b. Chondroma
   c. Osteoid osteoma
   d. Hemangioma

Answer: A, the picture depicts a classic sacral chordoma [4].

5. Which lesion is depicted in the picture below (see Fig. 9.3)?
   a. Chordoma
   b. Chondroma
   c. Osteoid osteoma
   d. Hemangioma

Answer: C, the picture depicts osteoid osteoma, with classic hypodense center with hyperdense rim.

6. What is the first line of treatment for pain related to osteoid osteoma?
   a. Surgery
   b. NSAIDS
   c. Narcotics
   d. Physical therapy

R. Nunna (✉) · M. Torres · W. Chen
Department of Neurosurgery, University of Missouri, Columbia, MO, USA
e-mail: ravisnunna@gmail.com

M. Torres
e-mail: ortiztorresm@health.missouri.edu

W. Chen
e-mail: wesley.chen@health.missouri.edu

S. Karuparti
School of Medicine, University of Missouri, Columbia, MO, USA
e-mail: srkdg2@health.missouri.edu

C. Gragnaniello et al. (eds.), *MCQs in Spine Surgery*,
https://doi.org/10.1007/978-3-031-69332-8_9

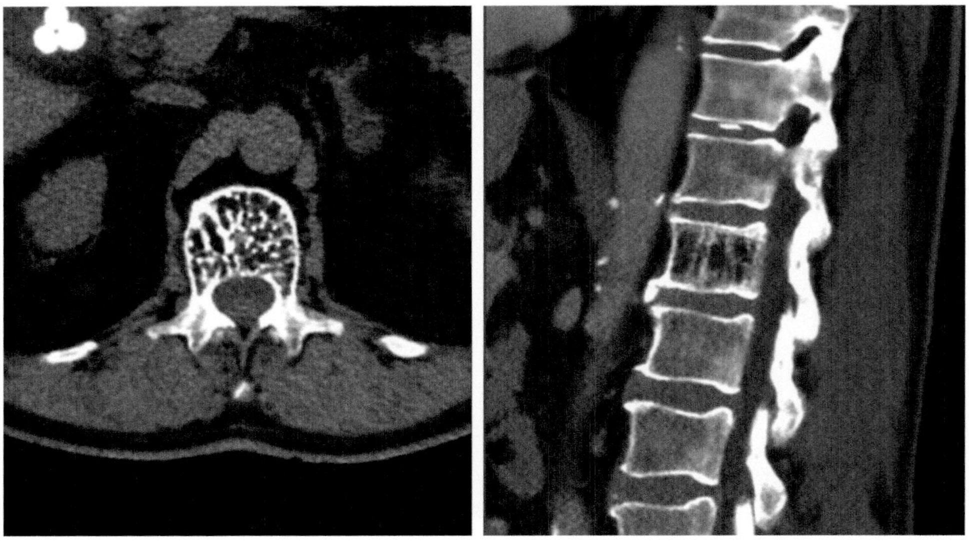

Fig. 9.1 Axial and sagittal CT of the midthoracic spine

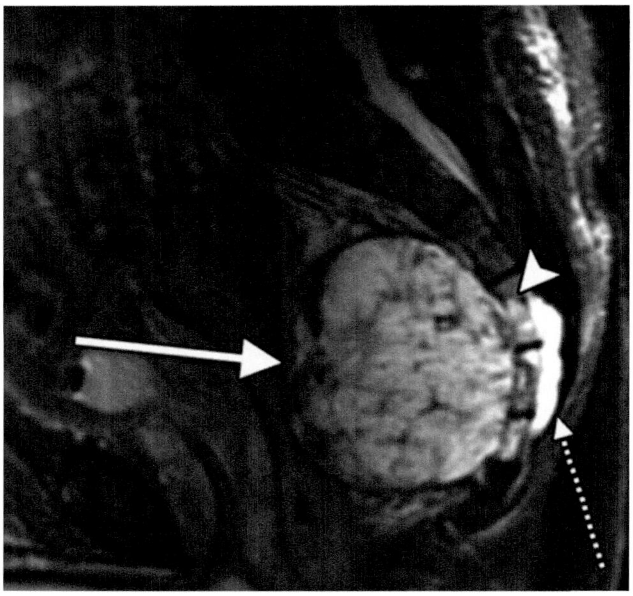

Fig. 9.2 Sagittal T1 post gadolinium image of the sacral spine

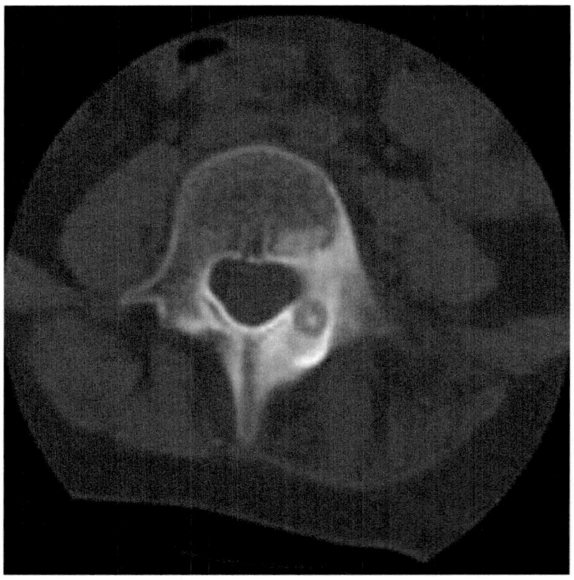

Fig. 9.3 Axial CT of lumbar vertebra [5]

Answer: B, NSAIDS are first line therapy for pain from osteoid osteoma, and a good portion of patients are able to manage the pain with these medications.

7. For sacral chordomas, what is the only independent factor that influences prognosis?
   a. Extent of resection
   b. Radiation
   c. Chemotherapy
   d. Pre-operative symptoms

Answer: A. Wide en-bloc resection is the only independent factor that contributes to reducing tumor recurrence and tumor related death.

8. A patient with axial back pain has MRI imaging showing a bony lesion at L4 with various fluid–fluid levels. What is the lesion most likely to be?
   a. Osteoblastoma
   b. Chordoma
   c. Aneurysmal bone cyst
   d. Hemangioma

Answer: C, the description fits the characteristic appearance of aneurysmal bone cysts.

9. Which of the following is NOT a benign lesion?
   a. Osteoblastoma
   b. Osteoid osteoma

c. Aneurysmal bone cyst
d. Chordoma

Answer: D, Chordoma is a malignant lesion.

10. A nerve sheath tumor is resected from a patient with known neurofibromatosis type 2. What is the lesion most likely to be?
a. Neurofibroma
b. Schwannoma
c. Oligodendroglioma
d. Lymphoma

Answer: B, Patients with NF2 and nerve sheath tumors often have schwannomas, whereas NF1 patients with nerve sheath tumors often have neurofibromas.

11. A patient with back pain presents with imaging showing a mass that protrudes from the T12 spinous process with a cartilaginous cap. Which of the following lesions is this most likely?
a. Osteochondroma
b. Osteoblastoma
c. Osteoid osteoma
d. Chordoma

Answer: A, Description fits osteochondroma of the spine.

12. A patient with a known osteochondroma has continued back pain and is found on repeat imaging to have widening of the cartilaginous cap, and additional osteolytic activity around the growing lesion. What will a biopsy of the lesion most likely reveal?
a. Transformation to osteosarcoma
b. Transformation to chordoma
c. Transformation to chondrosarcoma
d. No change in osteochondroma

Answer: C, transformation of osteochondroma to chondrosarcoma is typically indicated with widening of cartilaginous cap, increasing size and osteolytic activity, and size > 2.5cm.

13. A bony mass on the T11 lamina is resected from a 16-year-old and pathology is confirmed as Ewing's sarcoma. What is the pathological appearance of this mass?
a. Large GFAP staining cells with high mitotic activity
b. Small blue cells
c. Spindle cells
d. Layers of cuboidal cells

Answer: B, Ewing's sarcoma is among the lesions with small blue cells on pathology that can be isolated from bone, which include neuroblastoma, PNET, lymphoma, rhabdomyosarcoma.

14. What is the defining characteristic between osteoblastoma and osteoid osteoma?
a. Pathology
b. Location
c. Size
d. Shape

Answer: C, osteoblastoma is typically > 2cm in size. The remainder of the characteristics are similar between the two lesions.

15. What does this picture most likely depict (see Fig. 9.4)?
a. Chondrosarcoma
b. Chordoma
c. Hemangioma
d. Enostosis

Answer: D, vertebral enostosis is characteristically hyperdense round areas that do not have signal change on MRI or increased metabolic activity on PET scans.

16. Of the below, all are common primary pathologies that metastasize to the spine except

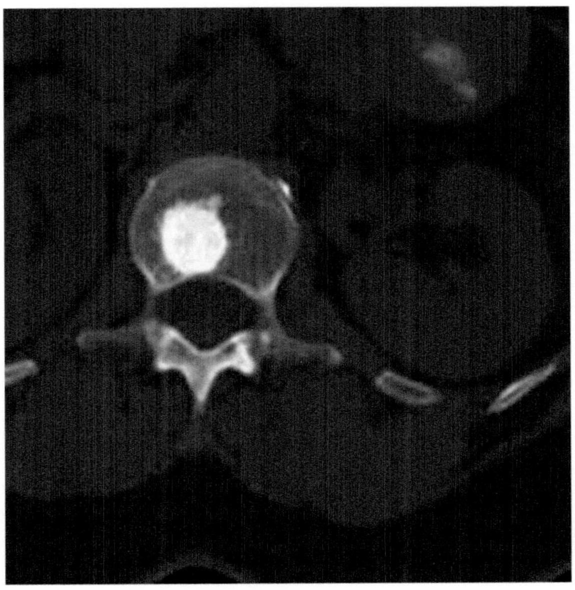

Fig. 9.4 Axial CT of thoracic vertebra

a. Breast cancer
b. Prostate cancer
c. Uterine cancer
d. Lung cancer

Answer: C, breast, prostate, and lung cancers are among the most common with metastases to spine.

17. Of the following, which of these is primarily osteoblastic?
    a. Medullary thyroid carcinoma
    b. Melanoma
    c. Lung cancer
    d. Renal cell carcinoma

Answer: A, medullary thyroid carcinoma and prostate cancer typically present as osteoblastic lesions.

18. Which of the following could present with mixed osteoblastic and osteolytic lesions?
    a. Urothelial carcinoma
    b. Multiple myeloma
    c. Osteosarcoma
    d. Melanoma

Answer: A, urothelial carcinoma, breast cancer, and lymphoma classically can present with both osteolytic and osteoblastic lesions.

19. Which of the following presents with osteolytic lesions?
    a. Melanoma
    b. Multiple myeloma
    c. Renal cell carcinoma
    d. All of the above

Answer: D, all of the above present with osteolytic lesions.

20. What part of the spine is typically involved in metastatic disease?
    a. Anterior vertebral body
    b. Spinous process
    c. Transverse process
    d. Pedicle

Answer: D, the pedicle is typically involved in metastatic disease, to the point where a "missing pedicle sign" is often an indicator of metastatic disease.

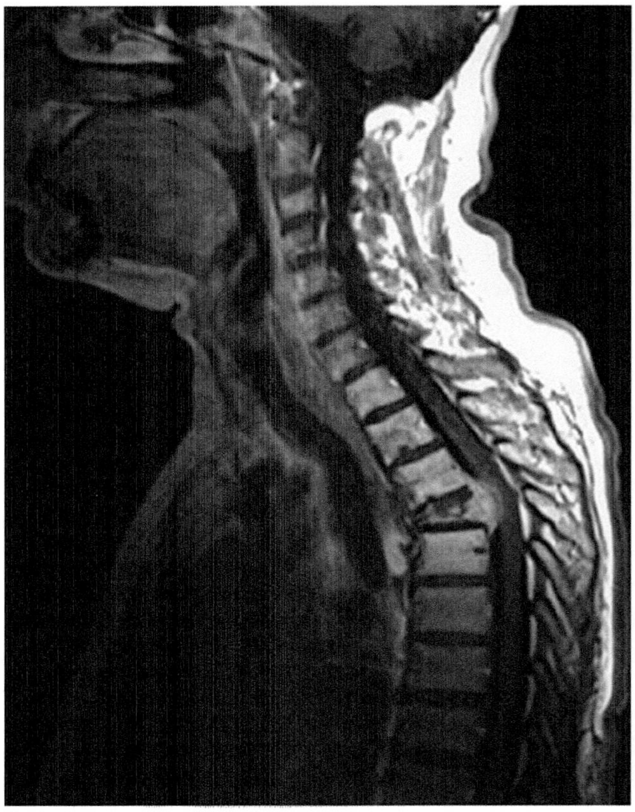

Fig. 9.5 Sagittal MRI post contrast image of the cervical and thoracic spine

21. A 55-year-old female with a history of breast cancer presents with burning pain in a stripe across the right side of her torso that worsens at night. She is otherwise neurologically intact on exam. Shown here is a sagittal T1W post contrast MRI (see Fig. 9.5). What is the next step in treatment for this patient?
    a. Decompression and fusion
    b. Focused radiation
    c. Chemotherapy
    d. IR biopsy of lesion

Answer: A, this patient has a thoracic spinal cord mass that is compressive on spinal cord with a kyphotic deformity as well. Surgical decompression and fusion are warranted.

22. An 85-year-old male with history of prostate cancer presents with diffuse back pain that is worse at night. Imaging reveals widespread metastatic disease in his spine with no spinal cord or spinal element compressions. What is the next step in treatment?
    a. Decompression and fusion
    b. Focused radiation

c. Physical therapy
d. IR biopsy of lesion

Answer: B, radiation is the modality of treatment for widespread metastatic disease of the spine if there is no neurological element involvement.

23. An 80-year-old male presents with diffuse back pain and the below imaging (see Fig. 9.6). What is the likely etiology of their disease?

    a. Prostate cancer
    b. Thyroid cancer
    c. Renal cell carcinoma
    d. Multiple myeloma

Answer: D, the image portrays diffuse bony osteolytic activity representative of multiple myeloma.

24. Which of these is most likely to occur in a 30-year-old male as multiple bony lesions in the spine?
    a. Testicular cancer
    b. Melanoma
    c. Breast cancer
    d. Prostate cancer

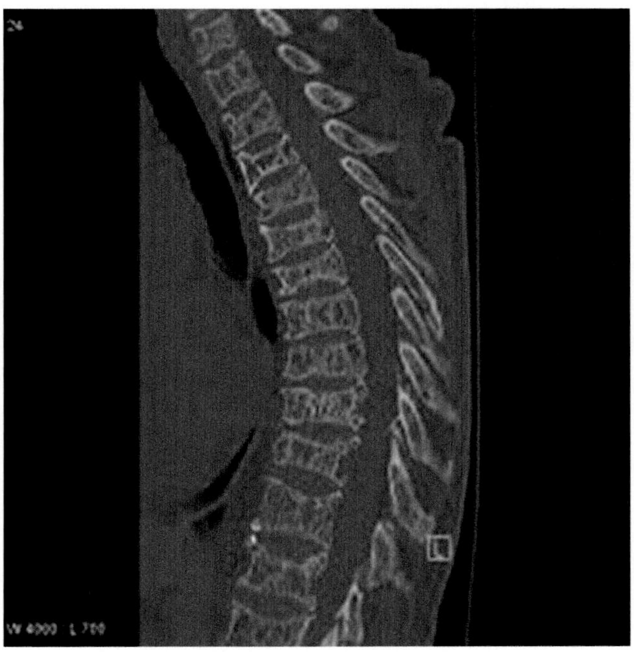

Fig. 9.6 Sagittal CT of the thoracic spine

Answer: B, melanoma has the highest predilection to spinal metastases in the younger population among those listed.

25. A 55-year-old male patient presents with hematuria, weight loss, and nonspecific leg weakness/numbness. What is the most likely diagnosis?
    a. Metastatic disease to the thoracic spine
    b. Thoracic osteomyelitis
    c. Traumatic fracture of the thoracic spine
    d. Osteosarcoma of thoracic spine

Answer: A, the patient likely has renal cell carcinoma with metastatic disease to the spine with neural element compression.

26. Which of the following is most likely to have spinal metastases?
    a. Breast cancer
    b. Lung cancer
    c. Prostate cancer
    d. Lymphoma

Answer: A, ~ 20% of patients with metastatic disease in the spine have breast cancer primaries.

27. A single osteolytic lesion in L3 is found in a 65-year-old male with back pain. Biopsy reveals a malignant process. What is the likely etiology of this lesion?
    a. Drop metastasis
    b. Primary bone lesion
    c. Osteomyelitis
    d. Hematogenous metastasis

Answer: D: The majority of spinal lesions especially in the aged population are derived from metastatic spread from other primary lesions.

28. Which characteristic on imaging helps to differentiate osteomyelitis from metastatic lesion?
    a. Metastases tend to be disc sparing
    b. Osteomyelitis tends to be disc sparing
    c. Metastases tend to involve the vertebral body
    d. Osteomyelitis tends to involve the vertebral body

Answer: A, though not true in all cases, metastatic disease tends to spare the intervertebral discs more often than osteomyelitis.

29. All of the following raise suspicion of metastatic disease to spine in a patient with known malignancy except:
    a. Back pain
    b. Neck pain
    c. Weight loss
    d. Urinary incontinence

Answer: D: Along with classic "B symptoms", metastatic disease to spine often causes back and neck pain without known trauma. Urinary incontinence is a non-specific symptom that is not readily attributable to spinal metastatic disease.

30. In the pediatric population, epidural metastatic disease that causes spinal cord compression is most likely secondary to:
    a. Medulloblastoma
    b. Neuroblastoma
    c. Retinoblastoma
    d. Hemangioblastoma

Answer: B, neuroblastoma and Ewing's sarcoma are the vast majority of epidural metastatic disease in the pediatric population.

31. What is the most common transmission avenue for bacterial osteomyelitis?
    a. Hematogenous
    b. Lymphatic
    c. Direct external contact with pathogen
    d. Ingestion

Answer: A, primary avenue for bacterial osteomyelitis is hematogenous transmission. Patients will frequently have positive blood cultures and potentially concurrent sepsis. However, negative blood cultures do not rule out bacterial etiology of osteomyelitis.

32. What is the expected ESR (erythrocyte sedimentation rate) in a patient who has undergone uncomplicated spine surgery 4 days ago?
    a. 0–20
    b. 20–40
    c. 40–60
    d. Above 60

Answer: D, ESR and CRP are both inflammatory markers utilized to track and diagnose potential infections post-operatively. However, it is important to remember that in the immediate post-operative period, both markers have significant elevations. CRP peaks in the first 2–3 days after surgery, and ESR peaks 4–5 days after surgery, typically to a range of 70–120. CRP will normalize within 2 weeks, and ESR will typically take anywhere between 2–6 weeks to normalize. Hence, an ESR value of above 60 is expected at POD4 and does not in any way raise suspicion for infection.

33. Which chronic medical condition is the single greatest risk factor for developing spinal epidural abscesses?
    a. COPD
    b. CAD
    c. Obesity
    d. Diabetes

Answer: D, Diabetes is the chronic medical condition with the highest correlated risk factor for spinal epidural abscess.

34. What is the most common bacterial organism seen in epidural abscesses?
    a. Staph Epidermidis
    b. Strep Pyogenes
    c. Staph Aureus
    d. Pseudomonas

Answer: C, Staph aureus is the most common organism seen in epidural abscesses.

35. A 70-year-old male with DM, presents with back pain radiating down to legs, urinary retention, perineal numbness, and diminished rectal tone. MRI imaging below (see Fig. 9.7). What is the most appropriate next step in management?

    a. Antibiotics and observation
    b. Physical therapy
    c. Urgent surgical decompression
    d. Epidural steroid injection

Answer: C, this patient has a lumbar epidural abscess with evidence of cauda equina syndrome. Urgent surgical decompression is warranted and should be pursued unless contraindicated.

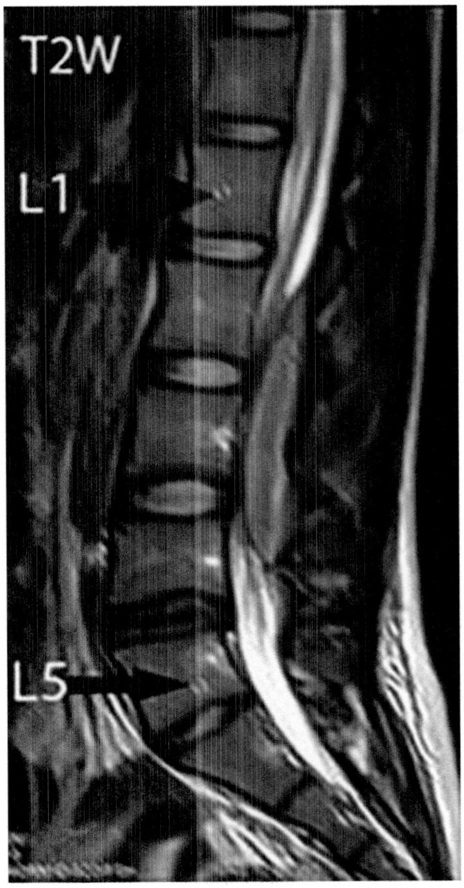

Fig. 9.7 Sagittal T2WI of the lumbar spine

36. A 5-year-old presents with neck stiffness and neck stuck turned to the left with no history of trauma. The patient had a recent respiratory infection. A CT scan shows 25-degree rotatory subluxation of C1 on C2. What is this syndrome called?
    a. POTS syndrome
    b. Lemierre's syndrome
    c. Grisel's syndrome
    d. Guillain Barre syndrome

Answer: C, Grisel's syndrome is a rare syndrome characterized by atraumatic rotatory subluxation of the atlantoaxial joint. This is thought to be secondary to inflammatory ligamentous laxity following infection. Lemierre's syndrome is a thrombophlebitis of the neck. Guillain Barre syndrome is characterized by ascending weakness. POTS is postural orthostatic tachycardia syndrome and is characterized by tachycardia with other symptoms when changing positions. This is thought to be secondary to relative hypovolemic states.

37. 30-year-old HIV + female presents with back pain, fevers, sweats, cough, cavitary lung lesion, with MRI imaging indicating T8 spondylitis without compressive etiology. Spine lesion does not exhibit bony collapse or evidence of instability. What is the best next step in management?
    a. Surgical decompression
    b. Physical therapy
    c. Antibiotics
    d. Biopsy of lesion

Answer: D, patient has risk factors and suspicion for possible spinal tuberculosis, however, many of these risk factors coincide with those of bacterial osteomyelitis. A biopsy would be able to determine this diagnosis. If the patient is neurologically intact and does not have compression on imaging, surgical decompression is not warranted. Antibiotics may be warranted, but a biopsy would be helpful in determining the pathogen.

38. What is the most common cause of spondylodiscitis worldwide?
    a. Staph aureus infection
    b. Tuberculosis infection
    c. Aspergillus infection
    d. Strep hominis infection

Answer: B, Tuberculosis infection is the most common cause of spondylodiscitis in the world. Though it is uncommon in the United States and developed nations, it still accounts for a majority of spinal infections.

39. A 65-year-old female IV drug user presents with back pain, bilateral lower extremity weakness, and fever. MRI obtained indicated below (see Fig. 9.8). What is the most likely responsible organism?
    a. Pseudomonas
    b. Streptococcus
    c. Candida
    d. E. Coli

Answer: A, though staph aureus remains the most common pathogen (in developed nations) involved in spinal epidural abscesses, pseudomonas is much more common in IV drug users than all of the other choices here.

40. 50-year-old male presents with back pain without any other symptoms. Patient had previously been diagnosed with L3-4 osteomyelitis/discitis and was treated with 6 weeks of antibiotics based on positive blood cultures.

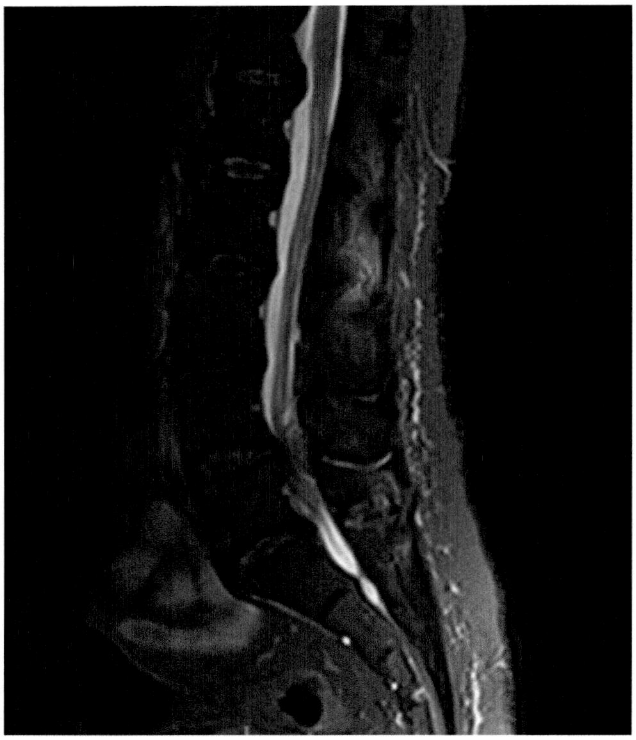

Fig. 9.8 Sagittal T1 post contrast MRI of the lumbar spine [38]

Recent MRI indicated progression of disease with endplate destruction. The patient does not have any neurological symptoms other than back pain. What is the most appropriate next step?
a. Physical therapy
b. Continue prior antibiotics
c. Biopsy
d. Surgical decompression and fusion

Answer: C, Prior diagnosis and treatment was based entirely on blood cultures, and patient displays continued symptoms with imaging findings of progression. It is entirely possible that the organism that is present in the spinal infection is not the same pathogen that was found in the patient's blood cultures, and thus the patient was not adequately treated. Though such a setting would be uncommon, this still warrants a biopsy of the infected area.

41. What cells of the spinal cord does polio affect?
a. Dorsal root
b. Oligodendrocytes
c. Schwann cells
d. Anterior horn cells

Answer: D, polio affects the anterior horn cells resulting in a characteristic weakness without sensory loss. Though it can often be accompanied by hyperesthesias or paresthesias.

42. Shingles is secondary to reactivation of latent zoster virus in what area of the nervous system?
a. Anterior horn cells
b. Dorsal root ganglion
c. Nerve root
d. Medulla

Answer: B. Zoster reactivation in the dorsal root ganglion creates the characteristic dermatomal distribution of hyperesthesias/paraesthesias with cutaneous manifestations.

43. A patient presents with malaise, back pain, fever, leg weakness, and urinary retention. What imaging modality is preferred to best obtain a diagnosis?
a. CT
b. Xray
c. Ultrasound
d. MRI

Answer: D, the patient likely has an epidural abscess, MRI is the imaging modality of choice for elucidation of any compressive etiology in the spine. If MRI is contraindicated, CT myelogram is an alternative.

44. A patient presents with back pain, fever, and MRI showing L4-L5 Discitis/osteomyelitis. A biopsy is obtained but is negative for growth on culture. Blood cultures are negative as well. You would like to start empiric therapy. Which combination of agents is most appropriate?
a. Cefazolin and Flagyl
b. Bactrim and clindamycin
c. Levofloxacin and metronidazole
d. Vancomycin and cefepime

Answer: D, combination of Vancomycin and a cephalosporin with good CNS penetration will cover the majority of pathogens responsible for osteomyelitis/discitis. It is important to keep in mind, though, that anaerobes, tuberculosis, and fungal infections, which make up a very small minority of spinal infections, are not covered by this combination.

45. A patient undergoes lumbar fusion and has a postoperative infection at the surgical site 6 months later.

Imaging reveals that bony fusion has occurred and the patient has back pain and fevers. Which of the following pathogens, if present during the initial infection, should sway decision making towards explanting the prior hardware at this point?
a. E. Coli
b. Tuberculosis
c. Staph Epidermidis
d. Pseudomonas

Answer: C: Many bacteria have the ability to form biofilms, but among the pathogens listed, Staph epidermidis is notorious for forming biofilms on indwelling medical devices that can harbor indolent infections that are resistant to treatment.

Use the following figure (see Fig. 9.9) to answer questions 46–48.

46. A 44-year-old male presents to your clinic for evaluation of neck pain. He has been having pain for several weeks. He is otherwise doing well clinically. No evidence of myelopathy. What is the next best step?
(a) initiation of high dose corticosteroids
(b) pain management referral
(c) biopsy of the C5-6 cord
(d) physical therapy and observation
(e) C5-C7 ACDF

Answer (d)

In a neurologically intact patient with a spinal cord lesion, observation with repeat imaging in 1–3 months is appropriate. Neurologic deterioration will result in acceleration of follow-up.

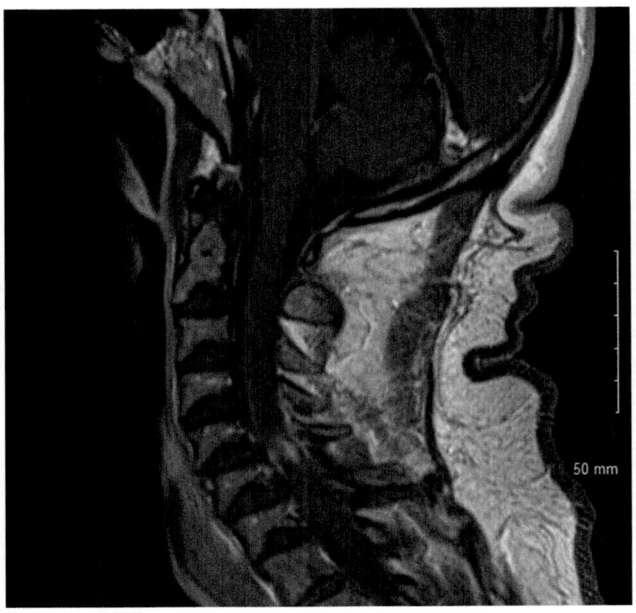

Fig. 9.9 Sagittal T1 post contrast MRI of the cervical spine

47. What is the following is not in the differential diagnosis for this lesion?
(a) astrocytoma
(b) ependymoma
(c) myelomalacia
(d) schwannoma
(e) hemangioblastoma

Answer (d)

Schwannoma is not an intramedullary spinal cord lesion, it is an intradural extramedullary lesion. Long standing myelomalacia can contrast-enhance. Notice the ill-diffuse contrast-enhancement just posterior to the herniated C5-6 disc.

48. The patient returns to clinic in 6 weeks with MRI evidence of an enlarging lesion. Still clinically asymptomatic. You perform a C5-6 laminectomy and biopsy of the lesion. Biopsy results are consistent with astrocytoma. Which of the following is part of the patients' post-operative course?
(a) flat bedrest
(b) chemotherapy
(c) radiotherapy
(d) steroid taper
(e) all of the above

Answer (e)

After resection of an intradural intramedullary tumor, such as an astrocytoma, the post-operative course consists of a steroid taper, approximately 24 h of flat bedrest to promote dural healing and care coordination for chemoradiation, if indicated.

49. Which of the following is the classic MRI description for spinal hemangioblastoma?
(a) homogenously contrast enhancing intradural extramedullary lesion
(b) diffuse intramedullary lesion with ill-contrast-enhancing pattern
(c) cystic lesion with mural nodule
(d) cord-expanding non-contrast enhancing lesion
(e) dumbbell-shaped homogenously enhancing lesion

Answer (c)

A cystic lesion with an associated, often contrast-enhancing, nodule is the classic description for hemangioblastoma.

50. Which if the following syndromes is associated with the development of spinal tumors?

(a) Neurofibromatosis type 1
(b) von Hippel-Lindau
(c) Von Recklinghausen's disease
(d) all of the above
(e) none of the above

Answer (d)

Both neurofibromatosis types 1 and 2 are associated with the development of spinal cord ependymomas and astrocytomas. Von-Hippel Lindau is associated with the development of multiple hemangioblastomas.

Use the following figure (see Fig. 9.10) to answer questions 51–52.

51. A 34-year-old male presents to your clinic with refractory, band-like right-sided chest pain and the above MRI findings. Which of the following is the most likely diagnosis?
    (a) sarcoma
    (b) meningioma
    (c) schwannoma
    (d) neurofibroma
    (e) myxopapillary ependymoma

Answer (c)

A diffusely contrast-enhancing lesion extending through the neuroforamen is classic for schwannoma.

52. What is the best next step in management of this lesion?
    (a) observation
    (b) radiation
    (c) thoracotomy and lateral approach for resection
    (d) laminectomy without costotransversectomy for resection
    (e) laminectomy with costotransversectomy for resection

Answer (e)

Single-level laminectomy with ipsilateral costotransversectomy is usually sufficient for resection of schwannomas with extraforaminal extension. Gross total resection is curative and should be the goal of surgery.

Use the following figure (see Fig. 9.11) to answer questions 53–54.

53. A 27-year-old patient comes to your clinic for MRI evaluation. She has a long-standing history of neck pain and has been getting worse at work with increased activity. A screening MRI was done. What is the most likely diagnosis?
    (a) Cobb syndrome
    (b) plexiform neurofibroma
    (c) metastatic disease
    (d) chordoma
    (e) none of the above

Answer (b)

The most likely diagnosis is plexiform neurofibroma. She has evidence of an extensive contrast-enhancing lesion, involving the neuroforamina, as well as paraspinal and subcutaneous lesions consistent with neurofibromatosis.

54. What is the next best step?
    (a) radiosurgery
    (b) observation
    (c) surgical resection
    (d) proton-beam therapy
    (e) laser interstitial thermal therapy

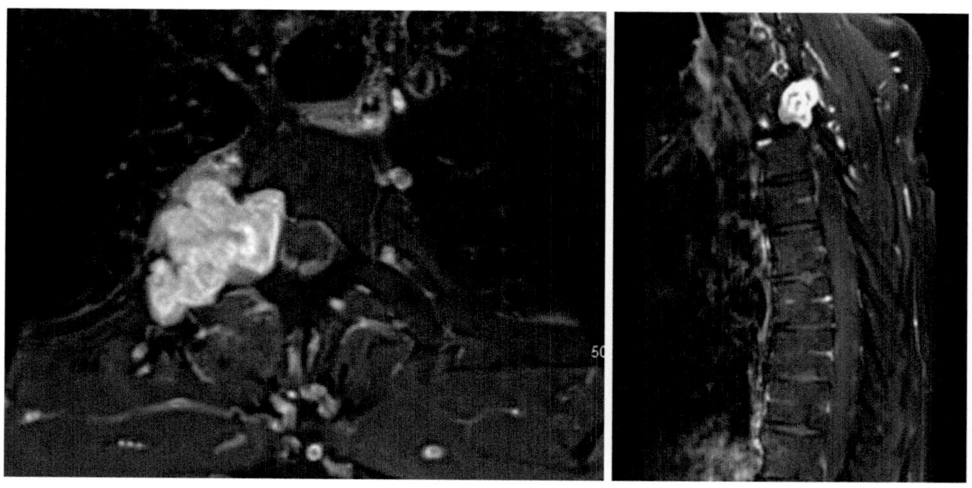

Fig. 9.10 Axial and Sagittal T1 post contrast MRI of the cervical spine

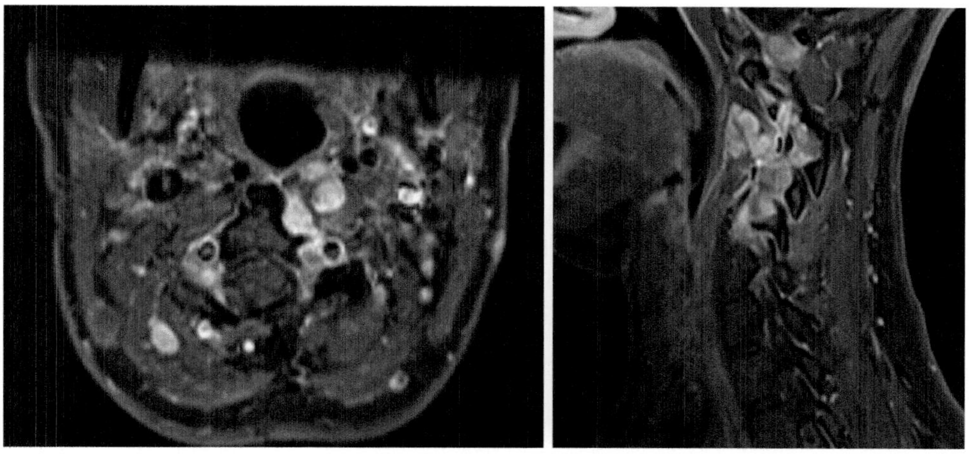

Fig. 9.11 Axial and Sagittal T1 post contrast MRI of the cervical spine [51]

Answer (b)

Unfortunately, plexiform neurofibromas are almost impossible to completely resect. Additionally, recurrence rates are high. The patient should be counseled and referred to genetic testing. Surgical intervention should be reserved for clearly symptomatic, resectable lesions on an as-needed basis.

55. A 14 y/o male presents to the emergency room with urinary retention and bilateral leg pain. MRI images are presented below (see Fig. 9.12). What is the most likely diagnosis?
    (a) tethered cord
    (b) astrocytoma
    (c) neurofibroma
    (d) meningioma
    (e) ependymoma

Answer (e)

A heterogeneously contrast-enhancing lesion of the filum terminale in a teenager is characteristic for myxopapillary ependymoma. Lipomas can also have similar appearance, but it can be noticed that there is an additional lesion at the L1-L2 level, compatible with CSF-seeding associated with ependymomas.

56. Which of the following is true regarding myxopapillary ependymomas?
    (a) they are intradural intramedullary tumors
    (b) they are common in adults
    (c) the classic location is the high cervical spine
    (d) they are highly malignant tumors
    (e) they can present with cauda equina syndrome

Answer (e)

Myxopapillary ependymomas are usually benign intradural extramedullary tumors with excellent prognosis after gross total resection. They can occasionally seed in the CSF and present with multiple lesions. They are most common in young adults and classically present in the filum terminale and/or conus medullary. Cauda equina syndrome

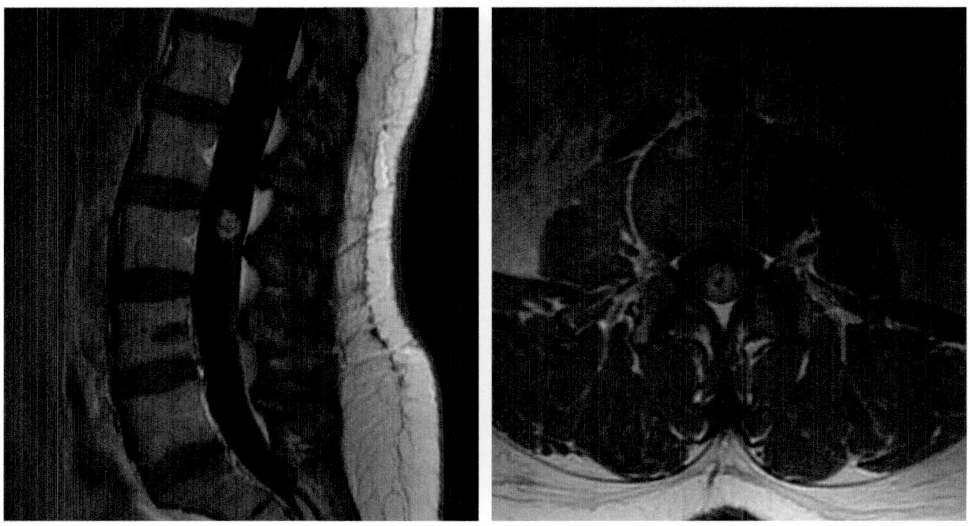

Fig. 9.12 Sagittal and axial T1 post contrast MRI of the cervical spine [53]

is commonly seen, particularly in the setting of tumor hemorrhage.

57. Which is of the following is true about intradural intramedullary spinal tumors?
    (a) are never associated with syrinxes
    (b) gross total resection is achievable for most subtypes
    (c) account for > 75% of all spinal cord tumors
    (d) may be associated with Sturge-Weber syndrome
    (e) none of the above

Answer (e)

Intradural intramedullary spinal tumors account for 20–50% of primary spinal cord tumors. Subtypes include astrocytoma, ependymoma and hemangioblastoma, along with other exceedingly rare tumors. Gross total resection is usually not feasible without neurological injury. Syrinxes can be associated with tumors and usually indicate CSF flow obstruction. Neurofibromatosis and von Hippel-Lindau are the most common genetic diseases associated with primary spinal tumors.

Use the following figure to answer questions 59–60.

58. A 63-year-old female presented to the ER with blurry vision and headaches. MRI revealed the findings shown below (see Fig. 9.13). What is the most likely diagnosis?

    (a) hemangioblastoma
    (b) pilocytic astrocytoma

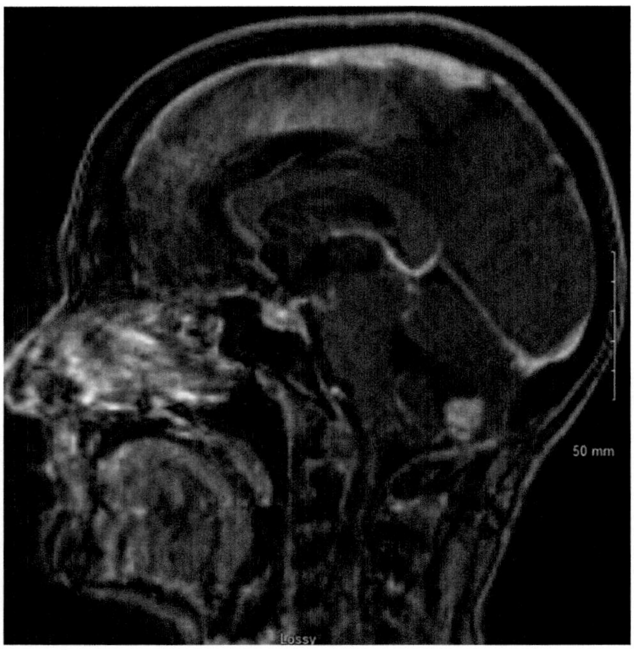

Fig. 9.13 Sagittal T1 post contrast MRI of the brain

    (c) medulloblastoma
    (d) cerebellar metastases
    (e) glioblastoma

Answer (a)

The patient has von Hippel-Lindau. A contrast-enhancing nodule with an associated cyst in the posterior fossa in an adult is classic for hemangioblastoma. The patient's blurry vision might be related to retinal hemorrhages from retinal hemangioblastomas.

59. The patient underwent surgery via a suboccipital craniotomy and gross total resection was achieved. The mass was hemorrhagic and pathology results confirmed hemangioblastoma. What is the best next step in the management of this patient?
    (a) genetic testing
    (b) MRI with and without contrast of the entire spine
    (c) ophthalmology evaluation
    (d) CT abdomen and pelvis with and without contrast
    (e) all of the above

Answer (e)

Gross total resection is often curative for hemangioblastoma. Ophthalmology evaluation for retinal hemangioblastomas is appropriate to identify retinal hemangioblastomas. Contrasted imaging of the spine and abdomen is appropriate to identify additional lesions. Genetic testing will confirm the diagnosis of Von Hippel-Lindau, which is characterized by an autosomal dominant inheritance pattern.

60. A 75 y/o female presents to the ER after multiple falls. She has hyperreflexia, clonus and Babinski's. MRI of the thoracic spine is shown below (see Fig. 9.14). What is the most likely diagnosis?
    (a) meningioma
    (b) schwannoma
    (c) neurofibroma
    (d) radicular artery aneurysm
    (e) ependymoma

Answer (a)

This clearly demarcated, avidly homogenously contrast-enhancing lesion in the thoracic spine is classic for meningioma. Notice the amount of compression and how the cord is displaced towards the right side.

61. What is the most common type of spinal vascular malformation?

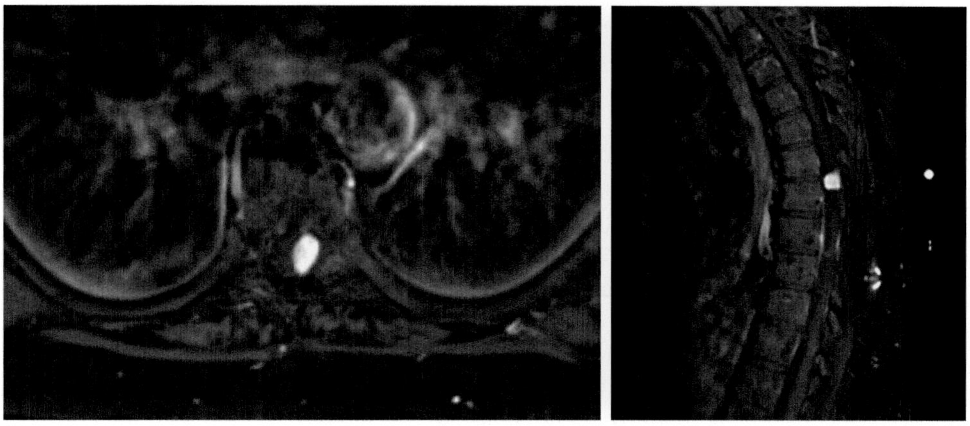

Fig. 9.14 Axial and Sagittal T1 post contrast MRI of the thoracic spine [58]

(a) true arteriovenous malformation
(b) arteriovenous fistula
(c) spinal artery aneurysm
(d) cavernous malformation
(e) spinal hemangioblastoma

Answer (b)

Spinal arteriovenous fistulas are the most common type of spinal vascular malformation and account for 50–85% of malformations.

62. The best imaging test for diagnosis of a spinal cord vascular malformation is:
    (a) CT angiography
    (b) MRI with and without contrast
    (c) Spinal angiogram
    (d) MR angiography
    (e) spinal cord biopsy

Answer (c)

The spinal angiogram is the goal standard imaging test for diagnosis of spinal cord vascular malformations. It provides information about anatomic location, associated vascular lesions, morphology and flow of the malformation.

63. Which of the following genetic syndromes is associated with spinal cord vascular malformations?
    (a) Multiple sclerosis
    (b) Osler-Weber-Rendu disease
    (c) Tuberous sclerosis
    (d) Sturge-Weber syndrome
    (e) Marfan syndrome

Answer (b)

Osler-Weber-Rendu disease, also known as hereditary hemorrhagic telangiectasia (HHT) is an autosomal dominant disease associated with central nervous system vascular malformations, pulmonary arteriovenous fistulas and mucocutaneous telangiectasis.

64. What is the classic configuration of a true spinal dural arteriovenous fistula?
    (a) located at the nerve root sleeve, connection between a spinal radicular artery and a perimedullary vein
    (b) intramedullary nidus with subpial shunting
    (c) anterior spinal artery shunt to pial vein
    (d) aberrant extramedullary spinal artery to nerve root sleeve vein
    (e) diffuse arteriovenous nidus including spinal cord, dura, bone, muscle and sometimes even skin

Answer (a)

Type 1 spinal dural arteriovenous fistulas, also known as angioma racemosum venosum is the classically described true spinal dural arteriovenous fistula. It is located at the nerve root dural sleeve and consists of an abnormal connection between a branch of a spinal radicular artery and a perimedullary vein. These are commonly associated with intradural venous hypertension.

65. What is the predominant pathophysiological mechanism for neurological injury associated with spinal arteriovenous fistulas?
    (a) spinal cord compression
    (b) obstruction of CSF outflow
    (c) hemorrhage, vascular steal and/or venous hypertension
    (d) perinidal aneurysm rupture
    (e) all of the above

Answer (c)

Hemorrhage, vascular steal related to shunting phenomena and mass effect from venous hypertension are the proposed predominant pathophysiological mechanisms for neurologic injury.

66. Which of the following is true regarding Foix-Alajounine syndrome?
    (a) is also known as subacute ascending necrotizing myelitis
    (b) is a result of symptomatic spinal dural arteriovenous malformations
    (c) symptoms include myelopathy, radiculopathy and sphincter dysfunction
    (d) treatment consists of fistula disconnection
    (e) all of the above

Answer (e)

All of the presented options are true.

Use the following figure (see Fig. 9.15) to answer questions 67–80.

67. A 55-year-old female presents to the emergency room with multiple falls, bilateral upper extremity weakness and bilateral positive Hoffmann signs. She has been using a walker for the past 2 weeks due to the increased falls. MRI of the cervical spine with and without contrast was performed (shown). What is the most likely diagnosis?
    (a) acute spinal cord injury
    (b) magnetic artifact- CSF flow voids
    (c) spinal cord arteriovenous malformation
    (d) acute disc herniation
    (e) epidural hematoma

Answer (c)

Notice the posterior epidural serpiginous blood vessels and the intradural nidus at the C5 level with surrounding myelomalacia, classic of true arteriovenous malformations, also known as Type 2 spinal vascular malformation or Glomus AVM.

68. What is the next best step for management of this patient?
    (a) start high dose corticosteroids
    (b) spinal angiogram
    (c) emergent fistula clipping/disconnection
    (d) close observation
    (e) endovascular embolization of associated spinal radicular artery

Answer (b)

A spinal angiogram is the next best step. It will provide additional information about nidus architecture, adjacent anatomy, associated vascular lesions and lesion flow. Corticosteroid use in this scenario is somewhat controversial. Observation in a myelopathic patient might not be in the patient's best interest. Emergent treatment is usually not necessary unless there is acute, compressive hemorrhage.

69. What is the gold standard for treatment of this lesion?
    (a) clipping of the fistulous connection
    (b) resection of the nidus

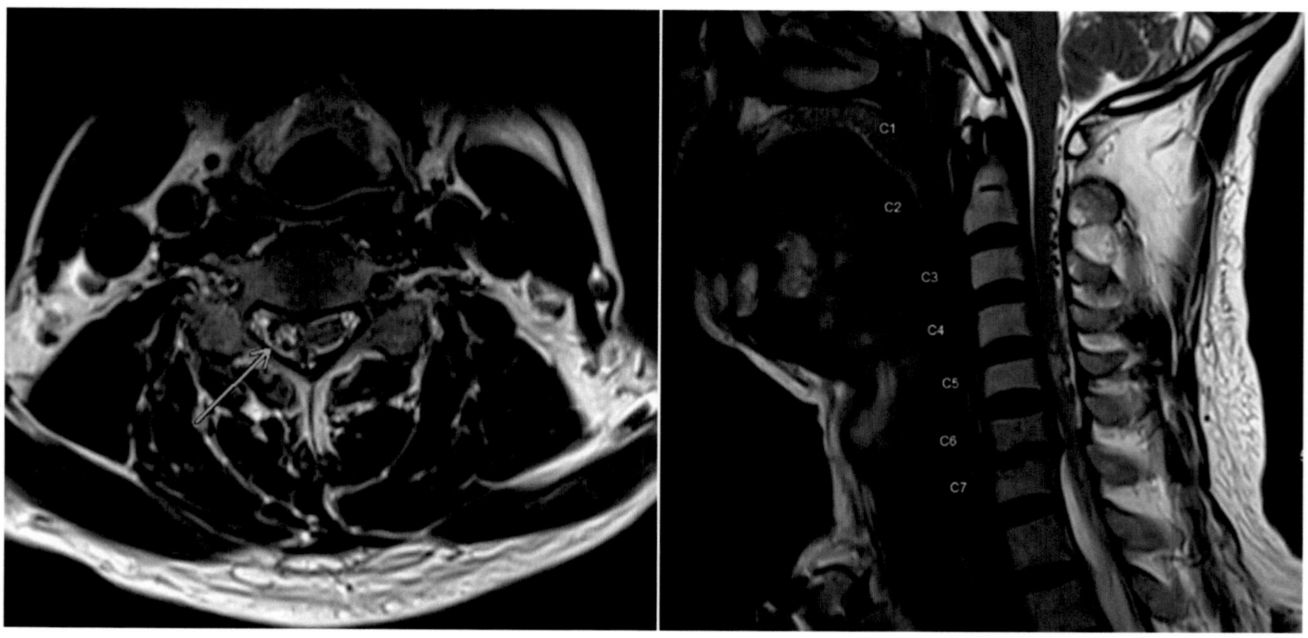

Fig. 9.15 Axial and Sagittal T2t MRI of the cervical spine

(c) high dose corticosteroids
(d) endovascular embolization
(e) none of the above

Answer (b)

In contrast with arteriovenous fistulas, which are treated with precise clipping of the fistulous connection, true arteriovenous malformations can be potentially cured with resection of the nidus. Embolization of feeding arteries may make the nidus smaller and reduce the risk of hemorrhage but is rarely curative and risks occlusion of the nidus' venous outflow and, consequently, AVM rupture.

70. What is the Aminoff-Logue Disability Scale grade for this patient?
(a) 0
(b) 1
(c) 2
(d) 3
(e) 4
(f) 5

Answer (e)

The Aminoff-Logue Disability Scale is a scoring system to stratify the functional status of patients with spinal dural arteriovenous fistulas. Grade 0 is normal. Grade 1 is weakness, gait disturbances but no restriction of activities. Grade 2 is restricted activity. Grade 3 is a patient who requires a cane, stick or some type of simple support for walking. Grade 4 is a patient who requires crutches or a walker. Grade 5 is a patient who cannot stand and is bed- or wheelchair-bound.

71. Which of the following is the reported annual risk of hemorrhage for a spinal AVM?
(a) 0.5–1%
(b) 1–3%
(c) 3–5%
(d) 5–10%
(e) > 10%

Answer (c)

The average annual risk of hemorrhage from a spinal AVM is estimated to be 4% and is markedly increased (two-fold) in patients with prior hemorrhage and associated aneurysms.

72. Spinal cord cavernous malformations account for what percentage of all central nervous system cavernous malformation?
(a) 1%
(b) 5%
(c) 10%
(d) 15%
(e) 25%

Answer (b)

5% of all cavernous malformations of the central venous system are spinal cord cavernous malformation. 20% of patients with spinal cord cavernous malformations also have an intracranial malformation.

73. A 27-year-old Hispanic patient presents to your clinic for evaluation of an abnormal spinal cord finding. MRI revealed T2 hyperintense, non-contrast-enhancing intramedullary lesion at the level of the conus medullaris. The lesion demonstrates a "popcorn" appearance. She also has a history of seizures but has never had a brain MRI performed. Which of the following is the most appropriate recommendation?
(a) obtain a brain MRI
(b) discuss genetic testing
(c) recommend open resection
(d) a & b
(e) a & c

Answer (d)

Familial Multiple Cavernous Malformation Syndrome (FMCMS) is an autosomal dominant disease that results in the occurrence of multiple brain and spinal cord vascular malformations. There is a high incidence in patients with Hispanic descent, classically Mexican descent. Patients with FMCMS are more likely to have spinal cord cavernous malformations.

74. The vascular supply for spinal arteriovenous malformations most commonly derives from which of the following?
(a) anterior spinal artery
(b) posterior spinal artery
(c) radicular arteries
(d) paraspinal arteries
(e) none of the above

Answer (c)

The radicular arteries are the most common source of vascular supply for these lesions. These arteries arise from the T6-L2 levels and are branches of the artery of Adamkiewicz.

75. Which of the following are common findings in patients with spinal cord arteriovenous malformations?
(a) progressive myelopathy
(b) paresthesia
(c) weakness

(d) back pain
(e) all of the above

Answer (e)

Progressive myelopathy, weakness, paresthesia and back are all symptoms attributable to these lesions. Neurologic deficits can sometimes be reversible, related to vascular steal phenomena, and can be the diagnosis elusive. A patient with any of the above symptoms and a suspicious spinal cord imaging finding should have an MRI of the entire spine with and without contrast for adequate diagnosis.

76. Of the following joints, which is frequently affected in rheumatoid arthritis (RA)?
    a. Distal interphalangeal joints
    b. First carpometacarpal joint
    c. Atlantoaxial joint
    d. Lumbosacral joint

Answer: (C) Atlantoaxial joint. The distal interphalangeal joints and the first carpometacarpal joints, unlike the other wrist joints and the proximal interphalangeal joints, are rarely affected in patients with rheumatoid arthritis. The axial skeleton is also rarely affected except for the cervical spine, which is affected in up to 90% of RA patients.

77. A 58-year-old woman presents to the clinic concerned about swollen and tender wrists and knees that are stiff primarily shortly after waking up. She also complains of an inability to completely extend her right index finger at the distal joint. On physical exam, nontender subcutaneous nodules about 5 mm in size were noted on the posterior surface of the left forearm. What pharmacologic agent would likely be indicated for long-term control in this patient?
    a. Methotrexate
    b. Hydroxyurea
    c. Tofacitinib
    d. Rituximab

Preferred Response: (A) Methotrexate. Methotrexate is a folate analog with anti-inflammatory properties and is recommended as the first-line treatment for patients presenting with moderate to severe rheumatoid arthritis. It has no contraindications for use. Hydroxyurea is a ribonucleotide reductase inhibitor that is used as a chemotherapy for myeloproliferative diseases and can be used to induce fetal hemoglobin synthesis in patients with beta-thalassemia or sickle cell disease. However, it has not been shown to benefit rheumatoid arthritis patients. Tofacitinib is a JAK inhibitor that is used as a second-line therapy for patients in which methotrexate does not satisfactorily alleviate symptoms. Rituximab is a tumor necrosis factor α inhibitor that is indicated after methotrexate fails to satisfactorily alleviate symptoms following at least three months of therapy.

78. What is recommended in rheumatoid arthritis patients prior to elective surgery?
    a. Discontinue methotrexate use
    b. Obtain flexion–extension x-rays of the c-spine
    c. Start adalimumab and continue through operation
    d. Discontinue daily glucocorticoids

Answer: (B) Obtain flexion-extension x-rays of the c-spine. Up to 90% of patients with rheumatoid arthritis will present with rheumatoid cervical spondylitis, and the diagnosis is often missed. Preoperative flexion-extension radiographs help evaluate the position of C1 relative to C2 and gauge the risk of spinal cord compression and injury. It is generally recommended to continue methotrexate and glucocorticoids throughout surgery. Tumor necrosis factor α antagonists such as adalimumab have the potential to lead to infections as they intervene in immunological processes. Thus, surgeries should be planned approximately 13 weeks after the last dose with the agent not being restarted until 10-14 days postoperatively.

79. What laboratory test is the strongest indicator of rheumatoid arthritis?
    a. Rheumatoid factor
    b. Anti-cyclic citrullinated peptide antibodies
    c. Anti-nuclear antibodies
    d. C-reactive protein

Answer: (B) Anti-cyclic citrullinated peptide antibodies. In the past, rheumatoid factor (RF) was used as a marker for rheumatoid arthritis. However, anti-cyclic citrullinated peptide (anti-CCP), although having similar sensitivity for RA ($\sim$70% compared to 60-80% for RF), is much more specific for the disease than RF (>90% for anti-CCP vs. 85% for RF). Anti-nuclear antibodies and C-reactive protein can also be elevated and reflective of the severity of the disease (especially CRP).

80. Which of the following is true regarding the etiology of rheumatoid arthritis?
    a. Autoimmune attack primarily occurs against cartilage and bone
    b. Mononuclear cells mediate tissue destruction

c. IL-1 receptor antagonists are ineffective in mitigating the disease process
d. Genetics is not believed to be a risk factor for developing the disease

Answer: (B) Mononuclear cells mediate tissue destruction. There is substantial evidence for a role for $CD4^+$ helper T cells in rheumatoid arthritis, which is characterized by autoimmune attack beginning in the soft tissues that then extends to cartilage and bone later in the course of the disease. T cells activated through interactions between the T cell receptor and class II MHC-peptide antigens can in turn activate B cells, some of which are destined to differentiate into autoantibody-producing plasma cells. This process leads to the formation of immune complexes that could include rheumatoid factors and anti-cyclic citrullinated peptide antibodies inside the joint, amplifying inflammation. Effector T cells stimulate macrophages and fibroblasts in the synovial joint to secrete proinflammatory mediators, including tumor necrosis factor α (TNF-α). TNF-α upregulates adhesion molecules on endothelial cells, promoting leukocyte influx and production of inflammatory mediators such as interleukin 1 (IL-1) and IL-6. Therefore, IL-1 receptor antagonists (such as anakinra) are effective in alleviating RA-associated inflammation. TNF-α also serves to inhibit bone formation and, with other pathways, induce osteoclastogenesis and therefore bone erosion. Major histocompatibility complex alleles HLA-DR1 and HLA-DR4 are associated with an increased risk for RA as well as a host of other autoimmune diseases including type I diabetes mellitus and Addison's disease.

81. Which of the following is true regarding rheumatoid arthritis therapies?
    a. Glucocorticoids are recommended for long-term symptom control
    b. Chosen DMARD therapy should be re-evaluated if minimal disease activity or remission is not achieved by six months
    c. Newer targeted and biologic DMARDs are now preferred to conventional long-term therapies
    d. Targeted DMARDs have fewer immunological side effects than conventional therapies

Answer: (B) Chosen DMARD therapy should be re-evaluated if minimal disease activity or remission is not achieved by six months. Glucocorticoids should be used at the lowest dose possible for the shortest amount of time possible due to its significant potential for toxicity. Conventional long-term DMARDs (such as methotrexate) is still the first line treatment for moderate to severe RA, and methotrexate monotherapy is strongly recommended over all other synthetic and biologic DMARDs in patients with severe disease. Furthermore, patients taking targeted DMARDs have the same potential to acquire severe infections as patients on traditional methotrexate therapy.

82. Which of the following is true regarding subaxial subluxation in rheumatoid arthritis?
    a. Lower c-spine instability is more common than atlantoaxial instability
    b. Atlantoaxial c-spine instability is typically not seen with subaxial subluxation
    c. Steroid therapy can help prevent lower c-spine instability
    d. Subaxial subluxation is often observed in patients with subcutaneous rheumatoid nodules

Answer: (D) Subaxial subluxation is often observed in patients with subcutaneous rheumatoid nodules. Lower c-spine instability is observed in approximately 20% of patients with rheumatoid arthritis while the incidence of atlantoaxial instability is 50-80%. Upper c-spine instability is often seen in patients presenting with lower c-spine instability. Steroid therapy can cause decreased bone mineral density resulting in c-spine instability and is a significant risk factor for subaxial subluxation.

83. Which radiographic finding is most consistent with cranial settling in rheumatoid arthritis?
    a. Superior tip of the dens is 5 mm above McGregor's line
    b. C2 is 15 mm below the line connecting the anterior and posterior arches of C1
    c. McRae's line is 2 mm above the superior tip of the dens

Answer: (A) Superior tip of the dens is 5 mm above McGregor's line. McGregor's line is defined as the line from the posterior edge of the hard palate to the caudal posterior occiput curve. Cranial settling is present when the superior tip of the dens is greater than 4.5 mm above this line. The Ranawat C1-C2 index is defined as the distance from the center of C2 pedicle to a line connecting the anterior and posterior C1 arches. Normal measurement in men is around 17 mm and 15 mm in women, and a distance of less than 13 mm is consistent with impaction. McRae's line defines the opening on the foramen magnum. The tip of the dens may protrude slightly above this line, but if the dens is below this line, then impaction is not present (see Fig. 9.16).

84. A 68-year-old woman with rheumatoid arthritis presents with a Ranawat C1-C2 index of 11 mm and an

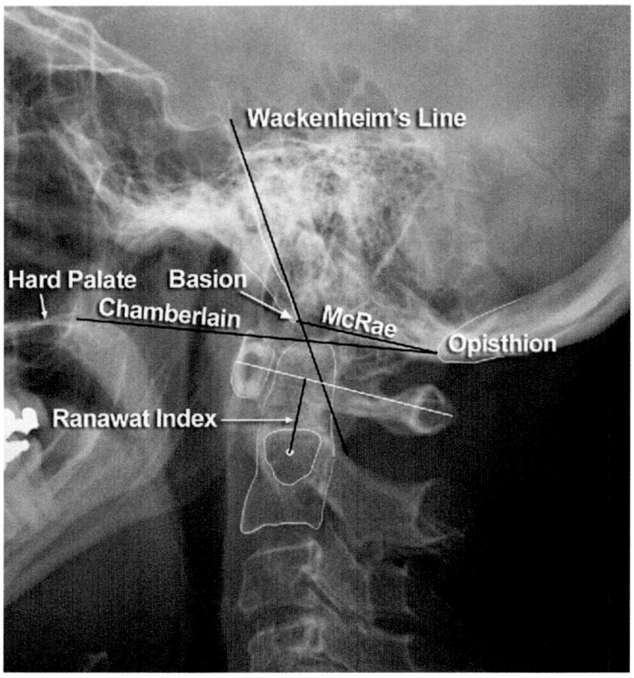

Fig. 9.16 Lateral XR of the cervical spine with depiction of cervico occipital parameters (from: Wasserman, Bradley R. et al. "Rheumatoid arthritis of the cervical spine–clinical considerations." *Bulletin of the NYU hospital for joint diseases* 69 2 (2011): 136–48) [93]

odontoid process protruding 2 mm above McRae's line on radiograph. What would be the next steps in management for this patient?
   a. C2 to occiput fusion
   b. Posterior fusion
   c. Start high dose glucocorticoid therapy
   d. Obtain CT and MR images

Preferred Response: (D) Obtain CT and MR images. A Ranawat index less than 13 mm and odontoid process above McRae's line are strongly suggestive of atlantoaxial subluxation with cranial settling. In such patients, occiput-C2 fusion is indicated. However, it is prudent to obtain further imaging prior to operating. CT is useful to better delineate bony anatomy. MRI will help evaluate the degree of spinal cord compression and identify myelomalacia, thus determining whether resection of the posterior C1 arch is necessary for complete decompression.

85. Which of the following is indicated in patients presenting with Ranawat class IIIB myelopathy?
   a. Posterior C1-C2 fusion
   b. Transoral retropharyngeal odontoid resection
   c. C2 to occiput fusion with resection of posterior C1 arch
   d. No surgical intervention is indicated

Preferred Response: (D) No surgical intervention is indicated. Ranawat classifications for cervical myelopathy range from I (pain, no neurologic deficit) to IIIB (objective weakness, long tract upper motor nerve signs, and an inability to ambulate). Patients with class IIIB myelopathy have severe basilar invagination. Surgical intervention is extremely risky and associated with a poor prognosis. C2 to occiput fusion or odontoid resection is indicated in patients with basilar invagination, and posterior C1-C2 fusion is indicated to resolve atlantoaxial instability. However, the three options would be contraindicated due to poor likelihood of success.

85. When should a resection of the posterior C1 arch be considered to resolve symptomatic atlantoaxial subluxation?
   a. Subaxial subluxation > 4 mm
   b. Anterior atlanto-dens interval > 10 mm
   c. Posterior atlanto-dens interval < 14 mm
   d. Ranawat C1-C2 index < 13 mm

Answer: (D) Ranawat C1-C2 index < 13 mm. Subaxial subluxation greater than 4 mm indicates cord compression and is treated by posterior fusion and wiring at the level of subluxation. An anterior atlanto-dens interval (AADI) greater than 10 mm and posterior atlanto-dens interval (PADI) less than 14 mm are general indications for surgery but are not in and of themselves an indication for resection of the posterior C1 arch. Often, a posterior C1-C2 fusion is sufficient to resolve symptoms and decompress the spinal cord. Subaxial subluxation does not call for decompression at the C1 level. A Ranawat index less than 13 mm suggests impaction due to basilar invagination. A C2 to occiput fusion is the recommended approach, but C1 posterior arch resection may be required if the atlantoaxial subluxation is not reducible.

86. Which of the following is not an indication for a posterior fusion?
   a. Anterior atlanto-dens interval of 11 mm between flexion and extension views
   b. Ranawat C1-C2 index of 7 mm and indications of brain stem compromise
   c. Subaxial subluxation of 5 mm
   d. Cervicomedullary angle of 120° on MRI

Answer: (B) Ranawat C1-C2 index of 7 mm and indications of brain stem compromise. Whenever there are indications of brain stem compromise with basilar invagination, a transoral, anterior retropharyngeal or endonasal odontoid resection is suggested. For atlantoaxial subluxation (as suggested by an AADI greater than 3.5 mm between flexion and extension views), posterior C1-C2 fusion is indicated. Posterior fusion of affected cervical levels is indicated with subaxial subluxations greater than 4 mm. A cervicomedullary angle of less than 135° in the context of basilar invagination suggests impending neurologic impairment which would be surgically treated by a C2 to occiput fusion or an odontoid resection.

87. What finding is most suggestive of neurologic compromise in subaxial subluxation due to rheumatoid arthritis?
    a. Cervical height index < 2.0
    b. Subluxation > 4 mm/20%
    c. Presence of > 1 subluxation
    d. Presence of subcutaneous rheumatoid nodules

Answer: (A) Cervical height index < 2.0. The cervical height index is a method for assessing subaxial subluxation that accounts for the contribution of subluxations at multiple levels along with the loss of disk height and bony collapse. It is calculated by first determining the distance from the center of the C2 sclerotic ring to the tip of the C2 spinous process. This distance is then divided by the distance from the center of the C2 sclerotic ring to the midpoint of the inferior border of the C7 vertebral body by the distance. A cervical height index less than 2.0 is almost 100% sensitive and specific for predicting neurologic compromise. Subluxation greater than 4 mm or 20% and the presence of more than one subluxation may increase the risk for neurologic compromise but are not particularly sensitive nor specific. The presence of subcutaneous rheumatoid nodules, while associated with subaxial subluxation, has not been shown to be associated with neurologic compromise.

88. When is conservative management **NOT** advised over surgical intervention?
    a. 5 mm subaxial subluxation without concomitant pain or neurologic symptoms
    b. Ranawat C1-C2 index of 15 mm with neurologic symptoms
    c. Posterior atlanto-dens interval of 12 mm without neurologic symptoms
    d. Lateral subluxation of C1 on C2

Answer: (C) Posterior atlanto-dens interval of 12 mm without neurologic symptoms. A PADI of less than 14 mm is an indication for posterior C1-C2 resection regardless of the presence of neurologic symptoms due to the significantly increased risk for injury. The other answer choices indicate alterations of the vertebral canal that may result in neurologic compromise but can be conservatively managed as long as evidence of compromise does not manifest.

89. A 65-year-old woman diagnosed with rheumatoid arthritis ten years ago comes into the ED with ataxia, headache, neck pain and stiffness. Physical exam reveals bilateral upper and lower extremity weakness, patellar hyperreflexia, and loss of sensation in the hands and toes although she is still ambulatory. Flexion–extension XR reveals a space available for cord (SAC) of 12 mm. She had a posterior C1-C2 fusion a little less than one year ago. What intervention would be recommended in this case?
    a. Occiput-C2 fusion with resection of posterior C1 arch
    b Odontoidectomy
    c. Posterior C1-C2 fusion
    d. Conservative management with steroid therapy

Preferred Response: (B) Odontoidectomy. Odontoidectomies are rarely indicated for simple atlantoaxial instability but are used as a secondary procedure when there is residual anterior cord compression following a posterior spinal fusion. In this case, the residual compression is likely due to pannus formation that failed to resolve with time as it usually would following posterior fusions. Occiput-C2 fusion is typically only indicated with basilar invagination. Posterior C1-C2 fusion, which failed once, is unlikely to work. Conservative management is not indicated in this patient as the space available for the spinal cord (SAC, which is equivalent to PADI) is less than 14, indicating a significant risk for neurologic injury without surgical intervention.

90. Which MHC allele is commonly found in patients with ankylosing spondylitis (AS)?
    a. HLA-DQ8
    b. HLA-DR4
    c. HLA-B27
    d. HLA-A3

Answer: (C) HLA-B27. Greater than 90% of patients presenting with ankylosing spondylitis present with the HLA-B27 allele of major histocompatibility complex (MHC) I. However, fewer than 10% of HLA-B27-positive patients have symptoms of AS. The exact mechanism by which HLA-B27 contributes to AS is unknown, but it is speculated that HLA-B27 can aggregate with peptides in the joints to lead to a degenerative cascade. Alternatively, it also has been speculated that HLA-B27 can cause a cytotoxic T-cell autoimmune reaction, leading to joint inflammation and degeneration. HLA-DQ8 is a MHC I allele associated with gluten-sensitive enteropathies–such as Celiac disease. HLA-DR4 is an MHC II allele that is associated with rheumatoid arthritis (RA), type 1 diabetes mellitus, pemphigus vulgaris, and Addison's disease. HLA-A3 is an MHC I allele associated with hemochromatosis.

91. Which is true regarding the pathogenesis of ankylosing spondylitis?
    a. Soft tissue, bone, and cartilage are destroyed in a TNF-mediated autoimmune reaction
    b. Decreased levels of endogenous bone morphogenetic protein (BMP)-inhibitors may contribute to syndesmophyte formation
    c. A hyperinsulinemic state may lead to an increase in calcium deposits leading to syndesmophyte formation
    d. Bony erosion occurs due to pervasive RANKL-expressing cells

Answer: (B) Decreased levels of endogenous BMP-inhibitors may contribute to syndesmophyte formation. Recent research has demonstrated that levels of sclerostin, DKK1, endogenous inhibitors of BMP are decreased in AS patients. In rheumatoid arthritis, a TNF-mediated autoimmune reaction results in the destruction of soft tissue, bone, cartilage. The TNF-mediated reaction leads to a signaling cascade that results in the infiltration of RANKL-expressing cells, resulting in non-osteoclast-mediated bony erosion. In diffuse idiopathic skeletal hyperostosis, hyperinsulinemia is believed to lead to an increase in calcium deposits which in turn leads to nonmarginal syndesmophyte formation.

92. What treatment is considered to be most vital in the treatment of ankylosing spondylitis?
    a. NSAIDs
    b. Regular physical therapy
    c. Infliximab
    d. Tofacitinib

Answer: (B) Regular physical therapy. Regular physical therapy best facilitates the maintenance of range of motion and posture—a critical goal for AS patients. NSAIDs are the first-line pharmacological therapy for AS; however, their utility is largely to help control joint pain and inflammation. Infliximab, a tumor necrosis factor (TNF) α inhibitor, is a second-line therapy used in AS that blocks TNF-α, a key protein in the inflammatory chain reaction that leads to joint inflammation, pain, and injury. Tofacitinib, a Janus kinase (JAK) inhibitor, has been shown to significantly increase the ASAS40 response rate (the rate at which patients achieve an improvement of at least 40% on the Assessment in Ankylosing Spondylitis). However, it typically only considered for use in patients who do not respond to NSAIDs, TNF-α inhibitors, or antiinterleukin-17 antibodies.

93. What labs are useful for establishing a diagnosis of ankylosing spondylitis?
    a. Erythrocyte sedimentation rate
    b. Rheumatoid factor
    c. Anti-nuclear antibodies
    d. Urine phosphoethanolamine

Answer: (A) Erythrocyte sedimentation rate. Labs generally have little diagnostic value for ankylosing spondylitis. Diagnosis of AS is primarily made from a clinical and radiographic standpoint. According to the Assessment of Spondyloarthritis International Society, diagnosis of AS can be made in a patient with lower back pain for greater than three months in patients less than 45 years of age and presenting with either: (1) sacroiliitis confirmed by XR or MRI and at least one typical clinical or laboratory finding or (2) a positive HLA-B27 test and at least two typical clinical or laboratory findings. Relevant clinical findings include inflammatory back pain, dactylitis, arthritis, enthesitis, uveitis, IBD, psoriasis, positive family history for AS, symptom relieved in 24-48 hours by NSAIDs. Laboratory findings include positive HLA-B27 and elevated ESR and CRP.

Rheumatoid factor and ANA are negative—which is why AS is often referred to as a seronegative spondyloarthropathy. Urine phosphoethanolamine is elevated in hypophosphatasia and is not useful for diagnosing AS.

94. A 40-year-old male presents with lower back stiffness and pain that has progressively gotten worse over the past year. A radiograph has already been obtained and is shown below (see Fig. 9.17). What additional finding would support a diagnosis of ankylosing spondylitis?
    a. Subcutaneous nodules
    b. Uveitis
    c. Type 2 diabetes mellitus
    d. Psoriatic lesions on the elbows and knees

Answer: (B) Uveitis. Acute anterior uveitis and iritis is a common systemic manifestation of ankylosing spondylitis. Subcutaneous nodules can be found in patients with rheumatoid arthritis but not in AS patients. Diffuse idiopathic skeletal hyperostosis is often found in patients with type 2 diabetes mellitus and in other conditions associated

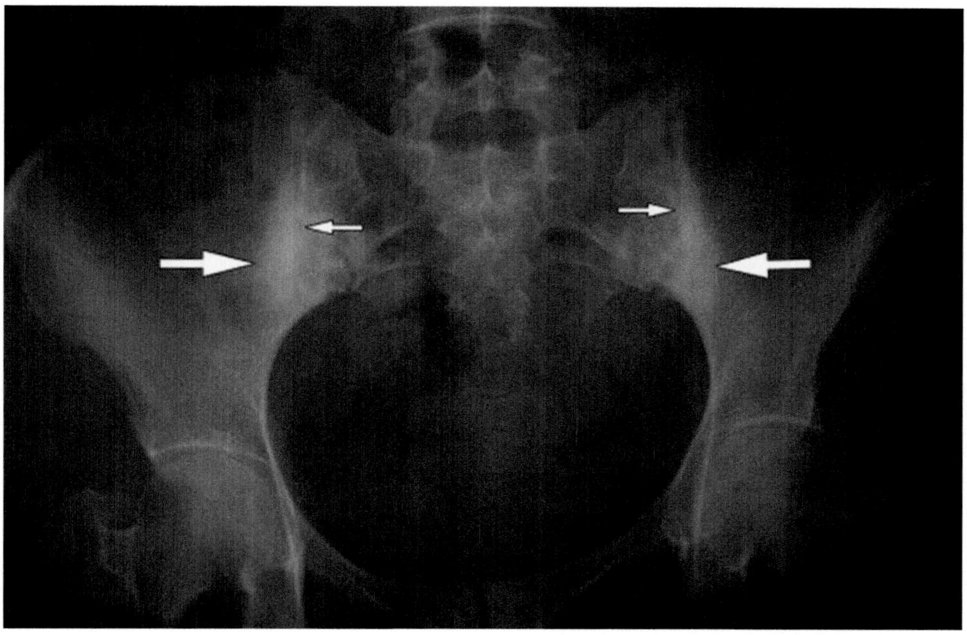

Fig. 9.17 AP XR of the sacro iliac joints. Credit to www.radiologykey.com

with increased insulin levels in the blood and can present similarly to AS. Type 2 DM has not been shown to be associated with AS. Psoriatic lesions indicate the presence of psoriasis which can cause psoriatic arthritis, which is distinct from AS.

95. Which finding is the most specific for diagnosing ankylosing spondylitis?
    a. Decreased spine flexion
    b. Positive Faber test
    c. Positive HLA-B27
    d. Limitation of chest wall expansion to < 2 cm

Answer: (D) Limitation of chest wall expansion to < 2 cm. In the context of inflammatory back pain with insidious onset in the 3rd decade of life, limitation of chest wall expansion to less than two centimeters is the most specific indicator of ankylosing spondylitis; it is even more specific than the presence of the HLA-B27 allele, which is present in 90-95% of AS patients. Decreased spine motion is often found in AS patients, and the Schober test can be used to evaluate lumbar stiffness. The Faber test, a sacroiliac provocative test in which the hip is flexed, abducted, and externally rotated, can be used to determine if there is inflammation of the sacroiliac joint. A positive Faber test, in which the flexion, abduction, and external rotation of the hip causes pain, is a typical finding in AS.

96. In patients with ankylosis spondylitis, spinal fractures can occur after minor trauma or even spontaneously. What should **NOT** be done in treatment following trauma in an AS patient?
    a. Place the patient in a cervical collar
    b. Perform a full neurological examination
    c. Perform CT to assess for spinal fractures
    d. Maintain the patient's preinjury spinal alignment

Answer: (A) Place the patient in a cervical collar. As many AS patients have a fixed kyphosis, attempting to reposition the spine into a neutral position by placing the occiput, shoulders, and hips in alignment can result in spinal cord injury. As a result, it is best to attempt to maintain the patient's preinjury alignment. This can be achieved using pillows or wedges underneath the head and upper back. Performing a full neurological examination and getting a CT or MRI to assess for fractures is standard protocol for trauma suspected to involve the spine. Spinal fracture should have a higher index of suspicion in patients with known AS.

97. A 35-year-old man comes into the ED after slipping while shoveling snow off his driveway. He reports new sharp, severe pain in his lower neck, but neurological exam reveals no deficits with + 2 DTRs throughout and strength 5/5. Past medical history is significant for ankylosing spondylitis for which he is taking meloxicam and etanercept. A CT was obtained which revealed an extension-type fracture at C8 with no evidence of an epidural hematoma. Twelve hours later, the patient reported feeling numbness in his arms and legs, and neurological exam revealed a decrease in strength of plantar and dorsiflexion. An MRI was emergently

obtained which revealed an epidural hematoma located posteriorly to the spinal cord. What is the appropriate next step in management?
a. Start high-dose IV methylprednisolone
b. Anterior decompression with fusion
c. Posterior laminectomy without fusion
d. Posterior laminectomy with fusion

Preferred Response: (D) Posterior laminectomy with fusion. High-dose methylprednisolone has been shown to have neuroprotective effects following spinal cord injury. It is believed that this effect is mediated by limiting posttraumatic oxygen free radical-induced lipid peroxidation. However, given that this patient is experiencing acute neurologic compromise due to spinal cord compression urgent surgical intervention is indicated in this situation. Given that the source of compression is located posteriorly to the spinal cord, the surgical approach should be posterior. Instrumented fusion is recommended in patients with AS due to long lever arms of the ankylosed spine and likely presence of osteoporosis.

98. A 67-year-old man presents with an inability to lift his head and look ahead. Radiographs reveal a severe cervicothoracic "chin-on-chest" deformity (see Fig. 9.18). He was diagnosed with ankylosing spondylitis ten years ago, but despite pharmacologic management with ibuprofen, infliximab, and tofacitinib, his condition progressively got worse. What is the most appropriate management for this patient?
a. Posterior fusion in situ
b. Anterior osteotomy with posterior fusion and instrumentation
c. Posterior extension osteotomy with fusion and instrumentation
d. Halo immobilization

Preferred Response: (C) Posterior osteotomy with fusion with instrumentation. This patient suffers from a progressively worsening kyphotic deformity of his cervicothoracic spine (see XR below). Posterior extension osteotomy will correct the deformity and subsequent fusion with instrumentation will prevent subluxation of the osteotomy site. It is recommended that the osteotomy be performed at the C7-T1 junction due to various anatomic advantages, including that the vertebral vessels are anterior to the spine and not located in the transverse foramina, and a wider spinal canal. Posterior fusion in situ would prevent further kyphosis but would fail to correct the existing deformity. An anterior approach to the osteotomy would be technically challenging and fail to allow access to the C7 pedicle which is essential to correct the cervicothoracic kyphosis. Halo immobilization would also fail to correct the kyphosis.

99. Which radiographic finding is most indicative of ankylosing spondylitis?
a. Nonmarginal syndesmophytes
b. Osteopenia
c. Scalloping of vertebral bodies
d. Subaxial subluxation

Answer: (C) Scalloping of vertebral bodies. Scalloping of vertebral bodies is a characteristic radiographic finding of AS and is referred to as "bamboo spine" due to the spine of patients with advanced AS having a striking resemblance to a bamboo tree (see Fig. 9.19). Although syndesmophytes are present in AS, they are marginal in nature (they originate from the margin between the intervertebral disc and the vertebral body). Nonmarginal syndesmophytes are seen in diffuse idiopathic skeletal hyperostosis. Osteopenia, although seen with AS, is a nonspecific finding. Subaxial subluxation does not typically occur in AS and is more commonly seen with rheumatoid arthritis.

100. A 71-year-old male diagnosed with ankylosing spondylitis 31 years ago comes into office with sagittal imbalance and an inability to stand straight. Until eight years ago, his condition was well-managed through ibuprofen initially with etanercept added to his treatment regimen later. Since then, he has been experiencing progressive stiffness and lower back pain. Radiographs reveal a thoracolumbar kyphotic deformity. What is the best choice in management for this patient?
a. Multi-segment opening wedge osteotomy
b. Single-level opening wedge osteotomy
c. Vertebral body resection
d. Closing wedge osteotomy

Preferred Response: (D) Closing wedge osteotomy. Over a multi-segment opening wedge osteotomy (multi-level OWO), single-level opening wedge osteotomy (single-level OWO), or a vertebral body resection, a closing wedge osteotomy (CWO) offer the greatest deformity correction–of 30 to 40 degrees per level versus 20–30 degrees with the other techniques. CWO also offers the best fusion and stability due to direct bony apposition. A multi-level OWO has advantages over a single-level OWO in that due to distributing the correction over multiple levels, a multi-level OWO has less bone loss than a CWO or a single-level OWO and preserves the anterior longitudinal ligament unlike a single-level OWO.

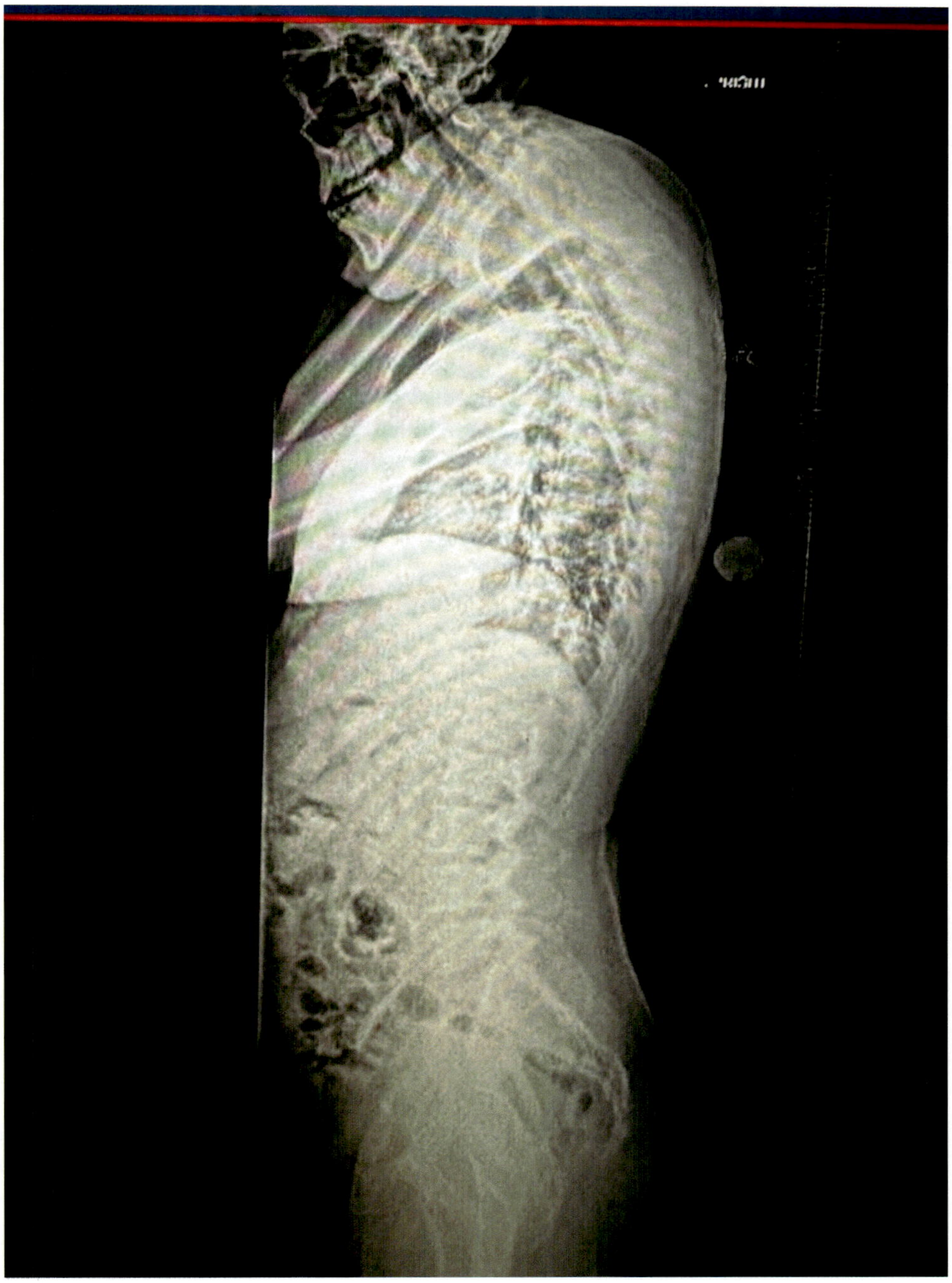

Fig. 9.18 Lateral XR demonstrating chin on chest deformity (from Dr. Gragnaniello's personal case)

101. Which of the following is the strongest indicator for surgical intervention for a kyphotic deformity caused by ankylosing spondylitis?
    a. Chin-brow-to-vertical angle of greater than 40°
    b. Dagger sign on AP XR
    c. Ankylosis of intervertebral joints
    d. Significant pain and physical disability

Preferred Response: (D) Significant pain and physical disability. The preferred surgical therapy for AS-induced kyphosis is spinal osteotomy, which is considered a relatively high-risk procedure. For most patients, the risks outweigh the potential benefits. Therefore, a compelling reason–such as unbearable pain or significant physical disability–is required to consider an osteotomy. A chin-brow-to-vertical angle > 40°, dagger sign on AP XR (indicating ossification of the vertebral ligaments), an ankylosis of intervertebral joints are all indicators of advanced AS, but in and of themselves, they are not indications for surgical intervention.

102. What imaging modality is preferred for the early detection of inflammatory changes in AS?
    a. CT
    b. MRI with gadolinium contrast

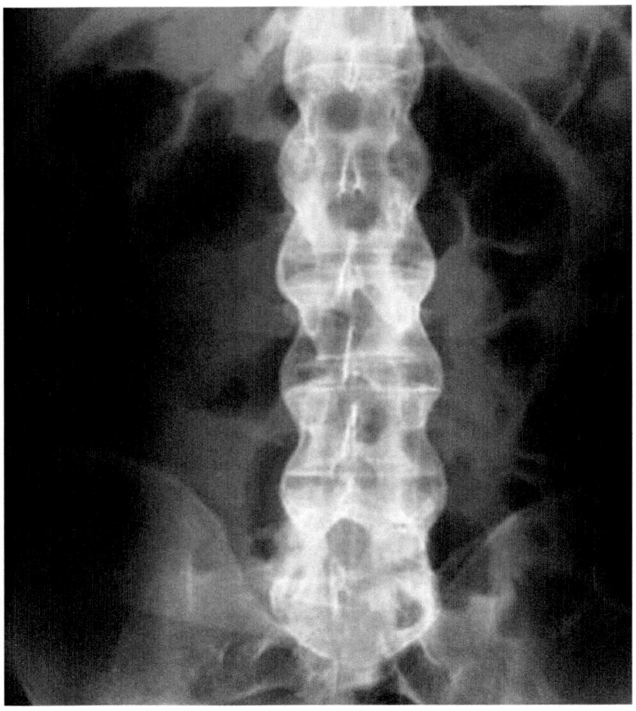

Fig. 9.19 AP radiograph of the spine showing classic bamboo spine (source www.radiopedia.org)

c. MRI
d. PA sacroiliac joint XR

Answer: (B) MRI with gadolinium contrast. MRI of the sacroiliac joints with gadolinium contrast is the most sensitive method for early detection of inflammatory changes of AS. With active inflammatory lesions, erosion of the sacroiliac joints and bone marrow edema (characterized by a high signal intensity in T2-weighted images) may be seen. Reparative changes due to older lesions include secondary bone formation (characterized by a low signal intensity in T1/T2). MRI (without contrast) can also be used if contrast is contraindicated. CT and XR are poor choices to detect acute inflammation.

103. A 71-year-old female previously diagnosed with ankylosing spondylitis comes into the ED after a fall. She presents with weakness and paresthesia in her upper and lower limbs and MRI reveals an anterior epidural hematoma and spinal fracture at C5. She also has a severe pre-existing chin-on-chest deformity for which she was scheduled for surgical correction next week. What is the next appropriate step in management?
   a. Anterior decompression with posterior fusion and instrumentation
   b. Anterior decompression at C5 with posterior osteotomy at C7-T1 with fusion
   c. Posterior osteotomy at C7-T1 with fusion and instrumentation
   d. Anterior decompression

Preferred Response: (A) Anterior decompression with posterior fusion and instrumentation. An anterior epidural hematoma at the level of C5 makes an anterior approach ideal for decompression. Fusion with instrumentation is recommended in patients with AS due to poor bone quality. Osteotomies to correct spinal deformities should not be attempted while correcting traumatic spinal injuries due high risk of adverse outcomes.

104. Which bones are most commonly fractured in Type I osteoporosis?
   a. Hip and pelvis
   b. Distal radius and vertebras
   c. Distal radius and pelvis
   d. Humerus and distal ulna

Answer: (B) Distal radius and vertebras. The distal radius and vertebral bones are commonly fractured in type I (post-menopausal) osteoporosis. The hip and pelvis are more commonly fractured in the Type II (senile) osteoporosis.

105. Which test is most sensitive and specific for detecting osteopenia and osteoporosis?
   a. DEXA of the lumbar spine
   b. AP XR of pelvis
   c. Serum 25-OH vitamin D
   d. Serum alkaline phosphatase

Answer: (A) DEXA of the lumbar spine. Dual Energy Xray Absorptiometry (DEXA) is the most accurate test to determine the presence of osteopenia or osteoporosis with the least radiation exposure. DEXA of the lumbar spine measures the bone mineral density (BMD) from L2 to L4 and compiles the scores. A T-score, which is defined as the number of standard deviations of the patient's BMD from the peak bone mass of a 25-year-old gender-matched individual. Osteopenia is defined as an L2-L4 T-score of -1 to -2.5. Osteoporosis is defined as L2-L4 T-score less than 2.5. AP radiograph of the pelvis or hip is recommended in patients suspected to have osteoporosis and there is a suspicion of fracture, the patient has lost height or is experiencing pain in the thoracic or lumbar spine. However, it is usually not helpful for diagnosis unless there has been bone loss greater than 30%. Serum 25-hydroxy vitamin D is useful for distinguishing between type I and type II osteoporosis. Serum alkaline phosphatase will be elevated in osteomalacia (except in osteomalacia due to hypophosphatasia in which ALP will be low-absent) and normal in osteoporosis. Therefore, ALP is useful for distinguishing between differential diagnoses of bone fragility but is not useful for establishing a diagnosis of osteopenia and osteoporosis.

106. Which of the following is true regarding osteoporosis?
    a. A decrease in estrogen-mediated osteoblast stimulation causes type II osteoporosis.
    b. Calcium and vitamin D therapy is ineffective for fracture prophylaxis type I osteoporosis.
    c. Long-term corticosteroid therapy is a common cause of iatrogenic osteoporosis.
    d. Raloxifene reduces the risk of vertebral and hip fractures in women with osteoporosis.

Answer: (C) Long-term corticosteroid therapy is a common cause of iatrogenic osteoporosis. Corticoid therapy stimulates osteoclastogenesis and increases the expression of RANK-L and CSF-1 and decreases the expression of osteoprotegerin. Corticoids also decrease osteogenesis by decreasing the number of osteoblasts secondary to a shift of progenitor cells away from the osteoblastic lineage. Corticoids also promote the death of mature osteoblasts. Corticoids also decrease the function of the remaining osteoblasts through the inhibition of IGF-1 expression. Type I osteoporosis, also known as postmenopausal osteoporosis, is caused by a decrease in estrogen-mediated osteoblast stimulation. Calcium and vitamin D therapy is effective prophylaxis for both type I and type II (senile) osteoporosis. Raloxifene has only been shown to reduce the risk of vertebral fractures in women with type I osteoporosis. It has not been shown to reduce the incidence of hip fractures.

107. Bisphosphonate therapy is the preferred pharmacologic therapy for patients with osteoporosis to reduce the risk of hip and vertebral fracture. For which of the following conditions are patients receiving bisphosphonate therapy at an increased risk?
    a. Coronary artery disease and MI
    b. Breast cancer
    c. Transient hypercalcemia
    d. Osteonecrosis of the jaw

Answer: (D) Osteonecrosis of the jaw. A rare but serious complication of intravenous (but not oral) bisphosphonate therapy is osteonecrosis of the jaw (ONJ). The exact etiology of bisphosphonate related ONJ is unknown, but it appears to be triggered by exposed bone and bacterial contamination. Therefore, it is recommended that patients receiving bisphosphonate therapy maintain good periodontal hygiene and avoid major dental procedures. Coronary artery disease and breast cancer are associated with hormone replacement therapy which is used to treat type I osteoporosis. Transient hypercalcemia is associated with teriparatide, a recombinant parathyroid hormone analog.

108. What pharmacologic agent used as fracture prophylaxis acts by inhibiting the binding of RANK-L to RANK?
    a. Romosozumab
    b. Teriparatide
    c. Raloxifene
    d. Denosumab

Answer: (D) Denosumab. Denosumab is a monoclonal Ig2 against RANKL and inhibits the binding of RANK-L to RANK, reducing bone resorption. Romosozumab is a monoclonal Ig2 that activates the Wnt pathway by sequestering sclerostin, serving to promote bone formation and inhibiting resorption. Teriparatide is a human recombinant parathyroid hormone and acts by activating osteoblasts and stimulates intestinal absorption of calcium and phosphate. Raloxifene agonizes bone estrogen receptors, inhibiting osteoclast activity, and antagonizes breast estrogen receptors.

109. A 77-year-old woman comes into the ED after slipping in the shower. She reports severe right-sided hip pain and is unable to walk. Radiographs reveal a transverse subtrochanteric noncomminuted fracture. She was previously diagnosed with osteoporosis twelve years ago for which she is taking calcium, vitamin D, and alendronate. She denies other medications. Her most recent DEXA scans indicate that her BMD is stable. After operative fixation, how should the patient be managed?
    a. Start romosozumab
    b. Discontinue alendronate
    c. Discontinue vitamin D supplementation
    d. Start teriparatide

Preferred Response: (B) Discontinue alendronate. Patients on long-term bisphosphonates such as alendronate are at a higher risk for atypical subtrochanteric transverse stress fractures as is seen in this patient. Such fractures are caused by extremely low bone turnover rates which is evidenced by reduced markers of bone resorption (including decreased urinary type 1 collagen cross-linked N-telopeptide). When patients experience an atypical femoral fracture, as long as BMD is stable and they are not on chronic corticosteroids, bisphosphonate drug holidays are recommended. Romosozumab, a monoclonal Ig2 that activates the Wnt pathway is also associated with atypical femoral fractures. Vitamin D supplementation is not associated with atypical femoral fractures. Teriparatide is indicated in patients with severe osteoporosis and a high fracture risk, but in this case, alendronate is the most likely cause of the atypical fracture.

110. A 63-year-old woman presents to the clinic with lower back pain. She has a five-year history of wrist fractures after low energy falls. A L2-L4 DEXA scan was conducted which revealed a T score of −2.6. Deep palpation at L2 resulted in considerable pain. What is the next appropriate step in management for this patient?
   a. L2 kyphoplasty
   b. Start pamidronate
   c. Start denosumab
   d. L2 vertebroplasty

Preferred Response: (B) Start pamidronate. Bisphosphonates such as pamidronate are the first line pharmacology therapy for osteoporosis. Indications for pharmacologic treatment include hip or vertebral fracture, T-score less than −2.5 at the femoral neck or spine, or a T-score between −1.0 and −2.5 with a 10-year probability of a hip fracture of at least three percent or a 10-year probability of a major osteoporosis-related fracture greater than 20%. Denosumab, a monoclonal antibody against RANK-L that decrease osteoclast activity, is typically only indicated for use in pates with impaired renal function or in whom bisphosphonate therapy has failed. Surgical intervention, including vertebroplasty and kyphoplasty, are somewhat controversial and are only indicated when the patient continues to have severe pain symptoms after 6 weeks of nonoperative treatment.

111. Which of the following is true regarding the aging spine?
   a. Primary disc degeneration begins in the fourth decade of life.
   b. Intervertebral disc degeneration typically occurs due to trunk and pelvic muscle weakness.
   c. Unlike with osteoarthritis in other joints, osteophytes are not typically seen in vertebrae.
   d. Angiogenesis in the nucleus pulposus is believed to be a cause of back pain associated with aging.

Answer: (D) Angiogenesis in the nucleus pulposus is believed to be cause of back pain associated with aging. The normal healthy adult intervertebral disc is avascular apart from a sparse vascularization at the superficial portion of the annulus. However, degenerated and herniated disc tissue exhibits significant vascularization. The invading vasculature is associated with increased nociceptive innervation. Primary disc degeneration is a common feature of aging, and the process begins in the second decade of life. This degeneration is considered as an initiating event that leads to the secondary deterioration of the articular facets, ligaments, and muscles. Osteophytes are commonly seen with osteoarthritis of vertebral facet joints as they are in any other synovial joint. The formation of osteophytes can impinge on spinal nerve roots, causing weakness and paresthesias to the affected dermatomes and myotomes.

112. A 38-year-old female presents to the ED with severe acute lower back pain. Palpation reveals localized pain in the lumbar spine. Lumbar spine XR is shown below (see Fig. 9.20). CBC is unremarkable, but serum chemistries are significant for high serum calcium, low phosphorus, and high alkaline phosphatase. A DEXA scan was performed which revealed a T-score of -2.4. Past medical history and family history is unremarkable, and the patient reports a regular 28-day menstrual cycle. What is the most likely cause of the patient's decreased bone mineral density?
   a. Decreased estrogen stimulation of osteoblasts
   b. Increased serum PTH levels
   c. Decreased RANK-L expression
   d. Decreased *SOST* expression in osteocytes

Answer: (B) Increased serum PTH levels. The patient's presentation is consistent with an osteopenia-induced vertebral compression fracture secondary to hyperparathyroidism. Elevated PTH levels will cause calcium to be released from bone into the blood, reducing bone mineral density and resulting in high calcium, low phosphorous, and high ALP. Decreased estrogen levels, which is most seen after menopause, is the major factor contributing to type I osteoporosis. However, this patient does not present with any clinical features suggestive of decreased estrogen levels (she reports a normal menstrual cycle). Decreased RANK-L expression would promote bone formation rather than bone breakdown. The *SOST* gene encodes sclerostin, an endogenous inhibitor of osteoblastic bone formation. Decreased *SOST* expression would similarly promote bone formation rather than bone breakdown.

113. Intervertebral disc degeneration is a common feature of aging. Which of the following is **NOT** true regarding disc degeneration?
   a. MRI is the best modality for assessing degenerative disc changes.
   b. Diffuse disc bulging occurs due to loss of mechanical competence and may result in spinal canal stenosis without herniation.
   c. The boundary between the nucleus pulposus and annulus fibrosis becomes more distinct throughout the aging process.

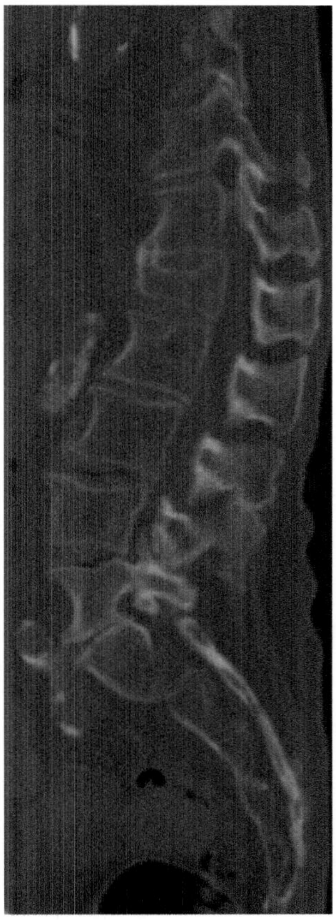

Fig. 9.20 Sagittal lumbar CT. (Dr. Gragnaniello) personal archive

d. A loss of aggrecan and water, decrease in collagen organization, and decrease in disc height are early changes seen in aging.

Answer: (C) The boundary between the nucleus pulposus and annulus fibrosis becomes more distinct throughout the aging process. During aging, the boundary between the nucleus and annulus becomes *less* distinct as there in an increase in collagen content of the nucleus. MRI is the modality of choice to detect degenerative changes in the intervertebral discs. Loss of disc height and darkening of disc signal are the most prominent changes seen with aging. Diffuse disc bulging can occur due to the loss of mechanical competence resulting from concentric fissuring and radial tears in the annulus that occur most often beginning in the third and fourth decades of life. This bulging can lead to spinal canal stenosis. A loss of aggrecan and water, decrease in collagen organization, and loss of disc height are among the earlies changes seen in aging, and these can have serious biochemical consequences. Such changes increase load bearing on the facet joints of the spine leading to facet hypertrophy, osteoarthritis, osteophyte formation, degenerative spondylolisthesis, and scoliosis.

114. A 74-year-old female presents to the clinic with persistent severe lower back pain. Seven weeks ago, she presented to the ED with back pain in the same location for which she was given calcitonin, alendronate, and ibuprofen. Radiographs show loss of vertebral height anteriorly of 4 mm at L2. What is the next appropriate step in management?
   a. Start estrogen-replacement therapy
   b. Percutaneous transpedicular kyphoplasty with PMMA injection
   c. Percutaneous transpedicular vertebroplasty with PMMA injection
   d. Posterior laminectomy with fixation

Preferred Response: (B) Percutaneous transpedicular kyphoplasty with PMMA injection. Kyphoplasty is the recommended surgical intervention indicated in patients presenting with severe pain secondary to vertebral compression fractures unabated by pharmacologic therapy. Estrogen-replacement therapy is only indicated to treat type I osteoporosis in the context of female patients who have undergone a hysterectomy. Vertebroplasties are generally not indicated due to increased risk of cement extravasation and associated complications. Surgical decompression and stabilization is generally not indicated in vertebral compression fractures unless the patient presents with progressive neurologic deficit or an unstable spine.

115. An 88-year-old woman presents to the clinic with moderate lower back pain that began two days prior. She was previously diagnosed with osteoporosis 25 years ago, and her most recent DEXA scan revealed a T-score of −2.8. She is currently taking alendronate, denosumab, and calcium and vitamin D supplements for her osteoporosis. Lateral spine radiograph reveals fractures and local kyphosis at L2 and L3. Physical exam reveals no neurological deficits. What is the best option for this patient at this time?
   a. Bedrest for ten days
   b. L2-L3 kyphoplasty with a percutaneous transpedicular approach
   c. Thoracolumbar orthosis and gradual return to activity
   d. MRI to evaluate for spinal cord compression

Answer: (C) Thoracolumbar orthosis and gradual return to activity. Most patients with vertebral compression fractures can be managed through observation, bracing, medical management, and a gradual return to pre-injury activity. Kyphoplasty is only indicated for severe symptoms not remitting after 4–6 weeks of medical management. Bed rest is not indicated for VCFs. An MRI is not indicated in this patient as she is not showing symptoms of acute spinal cord compression which is not common following VCFs.

116. A 58-year-old woman presents with upper back pain and sharp localized pain after deep palpation at the upper thoracic spine. Radiograph reveals a vertebral compression fracture at T4. The patient does not report any recent history of falls. In addition to osteoporosis, what other condition should be considered most in the differential diagnosis?
   a. Metastatic cancer to the bone
   b. Rheumatoid arthritis
   c. Osteomalacia
   d. Psoriasis

Answer: (A) Metastatic cancer to the bone. Metastases to the vertebral body are not uncommon and can cause vertebral compression fractures. Index of suspicion for bone metastases should be increased when the patient is younger than 55 years of age, fractures occur above T5, and abnormal radiologic findings are present. An MRI can be performed to differentiate between a malignant and osteoporotic VCF. MR signs suggestive of an osteoporotic VCF include fluid signal in the vertebral space and retropulsion of the vertebral fragment. MR signs suggestive of malignancy include complete replacement of normal marrow signal, an outward bulging of the posterior vertebral border, and epidural or focal paraspinal masses. Rheumatoid and psoriatic arthritis typically do not cause VCFs. Osteomalacia is more commonly associated with appendicular involvement while osteoporosis is associated with fractures of the axial skeleton.

117. Which of the following is a complication commonly associated with vertebral compression fractures?
   a. Compromised pulmonary function
   b. Epidural hematoma
   c. Spinal cord compression
   d. Fat embolism

Answer: (A) Compromised pulmonary function. VCFs and associated kyphosis can compromise pulmonary function with each fracture resulting in up to a 9% decrease in flow volume. Epidural hematomas, spinal cord compressions, and fat emboli can occur following vertebral fractures but are not commonly seen with VCFs.

118. Which of the following is true regarding age-related changes to the ligaments of the spine?
   a. The ligamentum flavum decreases in thickness with age.
   b. Increases in elastin concentration weakens the longitudinal ligaments, decreasing their ability to stabilize the spine.
   c. Decreases in elastin concentration weakens the longitudinal ligaments, decreasing their ability to stabilize the spine.
   d. Younger spinous ligamentous have a low collagen concentration.

Answer: (B) Increases in elastin concentration weakens the longitudinal ligaments, decreasing their ability to stabilize the spine. All spinous ligaments have high concentrations of collagen which contributes to their strength and function to restrain extremes of vertebral motion in all planes. As part of the aging process, ligaments undergo chemical and macroscopic changes, including a rise in the concentration of elastin, that result in ligamentous weakening. During aging and degeneration, the ligamentum flavum increases in thickness.

119. All of the following are common metabolic bone diseases that are associated with spinal pain and deformity EXCEPT:
   a. Osteoporosis
   b. Paget's disease
   c. Renal osteodystrophy
   d. Osteomyelitis and discitis

Correct answer: D. Osteomyelitis and discitis is an infectious process. Metabolic bone diseases are disorders of bone usually caused by abnormalities in minerals vitamin D, bone mass or bone structure, with osteoporosis being the most common.

120. "Rugger jersey" spine, pictured below (see Fig. 9.21), can be associated with which of the following conditions?
   a. Osteopetrosis
   b. Hypercalcemia
   c. Renal osteodystrophy
   d. Paget's disease

Correct answer: C. The "rugger jersey" spine describes alternating sclerotic-lucent-sclerotic appearance of contiguous vertebral levels that mimics a rugby jersey. This pattern of disease is secondary to hyperparathyroidism that is frequently encountered in renal osteodystrophy.

121. What is the most commonly affected site in Paget's disease?
   a. Spine
   b. Pelvis
   c. Long bones
   d. Skull

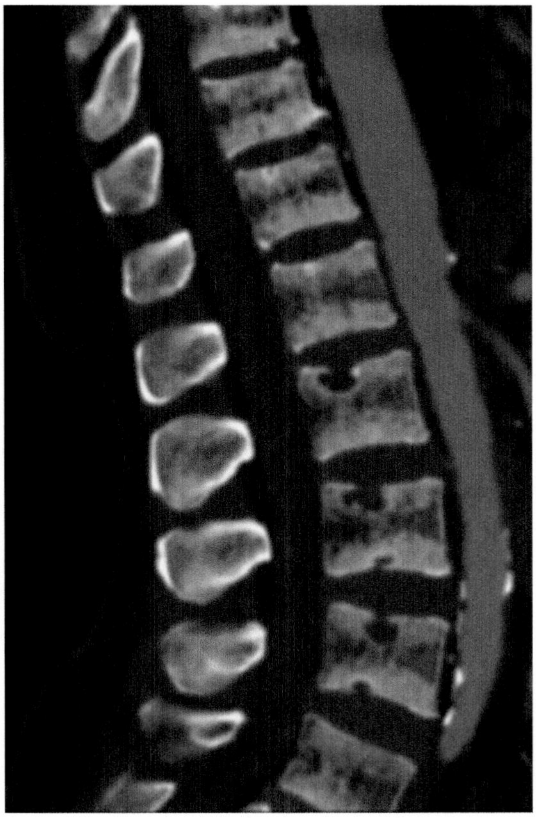

Fig. 9.21 Sagittal CT reconstruction of the thoracic spine

Correct answer: B. The pelvic is the most affected site, estimated to occur in ~ 70% of cases. The spine is the second most common, estimated to occur in about half of cases.

122. The pathophysiology of Paget's disease is which of the following?
    a. Disturbances in bone modelling and re-modelling due to an increase in osteoblastic and osteoclastic activity
    b. Vitamin D deficiency
    c. Hyperparathyroidism
    d. Chronic hypercalcemia

Correct answer: A.

123. Renal osteodystrophy, also referred to dialysis-associated destructive spondyloarthropathy (DSA), most commonly affects which segment of the spine?
    a. OC junction
    b. Lower cervical spine
    c. TL junction
    d. Lumbosacral spine

Correct answer: B. DSA patients can frequently present with atraumatic fractures in the lower cervical spine due to severe bone mineral density loss. They may also present with lumbar fractures.

124. Rickets, or osteomalacia, is a condition resulting from which of the following?
    a. Chronic kidney disease
    b. Vitamin D deficiency
    c. Hypercalcemia
    d. Poor bone mineral density

Correct answer: B.

125. The pathophysiology of renal osteodystrophy involves which of the following?
    a. Deposition of beta-2 microglobulin
    b. Hyperparathyroidism
    c. Osteomalacia
    d. Osteosclerosis
    e. All of the above.

Correct answer: E. All of these can play a part in the spinal complications associated with renal osteodystrophy.

126. Osteomalacia from renal osteodystrophy is the result of which of the following?
    a. Aluminum deposition
    b. Amyloidosis
    c. Decreased nutrient absorption in the gastrointestinal tract
    d. Intrinsic Factor deficiency

Correct answer: A. Most cases of osteomalacia are associated with aluminum accumulation in bone, and its incidence has decreased markedly with the decreased use of aluminum-containing phosphorus binders.

127. "Ivory vertebrae" pictured below (see Fig. 9.22) is associated with which of the following conditions?
    a. Renal osteodystrophy
    b. Paget's disease
    c. Rickets
    d. Osteoporosis

Correct answer: B. Progression of the sclerotic phase in Paget's disease leads to "ivory vertebra." This is secondary to an increase in the density of the vertebral body. There is no change in the density and size of the adjacent intervertebral disc.

128. Which of the following have been proposed as mechanisms of back pain in Paget's disease?
    a. Periosteal stretching
    b. Microfractures
    c. Facet arthritis
    d. Vascular engorgement
    e. All of the above.

Correct answer: E. All of the above have been proposed as hypothesized mechanisms for back pain in Paget's disease.

129. Malignant neoplastic transformation of the Paget's disease in the spine can result in which of the following?
    a. Chondrosarcoma
    b. Chordoma
    c. Osteosarcoma
    d. Osteoid osteoma

Correct answer: C. Neoplastic transformation in Paget's disease is very rare in the spine (0.7%). The majority of malignant transformations are osteosarcomas.

130. Which of the following has been proposed as frequent and underdiagnosed cause of adolescent idiopathic scoliosis?
    a. Paget's disease
    b. Rickets
    c. Hypocalcemia
    d. Cushing's syndrome

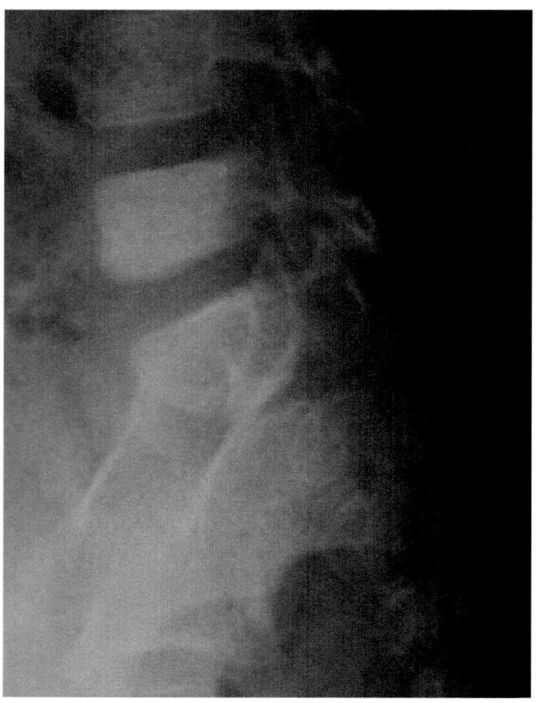

Fig. 9.22 Lateral XR of the spine

Correct answer: B. Several theories have been proposed to explain the etiology of adolescent idiopathic scoliosis (AIS). Many maintain that rickets is the cause of most cases of scoliosis, while others claim that rickets is only a secondary factor.

131. The inorganic matrix of bone mineral primarily consists of which of the following?
    a. Calcium hydroxyapatite
    b. Octacalcium phosphate
    c. Brushite
    d. Calcium triphosphate

Correct answer: A. Two thirds of the dry weight of bone consists of calcium phosphate in the form calcium hydroxyapatite.

132. Parathyroid hormone has an indirect effect on which organ in calcium homeostasis?
    a. Kidney
    b. Bone
    c. Liver
    d. Gastrointestinal tract

Correct answer: D. PTH directly affects the kidney and bones. It indirectly affects the intestines through the increased synthesis of the active metabolite of vitamin D.

133. The active form of vitamin D, calcitriol, works in which of the following ways?
    a. Increased expression of calcium-transport proteins
    b. Increased absorption of calcium and phosphate from the gut
    c. Mobilizes calcium from bone into the circulation
    d. All of the above.

Correct answer: D. All of the above are mechanisms by which vitamin D is critical in maintain calcium homeostasis in the body.

References

1. Aletaha D, Smolen JS. Diagnosis and management of rheumatoid arthritis: a review. JAMA. 2018;320(13):1360–72. https://doi.org/10.1001/jama.2018.13103.
2. Alvarez I, Collado J, Daura X, et al. The rheumatoid arthritis–associated allele HLA–DR10 (DRB1*1001) shares part of its repertoire with HLA–DR1 (DRB1*0101) and HLA–DR4 (DRB*0401). Arthritis Rheum. 2008;58(6):1630–9. https://doi.org/10.1002/art.23503.
3. Boden SD, Dodge LD, Bohlman HH, Rechtine GR. Rheumatoid arthritis of the cervical spine. A long-term analysis with predictors of paralysis and recovery. J Bone Joint Surg Am. 1993;75(9):1282–1297. https://doi.org/10.2106/00004623-199309000-00004

4. Chung KC, Kotsis SV, Wilgis EFS, et al. Outcomes of silicone arthroplasty for rheumatoid metacarpophalangeal joints stratified by fingers. J Hand Surg Am. 2009;34(9):1647–52. https://doi.org/10.1016/j.jhsa.2009.06.029.
5. Elliot MJ, Maini RN, Feldmann M, et al. Treatment of rheumatoid arthritis with chimeric monoclonal antibodies to tumor necrosis factor alpha. Arthritis Rheum. 2008;58(2 Suppl):S92–101. https://doi.org/10.1002/art.23362.
6. Fraenkel L, Bathon JM, England BR, et al. 2021 American college of rheumatology guideline for the treatment of Rheumatoid Arthritis. Arthritis Care Res. 2021;73(7):924–39. https://doi.org/10.1002/acr.24596.
7. Giles JT, Bartlett SJ, Gelber AC, et al. Tumor necrosis factor inhibitor therapy and risk of serious postoperative orthopedic infection in rheumatoid arthritis. Arthritis Rheum. 2006;55(2):333–7. https://doi.org/10.1002/art.21841.
8. Goodman SM, Springer B, Guyatt G, et al. 2017 American college of rheumatology/american association of hip and knee surgeons guideline for the perioperative management of Antirheumatic medication in patients with rheumatic diseases undergoing elective total hip or total knee arthroplasty. Arthritis Rheumatol. 2017;69(8):1538–51. https://doi.org/10.1002/art.40149.
9. Keith MP. Perspectives on rheumatoid arthritis for the orthopedic surgeon: overview of non-tumor necrosis factor biologic drugs and perioperative management. Am J Orthop (Belle Mead NJ). 2011;40(12):E272-275.
10. Kim DH, Hilibrand AS. Rheumatoid arthritis in the cervical spine. J Am Acad Orthop Surg. 2005;13(7):463–74. https://doi.org/10.5435/00124635-200511000-00006.
11. Kwong Y, Rao N, Latief K. Craniometric measurements in the assessment of craniovertebral settling: are they still relevant in the age of cross-sectional imaging? AJR Am J Roentgenol. 2011;196(4):W421-425. https://doi.org/10.2214/AJR.10.5339.
12. Monsey null. Rheumatoid Arthritis of the Cervical Spine. J Am Acad Orthop Surg. 1997;5(5):240–248. https://doi.org/10.5435/00124635-199709000-00002
13. Pan J, Huang D, Hao D, et al. Occipitocervical fusion: fix to C2 or C3? Clin Neurol Neurosurg. 2014;127:134–9. https://doi.org/10.1016/j.clineuro.2014.10.013.
14. Saag KG, Teng GG, Patkar NM, et al. American College of Rheumatology 2008 recommendations for the use of nonbiologic and biologic disease-modifying antirheumatic drugs in rheumatoid arthritis. Arthritis Care Res. 2008;59(6):762–84. https://doi.org/10.1002/art.23721.
15. Saleh KJ, Kurdi AJ, El-Othmani MM, et al. Perioperative treatment of patients with Rheumatoid Arthritis. J Am Acad Orthop Surg. 2015;23(9):e38-48. https://doi.org/10.5435/JAAOS-D-15-00014.
16. Schett G, Gravallese E. Bone erosion in rheumatoid arthritis: mechanisms, diagnosis and treatment. Nat Rev Rheumatol. 2012;8(11):656–64. https://doi.org/10.1038/nrrheum.2012.153.
17. Shah A, St. Clair EW. Rheumatoid Arthritis. In Jameson JL, Fauci AS, Kasper DL, Hauser SL, Longo DL, Loscalzo J, editors. Harrison's principles of internal medicine. 20th ed. McGraw-Hill Education; 2018. Accessed 22 Sept 2021. accessmedicine.mhmedical.com/content.aspx?aid=1157285895
18. Song YW, Kang EH. Autoantibodies in rheumatoid arthritis: rheumatoid factors and anticitrullinated protein antibodies. QJM: An Int J Med. 2010;103(3):139–146. https://doi.org/10.1093/qjmed/hcp165
19. Whiting PF, Smidt N, Sterne JAC, et al. Systematic review: accuracy of anti-citrullinated peptide antibodies for diagnosing Rheumatoid Arthritis. Ann Intern Med. 2010;152(7):456–64. https://doi.org/10.7326/0003-4819-152-7-201004060-00010.
20. Ankylosing spondylitis
21. Arun R, Dabke HV, Mehdian H. Comparison of three types of lumbar osteotomy for ankylosing spondylitis: a case series and evolution of a safe technique for instrumented reduction. Eur Spine J. 2011;20(12):2252–60. https://doi.org/10.1007/s00586-011-1894-3.
22. Belanger TA, Rowe DE. Diffuse idiopathic skeletal hyperostosis: musculoskeletal manifestations. J Am Acad Orthop Surg. 2001; 9(4):258–67. https://doi.org/10.5435/00124635-200107000-00006
.
23. Brent L, Patel A, Patel R. Ankylosing Spondylitis and Undifferentiated Spondyloarthropathy treatment and management: approach considerations, pharmacologic therapy, guideline-directed therapy. Published online 12 July 2021. Accessed 5 Oct 2021. https://emedicine.medscape.com/article/332945-treatment#d11
24. Chaudhary SB, Hullinger H, Vives MJ. Management of acute spinal fractures in ankylosing spondylitis. ISRN Rheumatol. 2011;2011: 150484. https://doi.org/10.5402/2011/150484.
25. Deodhar A, Sliwinska-Stanczyk P, Xu H, et al. Tofacitinib for the treatment of ankylosing spondylitis: a phase III, randomised, double-blind, placebo-controlled study. Ann Rheum Dis. 2021;80(8):1004–13. https://doi.org/10.1136/annrheumdis-2020-219601.
26. Enercan M, Ozturk C, Kahraman S, Sarıer M, Hamzaoglu A, Alanay A. Osteotomies/spinal column resections in adult deformity. Eur Spine J. 2013;22(Suppl 2):S254-264. https://doi.org/10.1007/s00586-012-2313-0.
27. Hall ED. The neuroprotective pharmacology of methylprednisolone. J Neurosurg. 1992;76(1):13–22. https://doi.org/10.3171/jns.1992.76.1.0013.
28. Haywood KL, Garratt AM, Jordan K, Dziedzic K, Dawes PT. Spinal mobility in ankylosing spondylitis: reliability, validity and responsiveness. Rheumatology. 2004;43(6):750–7. https://doi.org/10.1093/rheumatology/keh169.
29. Kerrigan MJ, Cooper JS. Venous gas embolism. In: StatPearls. StatPearls Publishing; 2021. Accessed 5 Oct 2021. http://www.ncbi.nlm.nih.gov/books/NBK482249/
30. Khalessi AA, Oh BC, Wang MY. Medical management of ankylosing spondylitis. Neurosurg Focus. 2008;24(1):E4. https://doi.org/10.3171/FOC/2008/24/1/E4.
31. Kim K-T, Park D-H, Lee S-H, Lee J-H. Results of corrective osteotomy and treatment strategy for ankylosing spondylitis with kyphotic deformity. Clin Orthop Surg. 2015;7(3):330–6. https://doi.org/10.4055/cios.2015.7.3.330.
32. Lukasiewicz AM, Bohl DD, Varthi AG, et al. Spinal fracture in patients with ankylosing spondylitis: cohort definition, distribution of injuries, and hospital outcomes. Spine. 2016;41(3):191–6. https://doi.org/10.1097/BRS.0000000000001190.
33. Maxwell LJ, Zochling J, Boonen A, et al. TNF-alpha inhibitors for ankylosing spondylitis. Cochrane Database Syst Rev. 2015;(4): CD005468. https://doi.org/10.1002/14651858.CD005468.pub2
34. Mundwiler ML, Siddique K, Dym JM, Perri B, Johnson JP, Weisman MH. Complications of the spine in ankylosing spondylitis with a focus on deformity correction. Neurosurg Focus. 2008;24(1):E6. https://doi.org/10.3171/FOC/2008/24/1/E6.
35. Nascimento FA, Gatto LAM, Lages RO, Neto HM, Demartini Z, Koppe GL. Diffuse idiopathic skeletal hyperostosis: a review. Surg Neurol Int. 2014;5(Suppl 3):S122–5. https://doi.org/10.4103/2152-7806.130675.
36. Sheehan NJ. The ramifications of HLA-B27. J R Soc Med. 2004;97(1):10–4. https://doi.org/10.1258/jrsm.97.1.10.
37. Sieper J, Rudwaleit M, Baraliakos X, et al. The assessment of SpondyloArthritis international society (ASAS) handbook: a guide to assess spondyloarthritis. Annals of the Rheumatic Diseases. 2009;68(Suppl 2):21–244. https://doi.org/10.1136/ard.2008.104018

38. Tam L-S, Gu J, Yu D. Pathogenesis of ankylosing spondylitis. Nat Rev Rheumatol. 2010;6(7):399–405. https://doi.org/10.1038/nrrheum.2010.79.
39. Taurog JD, Chhabra A, Colbert RA. Ankylosing spondylitis and axial Spondyloarthritis. N Engl J Med. 2016;374(26):2563–74. https://doi.org/10.1056/NEJMra1406182.
40. Vosse D, van der Heijde D, Landewé R, et al. Determinants of hyperkyphosis in patients with ankylosing spondylitis. Ann Rheum Dis. 2006;65(6):770–4. https://doi.org/10.1136/ard.2005.044081.
41. Weiss PF, Colbert RA. Juvenile Spondyloarthritis: a distinct form of juvenile arthritis. Pediatr Clin North Am. 2018;65(4):675–90. https://doi.org/10.1016/j.pcl.2018.03.006.
42. Werner BC, Samartzis D, Shen FH. Spinal fractures in patients with ankylosing spondylitis: etiology, diagnosis, and management. J Am Acad Orthop Surg. 2016;24(4):241–9. https://doi.org/10.5435/JAAOS-D-14-00149.
43. Yen Y-R, Luo J-F, Liu M-L, Lu F-J, Wang S-R. The anthropometric measurement of schober's test in normal taiwanese population. Biomed Res Int. 2015;2015: 256365. https://doi.org/10.1155/2015/256365.
44. Kallmes DF, Comstock BA, Heagerty PJ, et al. A randomized trial of vertebroplasty for osteoporotic spinal fractures. N Engl J Med. 2009;361(6):569–79. https://doi.org/10.1056/NEJMoa0900563.
45. Buchbinder R, Osborne RH, Ebeling PR, et al. A randomized trial of vertebroplasty for painful osteoporotic vertebral fractures. N Engl J Med. 2009;361(6):557–68. https://doi.org/10.1056/NEJMoa0900429.
46. McCalden RW, McGeough JA, Barker MB, Court-Brown CM. Age-related changes in the tensile properties of cortical bone. The relative importance of changes in porosity, mineralization, and microstructure. J Bone Joint Surg Am. 1993;75(8):1193–1205. https://doi.org/10.2106/00004623-199308000-00009
47. Okada E, Matsumoto M, Ichihara D, et al. Aging of the cervical spine in healthy volunteers: a 10-year longitudinal magnetic resonance imaging study. Spine. 2009;34(7):706–12. https://doi.org/10.1097/BRS.0b013e31819c2003.
48. Lyles KW, Gold DT, Shipp KM, Pieper CF, Martinez S, Mulhausen PL. Association of osteoporotic vertebral compression fractures with impaired functional status. Am J Med. 1993;94(6):595–601. https://doi.org/10.1016/0002-9343(93)90210-g.
49. McCarthy J, Davis A. Diagnosis and management of vertebral compression fractures. AFP. 2016;94(1):44–50.
50. Matzkin EG, DeMaio M, Charles JF, Franklin CC. Diagnosis and treatment of osteoporosis: what orthopaedic surgeons need to know. J Am Acad Orthop Surg. 2019;27(20):e902–12. https://doi.org/10.5435/JAAOS-D-18-00600.
51. Neer RM, Arnaud CD, Zanchetta JR, et al. Effect of parathyroid hormone (1–34) on fractures and bone mineral density in postmenopausal women with osteoporosis. N Engl J Med. 2001;344(19):1434–41. https://doi.org/10.1056/NEJM200105103441904.
52. Bogoch ER, Elliot-Gibson V, Beaton DE, Jamal SA, Josse RG, Murray TM. Effective initiation of osteoporosis diagnosis and treatment for patients with a fragility fracture in an orthopaedic environment. J Bone Joint Surg Am. 2006;88(1):25–34. https://doi.org/10.2106/JBJS.E.00198.
53. Huang Q-Y, Kung AWC. Genetics of osteoporosis. Mol Genet Metab. 2006;88(4):295–306. https://doi.org/10.1016/j.ymgme.2006.04.009.
54. Fraser WD. Hyperparathyroidism. Lancet. 2009;374(9684):145–158. https://doi.org/10.1016/S0140-6736(09)60507-9
55. Lehman RA, Kang DG, Wagner SC. Management of osteoporosis in spine surgery. J Am Acad Orthop Surg. 2015;23(4):253–63. https://doi.org/10.5435/JAAOS-D-14-00042.
56. Canalis E. Mechanisms of glucocorticoid-induced osteoporosis. Curr Opin Rheumatol. 2003;15(4):454–7. https://doi.org/10.1097/00002281-200307000-00013.
57. Benoist M. Natural history of the aging spine. Eur Spine J. 2003;12(Suppl 2):S86–9. https://doi.org/10.1007/s00586-003-0593-0.
58. Warriner AH, Saag KG. Osteoporosis diagnosis and medical treatment. Orthop Clin North Am. 2013;44(2):125–35. https://doi.org/10.1016/j.ocl.2013.01.005.
59. Kim DH, Vaccaro AR. Osteoporotic compression fractures of the spine; current options and considerations for treatment. Spine J. 2006;6(5):479–87. https://doi.org/10.1016/j.spinee.2006.04.013.
60. Spivak JM, Johnson MG. Percutaneous treatment of vertebral body pathology. J Am Acad Orthop Surg. 2005;13(1):6–17. https://doi.org/10.5435/00124635-200501000-00003.
61. Yokota K, Maeda T, Kawano O, et al. Progression of local kyphosis after conservative treatment for compressive cervical spine fracture with spinal cord injury. J Orthop Surg Res. 2019;14(1):98. https://doi.org/10.1186/s13018-019-1115-z.
62. Schlaich C, Minne HW, Bruckner T, et al. Reduced pulmonary function in patients with spinal osteoporotic fractures. Osteoporos Int. 1998;8(3):261–7. https://doi.org/10.1007/s001980050063.
63. Blake GM, Fogelman I. Role of dual-energy X-ray absorptiometry in the diagnosis and treatment of osteoporosis. J Clin Densitom. 2007;10(1):102–10. https://doi.org/10.1016/j.jocd.2006.11.001.
64. Lewiecki EM. Role of sclerostin in bone and cartilage and its potential as a therapeutic target in bone diseases. Ther Adv Musculoskelet Dis. 2014;6(2):48–57. https://doi.org/10.1177/1759720X13510479.
65. U.S. Preventive Services Task Force. Screening for osteoporosis: U.S. preventive services task force recommendation statement. Ann Intern Med. 2011;154(5):356–364. https://doi.org/10.7326/0003-4819-154-5-201103010-00307
66. Väänänen HK, Zhao H, Mulari M, Halleen JM. The cell biology of osteoclast function. J Cell Sci. 2000;113(Pt 3):377–81.
67. Gold DT. The clinical impact of vertebral fractures: quality of life in women with osteoporosis. Bone. 1996;18(3 Suppl):185S-189S. https://doi.org/10.1016/8756-3282(95)00500-5.
68. Kanis JA, Melton LJ, Christiansen C, Johnston CC, Khaltaev N. The diagnosis of osteoporosis. J Bone Miner Res. 1994;9(8):1137–41. https://doi.org/10.1002/jbmr.5650090802.
69. Capozzi A, Lello S, Pontecorvi A. The inhibition of RANK-ligand in the management of postmenopausal osteoporosis and related fractures: the role of denosumab. Gynecol Endocrinol. 2014;30(6):403–8. https://doi.org/10.3109/09513590.2014.892067.
70. Farfan HF. The pathological anatomy of degenerative spondylolisthesis. A cadaver study. Spine (Phila Pa 1976). 1980;5(5):412–418. https://doi.org/10.1097/00007632-198009000-00004
71. Esses SI, McGuire R, Jenkins J, et al. The treatment of symptomatic osteoporotic spinal compression fractures. J Am Acad Orthop Surg. 2011;19(3):176–82. https://doi.org/10.5435/00124635-201103000-00007.
72. Savage JW, Schroeder GD, Anderson PA. Vertebroplasty and kyphoplasty for the treatment of osteoporotic vertebral compression fractures. J Am Acad Orthop Surg. 2014;22(10):653–64. https://doi.org/10.5435/JAAOS-22-10-653.

Complications of Surgery of the Spine

10

Antonio Bocchetti, Ciro Mastantuoni, Valentina Cioffi, and Raffaele de Falco

(1) A 56 years-old man with history of Parkinson's disease (PD) and lumbar stenosis treated six months earlier at an outside institution with an L2-L5 posterior lumbar fusion and decompression, came to your attention. He has complained of severe low back pain for three weeks. What is the most frequent complication associated with spinal surgery in patients with PD?
   A. Infection
   B. Adjacent disk disease
   C. Progressive kyphotic deformity and screws pull out
   D. Cerebrospinal fluid leak
   E. Failed back surgery syndrome

Preferred Response: C: Several studies report that patients with PD harbor a higher risk of post-operative complications and surgical failure. Progressive kyphosis and screws pull out are the most frequent. Literature reports a failure rate ranging up to 29% [1].

(2) One of the following statements is true regarding vertebroplasty and kyphoplasty:
   A. Cement leakage, radiculopathy, spinal cord compression, adjacent-level vertebral body compression are the most common complications
   B. Overall complication rate is 0.5%
   C. Cement leakage occurs more frequently with balloon kyphoplasty than with vertebroplasty
   D. Adjacent-level vertebral body compression is a complication related only with osteoporotic vertebral fractures
   E. All of the above

Preferred response: A: The most common complications of vertebroplasty and kyphoplasty are cement leakage and neurological deficits related to that, radiculopathy, cord compression, adjacent-level vertebral body compression as well as lung and venous embolisms. Overall complications occurrence per vertebral body treated is around 6% with cement leakage occurring less frequently with balloon kyphoplasty than with vertebroplasty, whose rate is around 70% [2].

(3) Which lumbar spine level fusion is associated with lower risk of adjacent segment degeneration (ASD)?
   A. L4-L5
   B. L5-S1
   C. L4-S1
   D. L1-L2
   E. A + B

Preferred response: B: L5- S1 fusions showed a significantly lower risk of ASD (20%). L4-L5 fusions has an ASD rate of 46%. Bi-segmental L4-S1 fusions is associated with a risk of ASD of 24%. Junctional segments, like L1-L2 are associated with the higher risk of ASD [3].

(4) A 62 years-old woman presents with low back pain and bilateral S1 radiculopathies. She was treated with a L4-L5 PLIF 8 months earlier for a grade II spondylolisthesis. A radiologic investigation shows that the cage displaced posteriorly pushing on the nerve roots. What is the correct management?
   A. Removal of the whole implant via a posterior approach

A. Bocchetti (✉) · C. Mastantuoni · V. Cioffi · R. de Falco
Department of Neurosurgery, Santa Maria Delle Grazie Hospital, Pozzuoli, Italy
e-mail: Antonio.bocchetti74@gmail.com

C. Mastantuoni
e-mail: mastantuoniciro@gmail.com

V. Cioffi
e-mail: valentina.cioffi@aslnapoli2nord.it

R. de Falco
e-mail: Raffaele.defalco@aslnapoli2nord.it

C. Gragnaniello et al. (eds.), *MCQs in Spine Surgery*,
https://doi.org/10.1007/978-3-031-69332-8_10

B. Corticosteroids, physical therapy and strict follow up
C. 360° approach for posterior removal of the screws and rods and anterior removal of the cage
D. Anterior approach for cage removal and new cage placement
E. Lateral approach (XLIF) for cage removal and new cage placement and posterior surgery for extending the implant from L3-S1.

Preferred response: D: The ALIF rationale is to allow a safe cage removal, avoiding dural tears and nerve root damage, and indirect decompression of the spinal canal. The anterior route enables an extensive disk removal leading to a wider surface for the fusion. Furthermore, the higher cage implanted via this approach, allows for better restoration of lordosis and of disk height and shape [4].

(5) A 43 years-old man has been treated with a posterior stand-alone L3-L4 cage for a painful spondylolisthesis. Seven months after the surgery, he progressively developed L3 pain, hypoesthesia, and quadriceps weakness on the left side. What do you expect has Most likely happened?
A. Foraminal stenosis due to cage subsidence and vertebral slippage
B. Posterior displacement of the cage that pushes on L3
C. L2-L3 junctional disease
D. Foraminal stenosis due to insufficient disk height restoration
E. Spondylodiscitis

Preferred response: A: Posterior stand-alone cages, in most cases, do not provide enough biomechanical stability and are often associated with subsidence. Therefore, after an initial relief of symptoms, the underlying pathology may progress. In this case the symptoms are most likely due cage subsidence and vertebral slippage causing foraminal stenosis [5].

(6) Regarding the previous clinical case, what can be the most appropriate treatment?
A. Posterior L3-L4 fixation and compression
B. Posterior L3-L4 fixation and distraction
C. Posterior removal of the cage and short segment fixation
D. Posterior removal of the cage and long segment fixation
E. 360° approach: anterior approach for removal of the cage and new cage placement and posterior short segment fixation (L3-L4)

Preferred response: E: ALIF approach allows a safe removal of the subsided cage without the risk of dural tears and nerve roots damage. Furthermore, the placement of Taller cage restored the disk space height Providing indirect decompression. Lastly, the short segment posterior fixation provided greater stability to the whole construct [6].

(7) A 63 years-old-female with Cushing disease has been treated one month earlier in another hospital with a L5-S1 PLIF for grade II spondylolisthesis. She brings the post-op CT scan for review. This shows the correct placement of the implants and a complete reduction of the listhesis. She complains of low back pain and bilateral S1 radiculopathy since postoperative week two. Her blood tests are normal. Her physician told her that is normal post-operative pain and gave her NSAIDs. In your opinion, what may cause her symptoms?
A. Her physician is right. It is normal to have residual pain after a surgery. Moreover, Cushing's disease may cause emotional instability determining a higher perception of the pain.
B. L4-L5 adjacent segment disease. In fact, secondary osteoporosis due to Cushing's disease may increase the risk of its occurrence.
C. Failure of the construct, pull out of one or more screws and/or retropulsion or subsidence of one/both cages. In this case, secondary osteoporosis due to Cushing's disease may raise the risk of surgical failure.
D. Left L5 screw breaking due to the overcorrection. The cantilever forces applied to reduce completely the listhesis is the cause of the breaking of one or more screws.
E. Wound infection and spondylodiscitis. It is known that Cushing disease raises the infective risk inhibiting the immune response.

Preferred response: C: In this case the most likely explanation for the patient's symptoms is construct failure with screws pull out and retropulsion of both cages. Osteoporosis is associated with a higher risk of early complications (screws pull out, cage subsidence, adjacent segment disease). Answer B is not correct as a L4 fracture or slippage is not primarily associated with isolated bilateral S1 radiculopathies. Answer E is not correct because patient's blood work was normal. Answer D would have warranted left L4 or L5 radiculopathy, thus it is not correct.

(8) Regarding the previous clinical case, what would be the correct management?
A. Cage replacement via an anterior approach (ALIF). The compression forces applied by a taller cage

obviates the need of posterior repositioning of the screws.

B. Posterior replacement of pulled out screws with larger diameter screws and revision of the cage. Cranial extension of the implant to L4 and possibly to pelvis.
C. Control of Cushing disease, NSAIDs and psychiatric support. Next clinical and radiologic follow up in three months.
D. Contrast enhanced MRI and antibiotics.
E. Cage replacement via an anterior approach (ALIF). Posterior approach for screws removal and L5 laminectomy and foraminotomy.

Preferred response: B: In this case with a single approach the Pulled-out screws can be Upsized, and the cage revised. Moreover, extension of the construct is needed for increasing the stability of the construct, since the cause of failure was the poor bone purchase of the L5 and S1 screws.

(9) Which of the following is a patient's related risk factor for non-union in spine fusion?
A. Diabetes
B. Cigarette smoking
C. Age
D. None of the answers
E. A, B, C

Preferred response: E: A, B and C are correct. In fact, fusion rate has been reported To be significantly lower in diabetic patients. Moreover, diabetes is associated with higher pre- and post-operative VAS and ODI scores. Cigarette smoking is one of the most important risk factors for non-union. In heavy-smokers non-union rate range up to 30%. Alongside, age is reported as an important predicting factor of non-union in spine surgery [7].

(10) Most common ALIF complications are:
A. Vascular complications
B. Sympathetic nerve system injuries
C. Thromboembolic complications
D. A and C
E. A, B and C

Preferred response: E: Vascular complications in anterior approaches to the lumbar spine range from 0 to 12% and the most commonly involve the common iliac vein. Thromboembolic complications have a rate of 0–12%. Sympathetic nerve system injuries are the most common complication of ALIF determining retrograde ejaculation in 10–15% of cases [6].

(11) You are performing an ACDF on a 78-years-old patient with previous achalasia. During the closure you assistant rise the suspicion of esophageal injury. What would you do?
A. Check the surgical field. If any fistula is detected, it should be repaired immediately. After the surgery the patient will receive broad-spectrum antibiotics.
B. Close quickly the wound. Start prophylactic broad-spectrum antibiotic therapy and parenteral nutrition. Perform fiberoptic endoscopy to confirm the fistula. If after two weeks it is not repaired, the patients should undergo a revision surgery.
C. Primary repair, gastrostomy, and broad-spectrum antibiotics.
D. Normally, esophagus injury should not be treated since the esophagus is a muscular structure whose wall resistance is higher than internal pressure. Therefore, its content cannot exit its lumen. In this case it should be repaired during the surgery and the patient should receive antibiotics due to the pre-operative achalasia.
E. A + D

Preferred response: A: In cases of suspected esophageal injury the surgeon should meticulously check the surgical field. If any breach is found out, it should be primarily repaired, and the patient should be placed on broad-spectrum antibiotic therapy [8].

(12) Which of the following sentences is true about prevention of esophageal injury during anterior cervical spine approaches?
A. Sharp dissection should be preferred over finger dissection below the superficial cervical fascia
B. Preoperative esophageal dysmotility does not increase the risk of injury
C. Intraoperative detection of esophageal tear is impossible. Therefore, In case of suspicion the diagnosis is done post-operatively with fiberoptic endoscopic, esophageal motility films or making the patient drink methylene blue and looking for that color in wound drainage fluid.
D. During lengthy operations, it may be Useful to release the medial blades Of the retractor regularly to avoid esophageal necrosis.
E. Post-operative injury of the esophagus is not possible because the graft and the screws are smooth.

Preferred response: D: Esophageal injury may lead to disastrous consequences, including septicemia, mediastinitis, pneumonia, and meningitis. In order to prevent such occurrences, it has been proposed to use finger dissection, rather than a sharp dissection, below the superficial cervical fascia. Esophageal dysmotility (observed in 10% of patients, mostly in the elderly) may increase the risk of surgical injury. During lengthy operations, it may be Useful to release the medial blades Of the retractor regularly to avoid esophageal necrosis. During the latest stages of the surgery, the surgeon should inspect the esophagus and the trachea to detect inadvertent injury to these structures and eventually repair them. It has been reported that graft dislocations or implant failure may also cause perforation of the esophagus [9].

(13) Comparing conventional open surgery and minimally invasive approaches for the treatment of adult degenerative scoliosis:
   A. There are no differences between open surgery and minimally invasive approaches in terms of outcomes and complications.
   B. Minimally invasive approaches have less complications and morbidities.
   C. Even though conventional open surgery has higher risk and morbidities, it provides better clinical and radiologic outcomes.
   D. Minimally invasive approaches are not suitable for adult degenerative scoliosis, since it is often a rigid scoliosis that require extensive bony removal.
   E. Minimally invasive approaches have better outcomes then conventional open surgery.

Preferred response: B: Minimally invasive approaches have been proven to provide the same clinical and radiologic outcomes than conventional open surgery with lower rates of complications and morbidity (approximately 12%) as compared with conventional open surgery (>30%) [10].

(14) Why C1 lateral mass screws should be tilted 15° degree medially? (Chose the incorrect answer)
   A. The screws will gain bi-cortical bone purchase via medial tilting
   B. To reduce the risk of ICA damage into the retropharyngeal space
   C. To reduce the risk of damaging the vertebral artery
   D. To reduce the risk of damaging cranial nerve XII.
   E. To reduce the risk of complications even if this determines a monocortical bony purchase.

Preferred response: A: Tilting the C1 lateral mass screws 15° degree medially determines a monocortical bone purchase. This strategy, providing approximately 70% of Pull out strength, is chosen over straight C1 lateral mass screws, delivering 100% of Pull out strength, because it reduces the risk of ICA, vertebral artery and cranial nerve XII damage.

(15) Which of the following statements is false regarding lumbar pseudoarthrosis?
   A. The use of interbody devices reduces the risk of pseudoarthrosis.
   B. Risk of pseudoarthrosis is also related to patient's preoperative conditions (smoking, malnutrition, older age, osteoporosis).
   C. The use of bone morphogenetic protein-2 (bmp-2) reduces the rate of pseudoarthrosis
   D. The risk of pseudoarthrosis occurrence is inversely related to the graft contact surface on the plates.
   E. Pseudoarthrosis should be treated via the same route of the primary approach.

Preferred response: E: Treatment of lumbar pseudarthrosis includes a variety of surgical options such as replacing loose instrumentation, use of different biologic materials, and interbody fusion techniques. In order to bolster the effectiveness of revision surgery and reduce complications, it is advisable to employ a different approach [11].

(16) You are performing a C1-C2 fixation with a Magerl screw for a chronic Type II odontoid fracture. The pre-operative angio-CT scan showed no pathologic alteration in the vertebral arteries. During the placement of the left screw a deep bleeding occurred from the entry point. What would you do?
   A. It is a vertebral artery injury. I would continue inserting the screw since the screw itself act as a plug
   B. It is for sure a venous bleeding from the vertebral plexus. I would use a hemostatic agent and fibrin glue to stop it.
   C. It is a vertebral artery injury. I would remove the C2 posterior arch and open the vertebral foramen in order to ligate the vertebral artery.
   D. It is a vertebral artery injury. I would use a short plug screw to stop the bleeding
   E. It is a vertebral artery injury. I would stop the surgery and refer the patient to emergency endovascular embolization.

Preferred response: D: The optimal strategy for managing a close vertebral artery injury in the screw hole is to put a short plug screw or whenever possible tamponade. The endovascular embolization is preferred for the cases of vertebral artery injury in "open space" since the time span between the procedure may increase the morbidity or mortality risk. The choice of continuing the screw insertion may lead to the formation of a larger breach.

(17) Which consequences do you expect?
A. None. The Preoperative CT angiogram did not report any pathological alteration of either vertebral artery. Therefore, there are good possibility that the patients will not develop neurological deficit.
B. It depends on the anterior circulation compensatory mechanism.
C. Hemiplegia vegetativa alterna (HVA), a brainstem syndrome characterized by contralateral hemiplegia, hemisensory loss, hemi-hyperhidrosis and ipsilateral Horner's syndrome.
D. The consequences cannot be predicted because they depend on the configuration of the Posterior cerebral arteries (PCAs).
E. B + D

Preferred response: A: In a normal configuration of posterior circulation the contralateral artery is able to compensate the occlusion of one vertebral artery. Therefore, some form of vascular imaging is mandatory before performing posterior instrumented spine surgery.

(18) A 78-years-old male patients with severe tetra paresis came to your attention. He is obese and he has type II diabetes, hypertension as well as osteoporosis due to secondary hyperparathyroidism. His cervical lordosis is inverted (cervical kyphosis 11 degrees) and he has a circumferential stenosis from C3 to C7 determining intramedullary T2 hyperintense signal. Neurologic examination shows myelopathy signs. You decided to perform an open door laminoplasty. According to WFNS guidelines for cervical spine, is this choice proper?
A. Yes, it is. Laminoplasty is the gold standard for spondylotic myelopathy kyphotic cervical spine.
B. It cannot be stated since laminoplasty can be used in flexible kyphotic cervical spine and the question does not provide enough information.
C. No, it is not. In cases of cervical kyphosis, the most indicated approaches are the anterior or the posterior with fusion.
D. No, it is not. For elderly patients the anterior approach is the gold standard.
E. No, it is not. Osteoporosis is a major contraindication to laminoplasty.

Preferred response: C: WFNS guidelines for Cervical Spondylotic Myelopathy suggest the use of posterior decompression and fusion or anterior approaches in patients harboring both cervical spondylotic myelopathy and kyphosis. Furthermore, in elderly patients, like in this case, posterior approaches are preferred [12].

(19) The patient from the previous case example developed pain and tingling of the shoulder and weakness of the deltoid muscle, on the left side, one week after surgery. What do you think happened?
A. Laminectomy was not the proper approach, and the patient had a symptomatic worsening of cervical kyphosis.
B. C5-palsy
C. Incomplete decompression
D. All of the above
E. None of the above

Preferred response: B: C5 palsy incidence after laminectomy is highly variable, but it has been estimated around 4,8%. It can cause significant morbidity for the patient and can lead to dissatisfaction with the outcome of surgery. These injuries are usually motor-dominant but may also involve sensory and radicular pain. C5 dysfunction can occur immediately to 20 days postoperatively [12].

(20) Which approach to the cervical spine is related with the higher risk of C5-palsy?
A. Laminectomy
B. ACDF
C. Laminoplasty
D. ACCF
E. Laminectomy and fusion

Preferred Response: E. Recent series reported the rate of C5 palsy ranging up to 9,5%. Laminoplasty has the lower rate (4,8%) followed by ACCF (5,1%). Generally, the anterior corridors to the cervical spine are related with a lower risk of developing C5-palsy [13].

(21) Which of the following are predictors of post-operative kyphosis after laminoplasty?
A. T1 slope
B. C2 involvement
C. C2-C7 SVA
D. Pre-existing kyphosis
E. All of the above

Preferred Response: E: T1 slope is significantly associated with cervical kyphosis that has been proven to increase on a cut-off point of 29°. T1 slope can be a predictor of postoperative kyphotic changes in the cervical spine post laminoplasty. Moreover, T1 slope is related to C2-C7 SVA whose increment is related with a higher risk of post-operative kyphosis. C2 is the major site of extensor muscles attachment of the cervical spine. Therefore, its involvement along with the necessity of muscle detachment compromises the posterior tension band increasing the risk of developing kyphosis [14].

(22) A 77-year-old woman was operated through a transoral approach for the removal of anterior cervical spine osteophytes causing dysphagia. Before the surgery she was preventively tracheostomized. After the surgery she was admitted to the intensive care unit. Few days later, she developed a persistent a high WBC count (from 20,000 – 30,000 per microliter). She had no fever. 10 days later a nurse calls you during the night, because she has tachypnea with 57% saturation on room air. She has diffused reduction of vesicular murmur, and calves free from clubbing. What do you think it has happened?
   A. Tracheal edema due to infection of the superior airways
   B. Infection and breakdown of the wound that obstructed the superior airways
   C. Pulmonary embolization
   D. Lemierre's syndrome
   E. None of the above

Preferred Response: D: Lemierre's syndrome is featured by thrombophlebitis of the internal jugular vein and bacteremia following a recent oropharyngeal infection with septic embolization to the lungs or other organs. It is a rare but reported complication of transoral approaches to the cervical spine [15].

(23) What would you do?
   A. Neck and chest CT angiogram, antibiotic therapy and anticoagulation
   B. Eco doppler lower limb, chest CT scan, anticoagulation
   C. Surgical debridement of the surgical wound
   D. Checking and cleaning of the tracheostomy
   E. Empirical antibiotic therapy

Preferred Response: A: The correct diagnostic and therapeutic steps for Lemierre's syndrome are CT angiogram of the neck or CE-MRI, chest CT scan and prolonged antibiotic therapy and antigoagulation [15].

(24) What is the most important strategy for reducing risk of vertebral artery injury during subaxial cervical spine fixation?
   A. Performing the approach with a vascular surgeon
   B. Using the proper entry point and trajectory
   C. Performing and studying a preoperative CT-angiogram
   D. It is mandatory to use neuronavigation
   E. B + C

Preferred Response: E: The most important points to respect when performing posterior cervical fixation are: 1. Studying the vertebral arteries and their potential variations; 2. Respect the normal descriptive anatomy and the individual surgical anatomy [9].

(25) Which of the Following it is not a correct strategy for avoiding complications during vertebroplasty?
   A. Use a medial entry point for directing the trajectory of the needle from medial to lateral
   B. Viscous high-pressure delivery of the PMMA
   C. Use of the intraoperative CT scan
   D. A + B
   E. A + B + C

Preferred Response: E: None of the proposed answer are correct. The proper strategies for lowering complication rate during vertebroplasty are accurate needle placement, proper barium radio-opacification of polymethylmethacrylate (PMMA), viscous low-pressure delivery of PMMA under direct fluoroscopic visualization [2].

(26) How would you manage chylothorax?
   A. Diagnosis through milky pleural effusion
   B. Surgical ligation of the thoracic duct
   C. First line treatment is cessation of oral intakes
   D. A + B
   E. A + B + C

Preferred Response: E: Chylothorax is a condition featured by chyle accumulation in the chest cavity related to a thoracic duct lesion. It is a rare but severe complication of anterior cervical and thoracic approaches. Diagnosis is based on thoracentesis showing milky pleural effusion with chylomicrons and triglycerides on biochemical analysis. It is treated by cessation of oral intakes, as first line, and octreotide, if it fails. Surgical ligation of thoracic duct may be considered in cases of medical therapy failure [9].

(27) 64-year-old man harbors a lesion involving T11, which compresses the spinal canal. He has back pain and difficulties in mobilization. Symptoms have begun 4 months ago. Physical examination showed paraparesis. Laboratory work showed no abnormality. He is treated with anterior T9 corpectomy and instrumentation with cage. Microbiological diagnosis of the lesion was tuberculosis. Three days after the surgery the overall

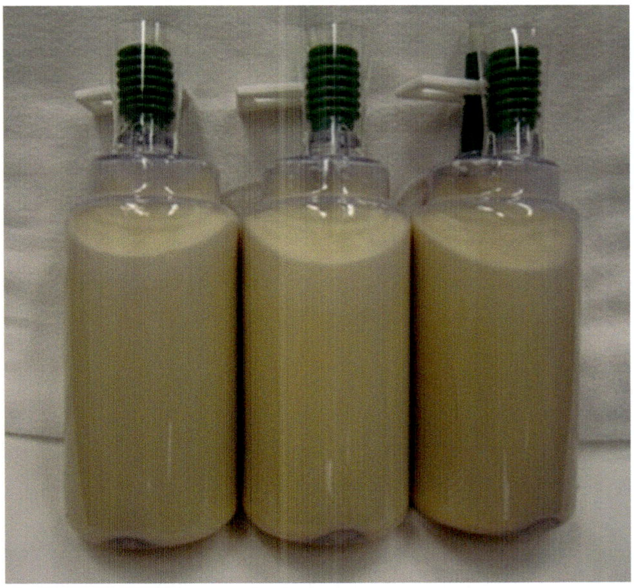

Fig. 10.1 Milky drainage as seen in the postoperative drain collection system

amount of the drainage was 4500 cc. The drainage liquid was milky (Fig. 10.1). What is the diagnosis?
A. Intrapleural dissemination of the tuberculosis
B. Bowel perforation and intrapleural dissemination of its content (the patient was receiving parenteral nutrition).
C. Chylothorax
D. Aerobic bacterial infection and pleuritis
E. Aseptic pleuritis

Preferred Response: The accumulation of milky pleural effusion in the drainage after a thoracic surgery indicated a chylothorax. This is a condition featured by chyle accumulation in the chest cavity related to a thoracic duct lesion. It is a reported complication of anterior thoracic spine surgery.

(28) You are planning an ACDF. What would your strategy be to lower the risk of recurrent laryngeal nerve injury?
A. In cases of repeated surgery change the side of the approach following ENT review for ipsilateral vocal cord palsy
B. Endotracheal cuff pressure release after retractor placement
C. Performing a rostral and caudal dissection greater than needed
D. Medial retractor insertion under the longus colli muscle
E. All of the above

Preferred Response: E: Repeated surgery has proven to be related to significantly higher risk of recurrent laryngeal nerve injury than the primary surgery. Therefore, changing the side of the approach is advisable, whenever possible. Endotracheal cuff pressure should be released after retractor placement and the pressure itself should be monitored. Extensive pressure is associated with higher risk of injury; therefore, the rostral and caudal dissection should be larger than needed to avoid soft tissue traction. The medial retractor should be inserted under the longissimus colli and both retractors should be released approximately every hour [16].

(29) Which of the following statement is incorrect regarding complications of anterior thoracic spine surgery?
A. Risk of complications Is higher in women
B. Risk of complications is in patients over age 60 years old
C. The overall complication rate attributed to anterior surgery is 11,5%
D. Deep wound infection is one of the most common complications
E. Risk of complication increase in patients with multiple pre-existing health problems

Preferred Response: D: Deep wound infection is a serious but rare complication of the anterior spine surgery, whose rate ranges up to 0,6%. Other severe complications as death and paraplegia are estimated around 0,3% and 0,2%. Woman, elderly patients and patients with multiple comorbidities have an higher risk of complications [17].

(30) After been treated with XLIF for grade II spondylolisthesis, a 57 years old man started to complain of having a "cold leg" contralaterally to the side of the approach. This feeling began immediately after the surgery. He visited a vascular surgeon that did not find any alteration to that leg. What could have happened?
A. The question does not provide enough information. The present symptom is not associated with XLIF.
B. Injury to the contralateral lumbar sympathetic plexus injury due to wrong positioning
C. Injury to the ipsilateral lumbar sympathetic plexus
D. Graft displacement and femoral artery occlusion
E. None of the above

Preferred Response: C: The lumbar sympathetic plexus may be injured during lateral interbody fusion. It occurs in up to 12% of XLIF. This may cause a "warm leg" on the ipsilateral site. Often patients report a contralateral "cold leg" instead of ipsilateral warm leg [18].

(31) What is the correct management of the patient in the previous scenario?
A. Neurorrhaphy

B. Stenting of the femoral artery and revision surgery for graft displacement
C. Physiotherapy
D. Corticosteroids
E. None of the above

Preferred Response: E: Lumbar sympathetic plexus injury has been reported to be transient. Therefore, no treatment is needed [18].

(32) Which of the following anterior cervical approaches has the lower incidence of C5 palsy?
A. ACDF
B. ACCF
C. Hybrid surgery
D. Oblique corpectomy
E. C5 palsy is a complication reported only for posterior cervical approaches

Preferred Response: A: The anterior approaches to the cervical spine have an overall rate of C5 palsy of 5,8%. ACDF have the better outcomes in terms of developing this complication. ACCF and Hybrid surgery have approximately the same rate of C5-palsy, even if hybrid anterior surgery proved to provide less complications than ACCF [19].

(33) Which of the following sentences is true regarding degenerative cervical myelopathy treatment:
A. Cervical lordosis and C2-C7 SVA worsen only in cases of straight or kyphotic cervical spine in patients treated with laminoplasty and laminectomy.
B. Anterior decompression and fusion is the first treatment choice in both young and elderly patients with straight or kyphotic cervical spine to avoid post-operative kyphosis.
C. Pre-operative smaller cervical lordosis is a major risk factor for poor recovery in posterior decompression and fusion surgery.
D. C2-C7 SVA worsens after both anterior and posterior spine surgery, but anterior decompression and fusion and posterior decompression and fusion grants the lowest modification of cervical curvature.
E. All of the above

Preferred Response: C: Posterior decompression and fusion is the preferred choice in elderly patients with a straight or kyphotic cervical spine in cases of more than 3 level correction. Nevertheless, the pre-operative cervical lordosis has proven to represent an independent risk factor for poor recovery. Therefore, posterior decompression and fusion should be carefully considered in those patients. Anterior decompression and fusion is discouraged in elderly patients due to the prolonged surgical time and the risk of dysphagia, even if it is not related with worsening of cervical lordosis and C2-C7 SVA. Laminoplasty and laminectomy are always associated with a worsening of the cervical lordosis, even in lordotic spine [12].

(34) Which of the following sentences is correct regarding adjacent disk disease in anterior cervical interbody fusion:
A. Cervicobrachial neuralgia with a distribution territory adjacent to the primary one (above or below) is reported in approximately 20% of cases of adjacent disk disease
B. In long term follow up radiologic adjacent segment degeneration can be found in up to 80% of cases and most times is asymptomatic
C. Radiologic adjacent segment degeneration is an early sign of adjacent disk disease, therefore should be treated to prevent symptoms and signs occurrence
D. A + B
E. A + B + C

Preferred Response: D: Radiologic adjacent segment degeneration may be found ranging up to 80%. The cause of degeneration of the degeneration of the level adjacent to discectomy/fusion is partly due to aging. Nevertheless, the literature agrees in indicating an accelerated degeneration of adjacent levels due to a redistribution of the shearing forces and the load. In most cases these modifications are asymptomatic. Symptoms occurred in approximately 20% of cases and they are represented mostly by cervicobrachial neuralgia with a distribution territory adjacent to the primary level [20].

(35) Sixty-four years old female with history of breast cancer and severe osteoporosis. She reported a rapidly progressive walking impairment. Radiologic evaluation showed C7 metastasis. The selected approach was one of anterior corpectomy and fusion. She did well and was discharged three days after surgery and referred back to her oncologist. Five days after surgery she developed progressive paraparesis, neck pain and bilateral C7 radiculopathy. Radiological evaluation in the form of a latera XR is shown here (Fig. 10.2). What happened?
A. The cage was placed too posteriorly. The symptoms were hidden by corticosteroids given immediately after surgery.
B. Posterior displacement of the cage
C. T2 fracture due to adjacent segment disease

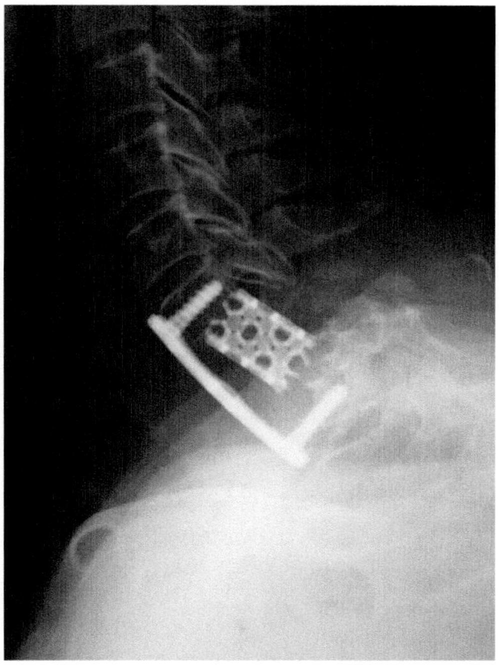

Fig. 10.2 Postoperative lateral cervical spine radiograph following C7 anterior corpectomy and fusion

D. Infection and spondylodiscitis
E. Bilateral iatrogenic injury of C7 root during surgery

Preferred Response: B: The image shows a posterior displacement of the cage due to construct failure. The reported history of severe osteoporosis and her oncological status suggest a higher risk of developing these complications.

(36) Two weeks after the posterior revision (posterior decompression and fusion) of previous surgery, she developed again the same symptoms. Radiologic evaluation showed a new construct failure (Fig. 10.3). What will be the following steps?
A. 360° revision: C5- T1 ACCF and posterior revision of C4-T3 construct
B. 360° revision: reposition of the cage and posterior extension of the construct cranially and caudally
C. Posterior removal of the construct. The patients should be referred to an endocrinologist for a proper therapy of the osteoporosis.
D. 360° revision: anterior removal of the cage and plate and posterior revision and extension of the construct with hooks
E. None of the above

Preferred Response: A + D: in case of multiple failure of the construct the hooks and pedicle screws proved to be a reliable method to provide further stability to the implant, a fortiori in cases of comorbidities impairing its strength. In the present case, removal of the anterior implant has been preferred because of the risk of further subsidence and progression of neurologic symptoms (Fig. 10.4) [21].

(37) Which of the following is not a potential complication of occipito-cervical fixation?
A. CSF leak
B. Wound breakdown and material exposure
C. Respiratory distress and swallowing
D. C2 radiculopathy due to its sacrifice
E. Restriction of the head movements

D: C2 root is not sacrificed during C0-C3/C4 occipito-cervical fixation as it is bypassed. (see Fig. 10.5).

(38) What are the potential "unique" risks of cervical total disc replacement?
A. Need of repeated surgery during a 4–5 years follow-up in 3–4% of patients
B. Immune reaction due to the generation of wear debris
C. Heterotopic ossification
D. Higher risk of adjacent segment surgery
E. A + B + C

Preferred Response: E: Cervical total disc replacement warrants some unique advantages over standard interbody fusion, such as fewer hardware related and post-operative complications, reduced risk of adjacent segment disease and maintaining of range of motion post-operatively. Nevertheless, this technique also presents unique risks, namely higher risk of repeated surgery at the same level, immune reaction due to generation of wear debris, such as metal ions generated by biocorrosion, and heterotopic ossification [22].

(39) What are recognized risk factors for heterotopic ossification in cervical total disc replacement?
A. Number of treated levels
B. Preoperative range of motion
C. Preoperative disc height
D. BMI (>30)
E. None of the above

Preferred Response: E: Recent studies on the occurrence of heterotopic ossification proved that the only factors related to the development of this complication are gender (male) and the percentage of endplate coverage. The other factors, such as number of treated levels, pre-operative range of motion and disc height, as well as BMI, were found to be not statistically significant [22].

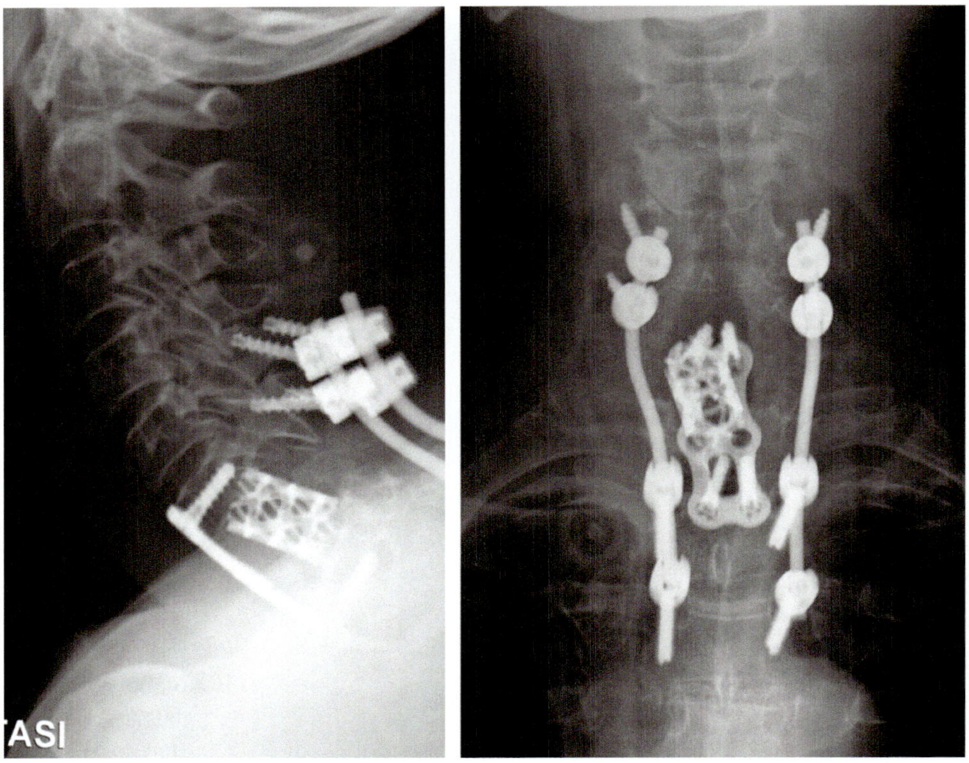

Fig. 10.3 Postoperative lateral (left) and AP (right) radiographs following revision surgery

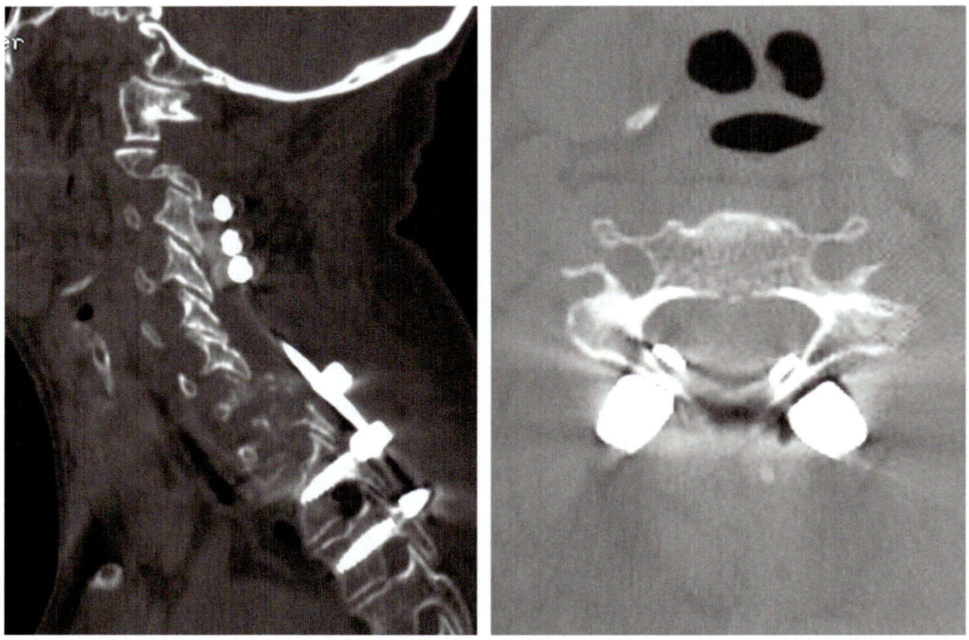

Fig. 10.4 Sagittal (left) and axial (right) CT scan images following second revision surgery demonstrating laminar hook fixation

(40) Which of the following sentences is true about Recurrent Laryngeal Nerve Injury?

A. The recurrent laryngeal nerve passes under the subclavian artery on the left side and under the aorta on the right side.

B. Hoarseness after surgery due to traction of the recurrent laryngeal nerve occurs from 3 to 11% of cases and it is usually transient

C. Left-sided approaches are at greater risk for recurrent laryngeal nerve injury

D. The most common cause of recurrent laryngeal nerve injury is its compression when it courses near the middle part of the outer lobes of the thyroid gland

E. All of the above

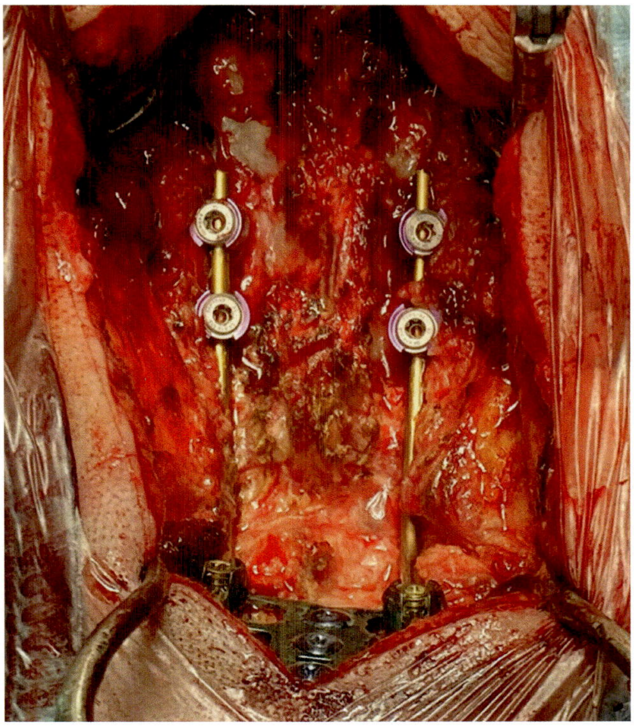

Fig. 10.5 Intraoperative picture demonstrating an occipito-cervical fixation with an occipital plate and subaxial lateral mass screws in C3 and C4

Preferred Response: B: Transient hoarseness due to recurrent laryngeal nerve traction has a rate ranging from 3 to 11%. The most common cause of its injury is compression within the endolarynx. Several studies report that the side of approach does not affect the incidence of recurrent laryngeal nerve injury. Of course, the recurrent laryngeal nerve courses under the aorta on the left side and under the subclavian artery on the right side [16].

(41) You are performing a percutaneous lumbar fixation. The intraoperative X-ray shows you the following images while introducing the Jamshidi needle (Fig. 10.6). What is happening?

A. The screw entry point is too lateral
B. The trajectory is too medial
C. The trajectory is following an anatomic route. It is proved that anatomic route has higher insertional torque than a straightforward route.
D. The trajectory of the screw is too lateral
E. None of the above

Preferred Response: B: In this case the trajectory of the screw is too medial. In fact, the Jamshidi needle is touching the medial pedicle contour in the AP X-ray while is passing the posterior wall of the vertebral body. Regarding the answer C, it is false because the anatomic route provides a lower insertional torque than the straightforward route.

(42) Which are the potential consequences of the previous clinical case?

A. CSF leak
B. Root injury
C. A + B + D
D. No consequences
E. A + B

Preferred Response: C: A medial screw may warrant several potential consequences. A patient may develop CSF leak with wound swelling, root injury with motor or sensory symptoms. Sometimes, lateral recess invasion by the screw may be asymptomatic.

(43) Ligation of the iliolumbar vein….

A. Is mandatory during OLIF and LLIF procedures when the side of the approach is the left

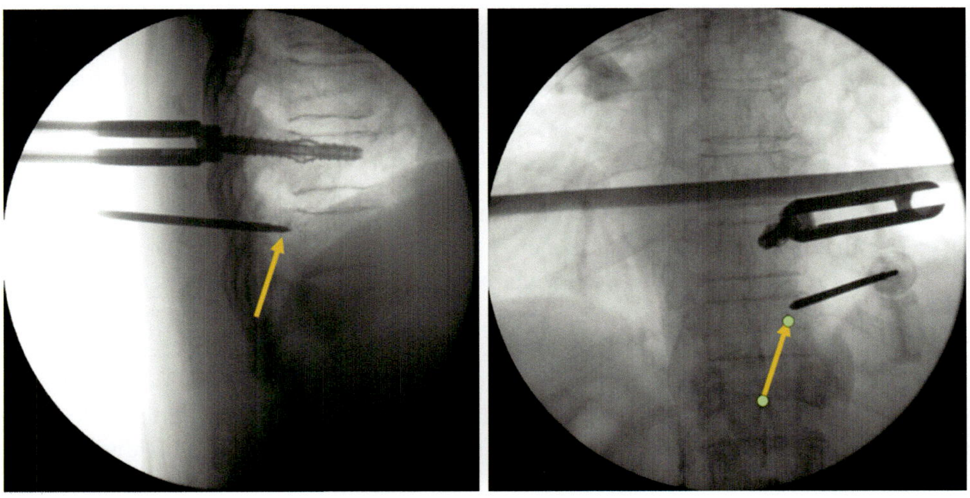

Fig. 10.6 Lateral (left) and AP (right) intraoperative XR demonstrating attempted placement of Jamshidi needle through the pedicle of a thoracic vertebra

B. Should be avoided whenever possible
C. It is mandatory, mostly for L5-S1 ALIF
D. It is mandatory, mostly for L4-L5 ALIF
E. All false

Preferred Response: D: Laceration of iliolumbar vein may result in deep and incontrollable bleeding due to the retraction of the vessel. Coagulation and hemostats are often insufficient. Therefore, when approaching L4-L5 during ALIF, identification and preventive ligation and division of this vessel is mandatory [23].

(44) You are performing a L4-L5 PLIF. During disc removal you had the feeling of the fibrous annulus breakdown, and deep anterior bleeding occurred. Such bleeding is controlled by floseal, fibrin glue and tamponade. It stops after cages insertion. After the surgery the patients complained an intractable abdominal pain. She was pale and her HR was 112 bpm. Hemoglobin was 7 mg/dl (preoperative Hb 12 mg/dl). Physical examination excluded acute abdomen. What is it happening?
A. Severe anemia and hypovolemic shock due to the intraoperative bleeding.
B. Bowel perforation
C. Iliac vein/artery injury and retroperitoneal hematoma
D. Anterior cage displacement due to fibrous annuls breakdown and lumbar sympathetic trunk irritation.
E. PLIF surgery is a long and complex surgery. Such symptoms and blood loss may be warranted by this procedure and will improve after few days.

Preferred Response: C: The present symptoms suggest the presence of anemia and hypovolemic shock due to current bleeding and retroperitoneal hematoma, determining the classical symptoms and signs of false acute abdomen. Iliac vein/artery injury justify this condition and it has been reported as a rare complication of posterior lumbar interbody fusion.

(45) What is the proper management of such situation?
A. Abdominal X-ray and refer the patient to a general surgeon
B. CT angiography abdomen and pelvis and refer the patient to vascular surgery
C. Anterior approach for cage revision
D. Hydration and blood transfusion
E. Paracetamol and tramadol for the pain

Preferred Response: B: Since the injury of the iliac vein/artery the correct steps for managing this situation are to perform an emergency CT angiography of abdomen and pelvis and to refer the patient to the vascular surgeon. Their choice may be either open surgery or endovascular stenting to stop the bleeding.

(46) Which of the following sentences about dural tear after anterior approaches to the subaxial cervical spine is correct?
A. Using good illumination, the operating microscope, and diamond-tip burrs in the vicinity of the dura mater may decrease the frequency of these complications.
B. OPLL increase the risk of dural tear after an anterior approach
C. OPLL is thinner laterally, thus the risk of dural tear increase during the removal of its lateral portion
D. Dura mater repair from a ventral approach is not always possible. Therefore, fascia hemostatic and sealants with or without lumbar drain may be effective solution.
E. All of the above

Preferred Response: E: The incidence of a CSF leak after anterior cervical OPLL resection has been reported to be between 6.7% and 31.8%. Proper surgical tools and techniques, such good illumination, the operating microscope, and diamond-tip burrs in the vicinity of the dura mater, reduce the occurrence of this complication. The posterior longitudinal ligament thins out laterally and dural tears occur mostly during lateral decompression.

In cases of dural tears, repair from a ventral approach is not always possible. Therefore, fascia lata with hemostatic agents (ORCs or gelatines) and fibrin glue application. Prophylactic insertion of a lumbar drain before surgery should be considered in high-risk patients [24].

(47) Which of the following is not a risk factor for adjacent segment degeneration (ASD) in spine surgery?
A. Fusion surgery
B. Anterior column support in lumbar interbody fusion
C. Modest increase of lordosis
D. Osteoporosis
E. All of the above

Preferred Response: B: Several studies with a long follow up showed that lumbar interbody fusion is not related to an increased risk of adjacent segment degeneration. Fusion surgery has a higher risk of ASD then non fusion strategies. Osteoporosis is related with higher risk of ASD, as well as surgical strategies gaining only a modest increase of lordosis. In fact, in this case, a greater range of motion of the superior vertebra has been detected as compared with surgeries providing greater increasing of lordosis [25].

(48) A thirty-five years old patient treated by means of a T12 vertebroplasty for an A3 fracture. After the surgery he developed paraplegia and bowel and urinary disfunction. What happened?
A. Adamkiewicz artery rupture due to bone fragment retropulsion
B. Wrong position of the patient determined fragmentation of the fracture that impinged the spinal cord
C. Cement leakage into the spinal canal and compression of the spinal cord
D. A higher fracture that was not noticed must be causing the symptoms
E. None of the above

Preferred Response: C: Cement leakage is one of the most serious complications of vertebroplasty and kyphoplasty. Its occurrence rate ranges up to 70% but its clinical significance can be detected only in less than 1% of cases.

(49) A thirty-six years old man treated with ALIF for severe discogenic pain at L5-S1. After surgery he presented retrograde ejaculation and bladder disfunction. What happened during surgery?
A. Using of monopolar for dissecting the ventral fascia
B. A transperitoneal approach was used
C. A left approach was used
D. A + B
E. A + B + C

Preferred Response: D: Retrograde ejaculation is one of the most dreaded complications of the ALIF. Its occurrence is estimated to range up to 1%. Using monopolar dissection of the ventral fascia increase the risk of superior hypogastric plexus injury. It has been proven that the use of transperitoneal approach is related with a greater risk of retrograde ejaculation as compared with retroperitoneal approaches (8,6% vs 3,2%). No difference in the side of approaches have been reported [6].

(50) Immediately after a C4-C5 ACDF with right sided approach, the patient is anisocoric (left > right). What would you do?
A. Nothing
B. I will carefully evaluate the patient: if he does not present any alteration of the consciousness or neurological deficit, I will do nothing else.
C. CT scan before waking up the patient
D. CT scan before sending the patient to the ICU
E. Exploration of the surgical field to rule out hematomas

Preferred Response: B: Bernard Horner syndrome is a rare complication of anterior cervical approaches. Its occurrence should be suspected in cases of anisocoria without consciousness alteration and neurological deficits [26].

(51) In the previous case, which is the most common cause of anisocoria?
A. Bernard-Horner syndrome due to injury to sympathetic chain ipsilaterally to the side of the approach
B. Pourfour du Petit syndrome contralaterally to the side of the approach
C. Spinal cord lesion due to hyperextension of the head
D. Epidural hematoma due to malpositioning of the head holder
E. None of the above

Preferred Response: A: Horner syndrome is made of blepharoptosis as well as ipsilateral pupillary miosis and facial anhidrosis. The reported rate varies between 0.06% and 3.8%. It can be caused by impairment to the sympathetic pathway. Pourfour du Petit syndrome is caused by irritation of sympathetic chain. It is featured by ipsilateral mydriasis, lid retraction and exophthalmos. Thus, in the present case its occurrence can be excluded since the anisocoria was left > right in a right sided approach [26].

(52) What are the strategies to avoid sympathetic chain injury in an anterior cervical approach?
A. Mobilize the longus colli muscle over the length of the exposure
B. The medial retraction blade should be inserted after the lateral blade
C. Longus colli muscle should not be detached
D. A + B
E. The lateral retraction blade should be inserted after the medial blade

Preferred Response: D: To avoid Bernard Horner syndrome, it is necessary to mobilize the longus colli muscle over the length of the exposure and insert the medial retraction blade after the lateral blades.

(53) How can you distinguish radiographically successful and failed fusion after surgery?
A. Absence of any movement on flexion and extension radiographs
B. Less than 6° of angular motion. Translational motion should be absent on flexion and extension radiographs.

C. Less than 3 mm of translational motion and less than 5° of angular motion on flexion and extension radiographs
D. The distinction is clinical and not radiological: failed surgery is defined when symptoms recurred in the same area in absence of any other cause
E. None of the above

Preferred Response: C: The FDA radiographic guidelines for successful lumbar fusion include less than 3 mm of translational motion and less than 5° of angular motion on flexion and extension radiographs [27].

(54) What is the major complication of intradural approach for posterolateral thoracic disk herniations?
A. Spinal cord injury
B. CSF leak
C. Incomplete resection of prolapsed disc
D. Instability
E. All of the above

Preferred Response: B: The intradural approach for thoracic disc herniation is a safe and effective technique that allow removal of the fragments under direct visualization. The major downside of this technique is the difficulty of ventral dura closure with some cases of postoperative CSF leaks [28].

(55) Which of the following are the morphological categories used by Heggeness and Esses in 1991 to classify posterolateral lumbar pseudarthrosis?
A. Anterior, posterior, anteromedial, anterolateral, posteromedial, posterolateral
B. Superior endplate, inferior endplate, anterior wall, posterior wall, complex
C. Non-union, anterior bridge, posterior bridge, circumferential, complex
D. Atrophic, transverse, shingle, complex
E. Atrophic, hypertrophic, non-union, shingle, complex

Preferred Response: D: In 1991, Heggeness and Esses described 4 unique morphological categories to help classify posterolateral lumbar pseudarthrosis: atrophic, transverse, shingle, and complex. The atrophic type is strongly associated with the presence of intact facet joints or spinal hardware [29].

(56) Which of the following is not an indication for early revision surgery of a spinal construct?
A. Suboptimal implant position, recognized immediately after surgery (for the OR without intraoperative CT scan)
B. Early failure
C. Inappropriate implant configuration for the mechanical environment
D. Pseudoarthrosis
E. All the answers are correct

Preferred Response: D: Answer A, B, and C are proposed by AO spine as indications for early revision surgery. Pseudoarthrosis is a late complication of spine fusion. It can be suspected when a patient presents with recurrent pain and/or neurological symptoms during the long-term follow-up. A fortiori, fusion is achieved 6 to 9 months after surgery. Lastly, diagnosis of pseudoarthrosis is not always an indication for revision surgery [30].

(57) A fifty-four years old man is treated for L4- L5 grade I spondylolisthesis via minimally invasive right lateral transpsoas approach (LLIF). The procedure was conducted without any relevant problem and lasted 33 min. During the surgery, no EMG activity was noted during the dissection of the psoas muscle. EMG of the distal muscles was activated only via direct stimulation posterior to the final retractor position. After the procedure the patient developed a 3/5 right hip flexor and quadriceps weakness and sensory paresthesia over the ipsilateral anterior thigh. What happened?
A. The approach was too posterior and there was a direct injury to the right L4 root
B. The opening of the posterior retractor may have compressed and stretched the lumbar plexus
C. The cage was too small, and it was displaced posteriorly compressing right L5 root
D. The surgery was too long, and lumbar plexus injury was due to the prolonged position
E. None of the above

Preferred Response: B: The lumbosacral plexus shows a progressive ventral migration from L2–3, L3–4, and L4–5. It is positioned most dorsally at the posterior endplate of L1–2. This configuration may result in nerve injury to the lumbosacral plexus, especially at the L4–5 level, when the dilator and/or retractor is placed in a posterior position along the disc space [31].

(58) A thirty-three years old patient came to the emergency room. He complained of severe orthostatic headache, vomiting, neck pain and photophobia. He has multiple sclerosis (MS) treated by immunosuppressive drugs (Fingolimod). He was treated surgically 7 months ago for a L3-L4 lumbar disc herniation with prompt resolution of the previous symptoms. Blood test showed a

mild lymphopenia, CRP and other inflammatory markers were normal. MRI showed a new right periventricular plaque, and a diffuse thickening of the dura mater. What is the next step?
A. MRI of the neck
B. Lumbar puncture (serologic and microbiologic test) and empiric broad spectrum antibiotics
C. Refer the patient to a neurologist to tweak the therapy for MS
D. NSAIDs
E. Contrast enhanced MRI of the brain and lumbar spine and hydration

Preferred Response: E: The patient's symptoms suggest intracranial hypotension. The history of previous lumbar surgery points to a iatrogenic cause. Therefore, the next step for the diagnosis are contrast enhanced MRI of the brain and lumbar spine, where a dural tear may be present. Moreover, hydration may relieve the symptoms further bolstering the hypothesis of intracranial hypotension.

(59) A thirty-three years old patient came to the emergency room. He complained severe orthostatic headache, vomiting, neck pain and photophobia. What could be the cause of patient symptoms?
A. Spondylodiscitis. The blood test does not show signs of infection due to the immunosuppressive drugs for MS
B. Meningitis. The immunosuppressive drugs increase the risk for aseptic meningitis (caused by viruses or bacteria like Borrelia and Treponema pallidum).
C. Relapsing MS
D. Intracranial hypotension
E. Cervical myelopathy

Preferred Response: D: Intracranial hypotension or craniospinal hypotension was first described by Schaltenbrand in 1938. It is defined as cerebrospinal fluid (CSF) pressure < 6 cm H_2O. Its clinical presentations are postural headache, nausea, vomiting, neck pain, visual and hearing disturbances, and vertigo. It results from a CSF leak somewhere along the neuraxis. Causes of spinal CSF leakage reported in the literature include, lumbar puncture, cervical bony spurs, meningeal diverticula, nerve root sleeve tears, thoracic disc herniation, trauma, and Tarlov cyst. Lumbar disc herniation surgery is a very rare cause of intracranial hypotension, but it should be considered when clinical history and symptoms match [32].

(60) Which of the following sentences is true regarding the treatment of adult scoliosis?
A. Combined anterior/posterior approaches (thoracotomies/thoracoabdominal) provide better results in terms of radiographic correction and alignment but are associated with higher complication rate.
B. Posterior-only surgery (pedicle screws/osteotomies/PLIF or TLIF) provides better results in terms of radiographic correction and alignment, but it is associated with higher blood loss, operative time and length of hospital stay.
C. Posterior-only surgery (pedicle screws/osteotomies/PLIF or TLIF) provides the same results of combined anterior/posterior approaches in terms of radiographic correction, alignment, clinical outcomes, and complications. Moreover, it is associated with lower blood loss, operative time and length of hospital stay.
D. Combined anterior/posterior approaches (thoracotomies/thoracoabdominal) provide worse results than posterior-only surgery (pedicle screws/osteotomies/PLIF or TLIF) in terms of correction, alignment, clinical outcomes, and complications. Nevertheless, it is related with lower blood loss, operative time and length of hospital stay.
E. Combined anterior/posterior approaches (thoracotomies/thoracoabdominal) is not an alternative to posterior-only surgery (pedicle screws/osteotomies/PLIF or TLIF). It depends on the preoperative coronal and sagittal alignment of the spine. Therefore, a comparison cannot be made between these approaches.

Preferred Response: C: Rigid adult scoliosis has been treated for decades with combined anterior/posterior approaches. Those approaches require long surgical times and are often performed in two steps. This increases the risks related to blood loss, operative time and length of hospital stay. Recently, posterior-only surgery (pedicle screws/osteotomies/PLIF or TLIF) arose as an alternative to the combined route. Several papers show that these corridors provide the same results of combined anterior/posterior approaches in terms of radiographic correction, alignment, clinical outcomes, and complications [33].

(61) Which of the following is not an adverse event related to the use of rhBMP-2 in spine surgery?
A. Symptomatic hypersensitivity and immunologic reactions
B. Increased risk of pseudoarthrosis
C. Ectopic bone formation
D. B + C
E. None of the above

Preferred Response: A: Symptomatic ectopic bone formation, pseudarthrosis and vertebral osteolysis, are complications associated with the use of rhBMP-2 in spine surgery. Improper dosage and postoperative BMP-2 fluid collection may be the potential causes. Besides, it has been proven that its use is not related with symptomatic immunologic reaction. Antibodies formation against rhBMP is transient and does not change clinical outcomes or safety parameters.

(62) Which of the following is a proper method for preventing infection after transoral surgery?
   A. Avoid transoral surgery in patients with rheumatoid or oncological diseases
   B. Self-rinsing the wound with diluted iodine solution
   C. A + B
   D. Post-operative parenteral nutrition for 7 days
   E. Preoperative microbiological swabs, significant cultures and sensitivities should be taken

Preferred Response: E: After trans-oral surgery the risk of wound infection rages from 1 to 4%. The patient should be nil-by-mouth for 5 days after surgery, and nutrition should be given by nasogastric feeding tube for 5 days (answer D incorrect). Professional oral nursing care decreases the possibility of oral wound infection and dehiscence (answer B incorrect). Although, oncologic and rheumatoid patients carry a higher risk of post-operative infections, they should undergo transoral approaches when required (answer A incorrect). Preoperative swabs should be taken from the oropharynx to exclude multiple-resistant pathogens. Other strategies are oral examination to exclude oropharyngeal infection and odontopathies, daily oral hygiene, and the use of Dobell's solution or chlorhexidine mouth wash. Odontopathies should be treated preoperatively. Oral hygiene should be maintained preoperatively to prevent the occurrence of wound infection [34].

(63) A sixty-seven years old patient complains of pain in right buttock and midline lower lumbar area that started 6 months earlier. During the last two weeks he developed sharp and stabbing pain and hypoesthesia radiating from the buttock down the leg to the outside of the ankle and into the top of the foot on the right. Neurological examination, with provocative tests for radicular pain, was negative. Two years prior to presentation the patient underwent a L3-L4 right TLIF surgery for foraminal stenosis due to scoliosis convex to the right with the apex at L3. After surgery he experienced symptoms relief and since then had no further problems. Lumbar MRI and CT scan showed the correct placement of the construct and a solid fusion. No foraminal stenosis or adjacent segment disease were detected. AP X-ray showed an exacerbation of the scoliosis. What could be the cause of patient symptoms?
   A. The exacerbation of the scoliosis.
   B. Failed back surgery syndrome
   C. Sacroiliitis
   D. Tandem spinal stenosis in cervical and lumbar segment
   E. None of the above

Preferred Response: C: The sacroiliac joint (SIJ) is a possible source of persistent or new onset pain after lumbar or lumbosacral fusion. Often it is a diagnosis of exclusion because its symptoms are similar to many other common sources of back pain. Its clinical presentation may vary from pain at ipsilateral buttock (94% cases) and at midline lower lumbar area (74%). Finally, up to 50% of cases have radiation to the lower extremity. X-ray of the pelvis/lumbar spine performed in an anteroposterior view shows sclerosis or other degenerative changes of the SI joint [35].

(64) What is the proper management of sacroiliitis occurred after spine surgery?
   A. Sacroiliac joint injection with methylprednisolone and local anesthetics
   B. Sacroiliac joint fixation/sacroiliac joint fusion
   C. NSAIDs
   D. B + C
   E. A + B + C

Preferred Response: E: In cases of sacroiliitis after lumbar spine fixation the proper management is NSAIDs followed by local injection of methylprednisolone and local anesthetics. The latter can be used as diagnostic blocks for diagnosis ex-adjuvantibus. Finally, if the patient has no relief, surgery with sacroiliac fixation or minimally invasive fusion [35].

(65) A sixty-seven years old male patient that underwent trans-thoracic corpectomy T12 and posterior T10-L2 fusion for a T12 vertebral fracture developed adjacent segment disease at L3 after three years. Decision was made to extend the construct further caudally to include the pelvis. Which of the following should be part of the planning/decision making to avoid long term failure of the pelvic construct?
   A. Sacral slope and pelvic incidence
   B. L5 disc height
   C. Using always monoaxial screws in the sacrum
   D. A + B
   E. A + B + C

Preferred Response: D: Sacral slope and pelvic incidence describe the shape of the spine and the position of the pelvis. In a straight pelvis (low sacral slope and low pelvic incidence) the forces going through L5-S1 junction are mostly axial whilst in patients with lordotic pelvis (high sacral slope and high pelvic incidence) force vectors are more tangential and pass through the disc. The L5-S1 disc height is an important factor influencing long term outcome. In fact, a tall L5-S1 disc may degenerate over time, increasing the risk of a progressive kyphosis, sagittal imbalance and screw pull-out with failure of the construct [36].

(66) A twenty-two years old patient harboring a T12 A4 (according to the AO Spine Classification) fracture and progressive neurological deficit was treated with a temporary short construct T11-L1. He returned 3 months later with back pain. The X-ray showed the following scenario (Fig. 10.7). What was the cause of the system failure?
- A. The screws have an anatomic route. For junctional construct, a straightforward trajectory is preferred
- B. The patient should have been evaluated for osteoporosis, also given the primary fracture
- C. The rods were too short
- D. Short constructs have to be avoided in thoracolumbar junction
- E. C + D

Preferred Response: C: in this case is clearly visible that the rods are too short, causing an aberrant lever arm determining the failure of the construct.

(67) Which of the following is the least frequent complication of transoral surgery for cranio-vertebral junction and upper cervical spine?
- A. Vertebral artery injury
- B. Wound infection
- C. Velopharyngeal insufficiency
- D. CSF leak
- E. Temporary quadriplegia

Preferred Response: A: Wound infection (3.1%), velopharyngeal insufficiency (3.1%), and CSF leak and temporary quadriplegia (both ranging up to 5%) are common complications of transoral surgery. Vertebral artery injury is reported to have a rate of 1% [37].

(68) A 12-year-old female patient with juvenile arthritis presents with complaints of cervical pain and progressive motor impairment. CT scan showed basilar invagination and dynamic cervical X-rays an increased atlantoaxial space (9 mm) and subluxation, which decreases in extension and increases in flexion. It was decided to perform an occipito-cervical fixation. Neuromonitoring, placed after the positioning, showed decreased motor and sensory evoked potentials. Data remained stable for the whole procedure. After the surgery the patient was quadriplegic, and she died few days later. What do you think happened?
- A. Posterior fossa hematoma due to misplaced occipital screws
- B. Wrong head positioning
- C. Vertebral artery rupture
- D. Sympathetic chain injury
- E. Thromboembolism

Preferred Response: B: Neurological injury can be avoided using proper stabilization before positioning, and obtaining neurophysiological monitoring data before positioning and then, just after head fixation before starting the procedure

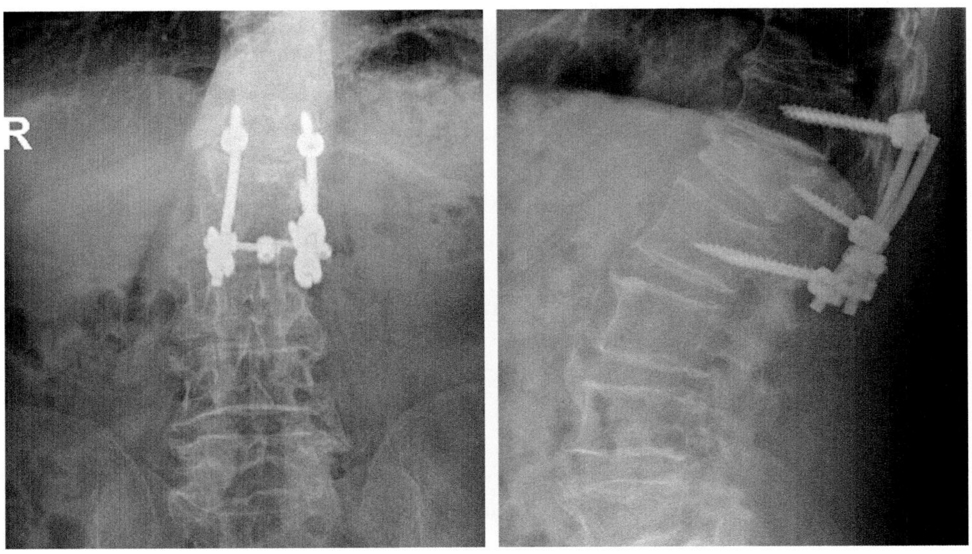

Fig. 10.7 Postoperative AP (left) and lateral (right) XR of T11-L1 construct at 3 months

itself. In fact, some patients may warrant head position adjustment due to decreased neuromonitoring signals [38].

(69) What is a true statement about standard iliac screws and S2-Alar-Iliac screws
   A. Standard iliac screws have a lower rate of implant failure due to more extensive bony purchase
   B. S2-Alar-iliac screws have a lower rate of implant failure due to more extensive cortical purchase
   C. There is no difference between Standard iliac screws and S2-alar-iliac screws in terms of implant failure
   D. Cross links in iliac screw construct reduces the rate of implant failure
   E. B + D

Preferred Response: E: S2-Alar-iliac screws have a lower incidence of implant failure as compared to iliac screws (27% vs. 57%,). Cross links in iliac screws construct may dramatically decrease the rate of standard iliac screws failure, making it comparable to the S2 alar-iliac screws [39].

(70) After C3-C7 cervical posterior decompression, a 69 years-old patient woke up quadriplegic. What would you do?
   A. Nothing. Transient quadriplegia is a common complication of posterior cervical decompression.
   B. High dose of corticosteroid
   C. Revision surgery
   D. CT scan and eventually revision surgery
   E. None of the above

Preferred Response: D: Quadriplegia is an uncommon but dramatic complication of posterior cervical decompression. Its cause may be epidural hematoma, CSF leak, ischemia. The proper management is to perform an emergency CT and eventually perform a revision surgery [38].

(71) A seventy-four years old patient with a T9 fracture (A2 according to AO Spine classification) is treated with a percutaneous kyphoplasty. After surgery he developed severe dyspnea (SpO_2 77%). What do you suspect?
   A. Atelectasis
   B. Pulmonary cement embolism
   C. Pulmonary embolism due to the fracture
   D. Hemorrhagic shock
   E. It is a normal complication due to the prone position

Preferred Response: B: The incidence of pulmonary cement embolism ranges from 2.1% to 26% after vertebroplasty and kyphoplasty. In its asymptomatic form, it is a common condition without permanent clinical sequelae. Nevertheless, if symptomatic it represents a severe clinical condition and warrants proper management of the respiratory and cardiovascular status in the intensive care unit [40].

(72) What is the most common peri-operative complication of pedicle subtraction osteotomy?
   A. Hypovolemic shock
   B. Neurological deficit
   C. Infection
   D. Screws pull out
   E. Pulmonary embolism

Preferred Response: B: The rate of neurologic deficit after PSO rages from 11 to 16%. Dural buckling and dorsal impingement, as well as manipulation of the nerve root, are the most common causes for the neurologic deterioration [41].

(73) What is the best augmentation material for reducing the rate of pulmonary cement embolism?
   A. PMMA, since there has not been reported any significant difference with new substitutes
   B. Polypropylene fumarate
   C. Calcium phosphate cement
   D. High-viscosity cements
   E. None of the above

Preferred Response: D: High-viscosity cements significantly decrease the incidence of leakage compared with low-viscosity cements. Furthermore, high-viscosity bone cement is associated with lower cement leakage rate. Calcium phosphate cement and polypropylene fumarate are interesting cement substitute for vertebral augmentation due to the cytocompatibility and osteoconductive behavior, nevertheless, they are associated with the same extrusion and pulmonary embolism rates than PMMA [42].

(74) During a revision surgery for a L4 adjacent segment disease in a patient operated 10 years earlier with L5-S1 TLIF, a dural tear occurs. You repair it with sutures and reinforce the closure with Tachosil and fibrin glue. After surgery, the patient is given therapy with fluids, antibiotics, and low molecular weight heparin (Enoxaparin). On the 3rd post-op day, he develops a fever (37,7 °C) that lasted for 8 days and has been never higher than 38 °C. His blood tests are normal. CT scan and MRI do not show any signs of acute infection. What can be the potential cause?

A. Immunogenic reaction to the new materials implanted
B. Pre-existing hematologic disease
C. Inappropriate administration of antibiotics
D. Aseptic meningitis
E. Enoxaparin

Preferred Response: E: Fever is reported as a potential adverse event related to the administration of Enoxaparin. Anecdotic cases are reported of prolonged persistent post-operative fever associated with the use of Enoxaparin. One of the possible explanations is that enoxaparin is typically derived from bovine or porcine intestines and lungs, potentially causing hypersensitivity reactions is perhaps unsurprising. Therefore, physicians should be aware of this occurrence.

(75) What is the proper management?
A. High dose of corticosteroids
B. Withdrawal of enoxaparin
C. Spinal tap and immunologic and bacteriologic tests
D. A + B
E. Protamine sulfate

Preferred Response: B: In the reported cases of enoxaparin induced fever, the discontinuation of the drug leads to symptoms relief. No other treatments is usually necessary.

(76) Fifty-five-years old male patient with a grade B (according to Schizas classification) L4-L5 lumbar stenosis. He reported back pain, difficulties in walking and in extending the spine. He does not report pain irradiating to the lower limbs. His other co-morbidities are Lyme arthritis, atrial fibrillation, Parkinson's disease, chronic obstructive pulmonary disease and right convex scoliosis with L2 as apical vertebra. His neurological physical examinations showed diffuse hyperreflexia (+3) and the other signs of his neurologic comorbidities. He underwent L4-L5 McCulloch laminectomy (also known as lumbar laminoplasty or unilateral laminectomy with bilateral decompression). You see the patient 7 months after surgery. He complains that his symptoms have not improved. Why did the surgery fail?
A. The symptoms were caused by Parkinson's disease, thus there was no need for surgery.
B. The patients may have a tandem stenosis. In this case he should perform a cervical MRI and eventually cervical spine decompression.
C. In case of scoliosis the first treatment is aimed at restoring the coronal alignment with long implants and anterior decompression or posterior osteotomies.
D. The symptoms are caused by the Lyme arthritis. The patient should receive long term therapy with antibiotics.
E. Schizas B stenosis is associated with a low rate of symptoms improvement after surgery.

Preferred Response: A: Parkinson's disease is characterized by cardinal motor signs: 4–6 Hz resting tremor, rigidity and bradykinesia as well as camptocormia, an abnormal forward flexion of the thoracolumbar spine in 3–18% of cases. Such symptoms may often mimic lumbar stenosis clinical scenario. Therefore, physicians should carefully consider the clinical history of the patient before deeming him suitable for surgery. In this case, the slight hyperreflexia (accompanied by plastic paresis) is a typical Parkinson sign and should not be confused for a mark of myelopathy.

(77) Which of the following is not a predictor of high risk of adverse events after percutaneous screws placement after single-segment thoracolumbar burst fractures?
A. Intervertebral disc injury
B. Preoperative Cobb angle
C. Type of fracture
D. Surgically corrected Cobb angle
E. Interpedicular distance (IPD)

Preferred Response: C: Radiological predictors for adverse events in patients with thoracolumbar burst fractures one year after percutaneous screws placement Include intervertebral disc injury, preoperative cobb angle, surgically corrected Cobb angle, and IPD were independent risk factors. The type of fracture is not a predictor of poor outcome [43].

(78) Cervical pedicle screws provide…
A. higher resistance to pull-out forces than lateral mass screws and lower rate of mispositioning
B. same resistance to pull-out forces than lateral mass screws but higher rate of mispositioning
C. higher resistance to pull-out forces than lateral mass screws and same rate of mispositioning
D. higher resistance to pull-out forces than lateral mass screws but higher rate of mispositioning
E. same resistance to pull-out forces than lateral mass screws and same rate of mispositioning

Preferred Response: D: Cervical pedicle screws demonstrated a significantly higher resistance to pull-out forces than did lateral mass screws. Nevertheless, the rates of pedicle screw mispositioning and related neurovascular complications and neurological deterioration is high. Pedicle screws insertion is more challenging than lateral mass screws, consequently, they should be used only after thorough preoperative evaluation of cervical anatomy [44].

(79) What is the most frequent complication of harvesting iliac crest bone grafting in spine surgery in children?
A. Sacroiliac penetration
B. Local pain
C. Infection
D. Skin irritation
E. B + D

Preferred Response: B: Complication rates in iliac crest bone grafting in children spine surgery is low (<2%). Among those, pain (24%) and pain that is severe enough to interfere with daily activity (15%) is an underrecognized condition that impact significantly with surgery outcomes [45].

(80) What is the most consistent risk factor for recurrent disc herniation?
A. Diabetes mellitus
B. Shape and size of the disc
C. Incomplete discectomy
D. L3-L4 and L5-S1
E. A + B

Preferred Response: E: A recurrent disc herniation is defined as a herniated disc material at the same level and site in a patient that has experienced a pain free interval after discectomy. Its incidence varies between 5 and 23%. The only risk factors that have consistently shown a strong association are diabetes mellitus and the shape and size of the herniation [46].

(81) What of the following sentences is true?
A. Minimally invasive discectomy such as fully endoscopic discectomy and microdiscectomy have no differences in terms of rates of disc removal and pain relief
B. Minimally invasive discectomy is associated with lower risk of surgical site and other infections as compared with microdiscectomy
C. Higher hazard of re-hospitalization due to recurrent disc herniation in minimally invasive discectomy as compared with microdiscectomy
D. A + B
E. All of the above

Preferred Response: E: A recent Cochrane review about comparison between minimally invasive discectomy and microdiscectomy was not able to demonstrate differences in clinical outcomes, such as pain and disc removal rate. Besides, the analysis of secondary outcomes, demonstrated that minimally invasive discectomy is associated with lower risk of surgical site and other infections, but higher hazard of re-hospitalization due to recurrent disc herniation [47].

(82) Which one is the correct Yeom classification for cement leakage:
A. Type B (leakage via the basivertebral vein), type S (leakage via the segmental vein), and type C (through a cortical defect)
B. Type I (intervertebral-extradiscal leakage), Type II (intradiscal leakage) and Type III (combined).
C. Type A (intracanalar), Type B (intraforaminal), Type C (Intervertebral), Type D (paravertebral)
D. Type I (<1 mm maximum width on axial CT scan), Type II (1 – 4 mm maximum width on axial CT scan), Type III (> 5 mm maximum width on axial CT scan)
E. None of the above

Preferred Response: A: Yeom And his colleagues, in 2003, classified cement leakage into three types: those via the basivertebral vein (type B), via the segmental vein (type S), and through a cortical defect (type C) [48].

(83) Which of the following complications increases specifically in spine surgery for the treatment of flaccid neuromuscular scoliosis in Duchenne's muscular dystrophy (DMD)?
A. Implant failure
B. Excessive intraoperative bleeding
C. Progression of deformity above or below the instrumented segments
D. Infections
E. All of the above

Preferred Response: E: Patients with neuromuscular diseases, especially DMD, are prone to excessive intraoperative bleeding and postoperative wound infections. Alongside, generalized osteopenia increases the risk of implant failure. Finally, risk of progression of deformity is increased due to the biomechanical impairment related to the pathology itself.

(84) What is the most frequent complication after Gaines' procedure for L5 spondyloptosis?
A. Sympathetic chain injury
B. Hypogastric plexus injury
C. Neurologic complications
D. Retroperitoneal hematoma
E. Implant failure

Preferred Response: C: The Gaines procedure was first described in 1985. It consists in complete anterior removal of the body of L5 anteriorly followed by posterior reduction of L4 into the sacrum. It has been reported to have a neurologic complication rate (transient or permanent) as high as 77% [49].

(85) Which are the most frequent complications of transsternal approaches to the cervical-thoracic spine?
  A. Right recurrent laryngeal nerve palsy
  B. Post sternotomy mediastinitis
  C. Left recurrent laryngeal nerve palsy
  D. A + B
  E. A + B + C

Preferred Response: D: The nerve that may be injured during surgical exploration and management of the lower neck is the right recurrent laryngeal nerve that passes under the right subclavian artery and ascends obliquely toward the medial aspect of the neck, travelling in the avascular plane between the right common carotid and the tracheoesophageal complex, at C7 level. Contrariwise, the left recurrent laryngeal nerve, turns under the aortic arch and ascends medially in the tracheoesophageal groove. The rate of right recurrent laryngeal nerve palsy is reported ranging from 3 to 7% after transsternal approaches for the cervical-thoracic junction. Finally, deep sternal wound infection, known as post-sternotomy mediastinitis, occurs in 1% to 3% of patients, leading to serious morbidity and mortality of up to 25% [50].

(86) Which of the following is not a factor for considering prophylactic inferior vena cava filter placement before anterior approaches to the lumbar spine?
  A. History of thromboembolism
  B. Thrombophilia
  C. expected need for significant iliocaval manipulation
  D. Malignancies
  E. None of the above

Preferred Response: E: All of these factors increase the risk of proximal deep venous thrombosis and pulmonary embolism. In such cases, consideration should be given to prophylactic inferior vena cava filter placement. The use of routine chemical deep venous thrombosis prophylaxis is controversial, and the risk of bleeding versus thrombosis should be weighed for each individual patient [51].

(87) What is the most common isolated microorganism during the perioperative period in cases of spinal wound infection?
  A. Enterobacter cloacae
  B. Pseudomonas aeruginosa
  C. Staphylococcus aureus
  D. Staphylococcus epidermidis
  E. Streptococcus B haemolyticus

Preferred Response: C: Data from the National Nosocomial Infections Surveillance (NNIS) system reported rates of wound infection of 1.25% after laminectomy and a 2.1% after spinal arthrodesis. In the perioperative period, Staphylococcus aureus is the most common isolated microorganism from both deep and superficial spinal wounds [34].

(88) Which of the following sentences is false about reconstruction strategies for wounds of the distal third (L3-S5)?
  A. Superior gluteal artery perforator flaps can be turned safely for covering wound dehiscence in the lower third.
  B. "Gluteal muscle advancement flaps" is one of the most common strategies for wound reconstruction in the distal third.
  C. Bilateral gluteal artery advancement flap is the gold standard to reconstruct wounds that have been previously irradiated.
  D. The transpelvic vertical rectus abdominus myocutaneous (VRAM) flap should be employed when the gluteal arteries have been sacrificed
  E. The transpelvic vertical rectus abdominus myocutaneous (VRAM) flap should be employed in patients that had previous radiation to the pelvis.

Preferred Response: C: Spinal wounds can be localized by dividing the back in thirds: cervical, thoracic, and lumbosacral. Lumbosacral third, or distal third, embeds wounds extending from L3 to S5. The choice rationale for the proper flap relies on the patency of gluteal vessels. Therefore, in cases of either nonirradiated patient with compromised gluteal vessels or patients who received pelvic irradiation the VRAM flap (or free flaps) should be preferred over bilateral gluteal artery advancement. The latter is used only in cases of non-irradiated patients and patients with spared gluteal vessels [9].

(89) Which of the following sentences is false about slip progression after surgical treatment in lumbar spondylolisthesis?
  A. Posterior-only fusion in the presence of a high-grade listhesis are at risk of slip progression due to the tension that occurs across the kyphotic

deformity and the non-physiologic orientation of the fusion mass
   B. Risk of further slippage is related to the type of slip and the amount of initial sagittal plane deformity.
   C. Disc degeneration may increase the risk of slip progression
   D. Decompression alone by removing all the posterior elements (Gill's procedure) can be performed alone in grade II and III spondylolisthesis, because it provides fast symptoms improvement and the same rate of slip progression of posterior instrumented surgery.
   E. B + D

Preferred Response: D: Surgical technique plays a pivotal role in determining the risk of slip progression after the treatment of spondylolisthesis. In situ fusion with removal of posterior elements for decompression is associated with a higher rate of slip progression and kyphosis. A fortiori, complete removal of the posterior elements at the slipped, lytic level, known as the Gill procedure, increases the risk of slippage. Even if this procedure is associated with good short terms clinical outcomes, its biomechanical long terms results are much worse than the other procedures [52].

(90) After a L2 vertebroplasty you detect an intradiscal cement leakage. What will you expect regarding patient's clinical outcomes?
   A. Higher risk of adjacent vertebra collapse
   B. Higher risk of delayed neurological deficits
   C. Delayed pain relief
   D. A + B
   E. A + B + C

Preferred Response: C: Intervertebral cement leakage has been classified in three types: Type I intervertebral extra-discal leakage, Type II intradiscal leakage and Type III combined. It has been proven not to be related with an increased risk for adjacent vertebral fractures, and impaired outcomes in terms of pain relief or improvement of physical function. Intradiscal leakage is the most common type of cement leakage, and it is related to delayed pain relief [53].

(91) Which of the following sentences is false regarding post-operative kyphosis after cervical laminectomy?
   A. The correlation between the development of post-operative kyphosis and neurologic outcomes has not been demonstrated.
   B. Long term deterioration results from the draping and compression of the spinal cord over the ventral kyphotic deformity.
   C. The incidence of late deterioration following cervical laminectomy varies from 10 to 39%.
   D. Post-operative kyphosis is caused by the loss of the posterior tension band and the loss of the posterior cervical musculature.
   E. The incidence of post-laminectomy kyphosis is higher in adults then in children

Preferred Response: E: The incidence of post-laminectomy kyphosis ranges from 6 to 47% in adults and up to 100% in children. In children, there are two types of postoperative cervical laminectomy kyphosis: wedging of the vertebral bodies and subluxation with excessive motion between vertebrae. Several studies found a rate of post-laminectomy kyphosis near to 100% in children; therefore, fusion is required after posterior cervical decompression [54].

(92) What is the correct definition of pseudomeningocele?
   A. Pseudomeningocele is a postoperative extravasated collection of extradural CSF that communicates with the subarachnoid space through a breach in the dura mater and arachnoid.
   B. Pseudomeningocele is a cystic dilatation of the meninges containing cerebrospinal fluid without any neural tissue.
   C. Pseudomeningocele is a birth defect in which the spinal canal does not close before birth.
   D. Pseudomeningocele is an extradural CSF communication with the subcutaneous space or a direct communication with the outside through the skin.

Preferred response: A: Pseudomeningocele is defined as a postoperative extravasated collection of extradural CSF that communicates with the subarachnoid space through a breach in the dura mater and arachnoid. CSF fistula relies on the same mechanism and occurs when there is a direct communication of the CSF with another cavity or with the outside.

(93) A twenty-two years old patient with rheumatoid arthritis has been treated with a C0-C4 occipito-cervical fixation for basilar invagination. After implant failure and revision surgery with the removal of the articular mass screws and placement of C3-C4 laminar clamps, she developed CSF leak and fever. Pseudomonas aeruginosa was isolated from the wound. She was treated with broad spectrum antibiotics, and she underwent surgery for debridement, CSF leak Repair with fibrin glue and meticulous reconstruction of the superficial layers. Nevertheless, after 10 days the wound presented a cranial dehiscence with hardware exposure (Fig. 10.8). What could be the proper management?
   A. Hardware removal and VAC therapy

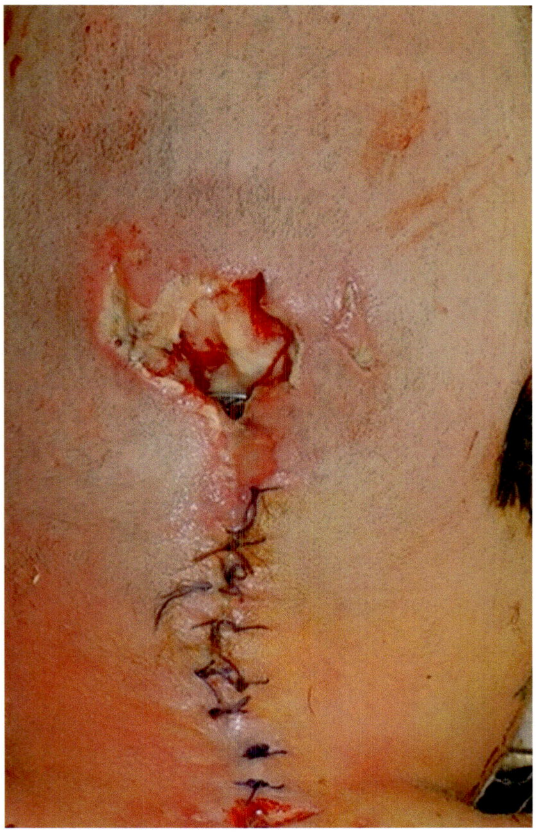

Fig. 10.8 Postoperative photograph of the occipito cervical region demonstrating dehiscence with exposure of the superior aspect of the occipital plate

B. Stand-alone rotation scalp-flap
C. Pericranial and scalp rotation flap
D. Hardware removal, stand-alone rotation flap and transoral surgery for the basilar invagination
E. New debridement and local instillation of rifampicin

Preferred Response: C: Pericranial and scalp rotation flap offers a double-layer barrier for preventing recurrent CSF leakage and separating the occipital plate from the skin. Furthermore, it reduces the wound pressure, and improves vascularization to the surrounding tissues [21].

(94) Which of the following is the best strategy for avoiding cage subsidence after ACDF?
A. Using the smallest cage that suites the intradiscal space
B. Sparing the endplates avoiding the use of the drill
C. Extensive using of the drill for opening the Luschka's joints
D. Insert the cage after removal of cervical distractor
E. None of the above

B: Cage subsidence may be cause by several factors, such as shape of endplates and, cage materials and shape. Nevertheless, sparing the endplates Remains the mainstay of a proper strategy aimed at avoiding this occurrence [55].

(95) A 58 years-old patient was treated with a two stages approach: L3-L4 XLIF (left side) and L3-L4 posterior fixation with percutaneous pedicle screws insertion. He had a long history of low back pain and neurogenic claudication. MRI showed a central and left paracentral disc herniation leading to sever critical canal stenosis with foraminal narrowing due to disc height loss At L3-L4. Neurological examination Showed only bilateral hypoesthesia (left > right) In the L3 distribution. After surgery he was placed on enoxaparin 6000 units subcutaneously per day and his coagulation profile pre-operatively was normal. Six days after surgery he developed groin pain and numbness and weakness of quadriceps femoris with loss of knee extension on the left side. Hip flexion was Pain limited. Furthermore, he was found to have lateral flank bruises and a drop in hemoglobin from 11 to 7.2 g/dL. What do you suspect?
A. Retroperitoneal hemorrhage due to left internal iliac artery injury
B. Retroperitoneal hemorrhage due to left common iliac artery injury
C. Femoral nerve palsy due to XLIF approach and normal hemoglobin drop after two steps approach
D. Retroperitoneal hemorrhage due to left psoas hematoma
E. L3 root injury due to misposition of left L3 screw

Preferred Response: D: Ileopsoas hematoma is a rare complication (reported from 0,18% to 1,7% of cases) of lateral lumbar interbody fusion. It can be caused by segmental artery injury, whose bleeding can be undetected during surgery. Moreover, coagulation disorders or use of anticoagulants may increase the risk of its occurrence. This complication may lead to lumbar plexus palsy, hemoglobin dropping and can be life-threatening if the bleeding leads to hypovolemic shock. Therefore, even if rare, its occurrence should be taken into account by physicians [56].

(96) What is the proper management of psoas hematoma?
A. Patients should always undergo emergency evacuation surgery
B. Intervention is always recommended. Surgeons may choose between surgery or CT guided drainage, according to the size of the hematoma.
C. Iliopsoas hematomas can be managed conservatively if there is no clinical and hemodynamic deterioration

D. Conservative treatment is always recommended since neurological deficit will be transient.
E. None of the above

Preferred Response: C: Treatment strategy of iliopsoas hematoma is controversial. The state of the art suggests managing conservatively patients that do not show signs of clinical or neurological deterioration. Conservative management consists of stopping anticoagulants, fluid and blood (if needed) administration and Serial evaluation of hemoglobin and coagulation profile. Surgical intervention is warranted in case of hemodynamic instability and progressive neurological deficit [56].

(97) Which of the following is a proper method to reduce the risk of sacral instrumentation bulkiness in high grade spondylolisthesis?
A. In high grade spondylolisthesis the sacrum should not be included in the construct
B. Patient in prone decubitus for three days after surgery
C. Distal rods as short as possible
D. Using only S2 alar screws
E. None of the above

Preferred Response: C: In cases of high-grade spondylolisthesis, the posterior cortex of the sacrum is close to the skin. Therefore, the rod caudal extremity lays just below the skin and can Be protruding after edema resorption. Thus, it is be better to leave the distal rods, below the sacral screws, as short as possible to reduce the risk of such occurrence.

(98) Which of the following sentences is true about pedicle subtraction osteotomy (PSO)?
A. In adult rigid scoliosis, PSO alongside posterior lumbar and sacropelvic fusion provides better sagittal and coronal correction than two stages (anterior/lateral + posterior) approaches and similar complication rates.
B. In adult rigid scoliosis, PSO alongside posterior lumbar and sacropelvic fusion provides Similar sagittal and coronal correction of two stages (anterior/lateral + posterior) approaches and lower complication rates.
C. In adult rigid scoliosis, PSO alongside posterior lumbar and sacropelvic fusion provides Similar sagittal and coronal correction of two stages (anterior/lateral + posterior) approaches and higher complication rates.
D. In adult rigid scoliosis, PSO alongside posterior lumbar and sacropelvic fusion provides better sagittal and coronal correction of two stages (anterior/lateral + posterior) approaches and higher complication rates.
E. In adult rigid scoliosis, PSO alongside posterior lumbar and sacropelvic fusion provides better sagittal and coronal correction of two stages (anterior/lateral + posterior) approaches and lower complication rates.

Preferred Response: A: The current trend in adult rigid scoliosis foresees the preferred employment of posterior only approaches instead of two stages surgery. In this scenario where these strategies provide same clinical results, the pedicle subtraction osteotomy along with posterior fusion increases sagittal and coronal plain correction having an overall complication rate similar to the two stages approaches [57].

(99) Which of the following sentences is false regarding complications of dynamic stabilization of the lumbar spine?
A. The complications with the dynamic systems are similar to those seen with standard fusion systems
B. Loss of bone screw interface is a late complication (> 6 months)
C. In case of failure, revision surgery should be aimed at performing a bony arthrodesis
D. A + B
E. A + B + C

Preferred Response: B: Dynamic stabilization for lumbar spine is an attempt to push spine surgery beyond its previous limits. Its goals are to maintain control of segmental motion, neutralizing excessive forces, improving spinal alignment, preserving motion, and preventing adjacent-level disease. This technique carries the same complications of standard fixation. Therefore, complications as dural tears are the most common occurrence and symptomatic loss of bone–screw interface is an early (less than3 months) postoperative complication [58].

(100) What is the "fusion disease" referred to transverse process fusion?
A. A unique type of pseudoarthrosis that occurs after transverse process fusion
B. Unilateral fusion failure that leads to coronal imbalance
C. Retroperitoneal hematoma due to injury of the segmental vessels
D. Postoperative back pain
E. Unilateral sympathetic chain injury

Preferred Response: D: Fusion syndrome in the context of transverse process fusion is characterized by postoperative pain resulting from excessive retraction or devascularization of the paraspinal muscles during lengthy fusion operations.

(101) How is it possible to reduce the risk of "fusion disease" after transverse process fusion?
A. Correct choice of the patients (e.g., obese, smoker patients, as well as patients with high grade scoliosis should be considered not suitable for this surgery)
B. Familiarity with segmental vessels anatomy and their early identification and coagulation
C. Using the neuromonitoring for early identification of the lumbar plexus
D. Avoiding monopolar electrocautery
E. Periodic release of self-retaining retractors

Preferred Response: E: Periodic release of self-retaining retractors should be carried out to avoid paraspinal muscles compression leading to injury and ischemia that are the cause of "fusion disease".

(102) Profuse venous bleeding during AxialLIF procedure…
A. …can occur frequently while creating the sacral channel with the drill and during the diskectomy
B. … can be controlled effectively using Flo-Seal or other hemostatic agents at the entry point
C. … tamponades with placement of the device.
D. …it is never caused by vascular injury due to the trajectory of the implant
E. A + B + C

Preferred Response: E: During AxialLIF profuse bleeding is rare. Of course, a proper evaluation of vessels anatomy should be performed before surgery to rule out vascular abnormalities. Nevertheless, venous bleeding can frequently occur when drilling the sacrum and when performing the discectomy. The use of floseal of other hemostatic agents, as well as the placement of the implant, are good strategies to stop the bleeding. Leaving a small portion of the device protruding from the sacrum adds further strength to the construct and seals sacral bleeding. Even if rare, vascular injuries are reported during AxialLIF and thus, if the bleeding cannot be stopped or in cases of development of cardiovascular instability, an emergent vascular consultation is recommended [59].

(103) What is the range of vertebral artery injury after posterior cervical spine non instrumented decompression?
A. < 0.5%
B. 0.5–1%
C. 1–5%
D. 5–10%
E. 10–15%

Preferred Response: A: Vertebral artery injury is a very rare complication of posterior spinal surgery, occurring reportedly around 0.07%. Nevertheless, it is more common with inexperienced surgeons. It carries a 10% risk of neurologic sequelae or death [60].

(104) Which of the following sentences is true regarding Smith Petersen Osteotomy (SPO)?
A. Vascular complications are due to lengthening of the anterior column
B. Neurologic complications rate is higher than with pedicle subtraction osteotomy
C. Foraminotomy should be avoided at level of SPO
D. A + B
E. A + B + C

Preferred Response: D: Most of the complications related to SPO are due to lengthening of the anterior column. A fortiori, the risk of vascular complication is higher in cases of either elderly patients or patients with ankylosing spondylitis because of calcified vessels. Neurologic complications (30% after SPO and 11–16% after PSO) are mostly featured by radiculopathy due to foraminal narrowing. Therefore, wide foraminotomy is warranted at the level of a SPO [61].

(105) Which of the following conditions increases the risk of neurological injury during intubation?
A. Rheumatoid arthritis
B. Cervical spinal stenosis
C. Ankylosing spondylitis
D. Down syndrome
E. All of the above

Preferred Response: E: Several conditions may increase the risk of neurological injury with intubation (e.g., cervical spondylosis with spinal canal stenosis, congenitally narrow spinal canal, ankylosing spondylitis, rheumatoid arthritis). Down syndrome increases both the risk of neurological deficit due to the high rate of atlantoaxial instability (20% approximately) and issues related to the intubation itself (microcephaly, macroglossia, subglottic stenosis, airways obstruction, respiratory tract infections).

(106) Which of the following is not a major risk for posterior cage migration in posterior lumbar interbody fusion?

A. Bullet shaped cages
B. Preoperative spine mobility
C. A + B
D. Undersized cages
E. Posteriorly located cages

Preferred Response: C: Posteriorly located cages and undersized cages significantly increase the risk of posterior cage migration. Other factors, such as cage shape and high preoperative spine mobility, do not increase the odds of such occurrence. Thus, cage height should be equal or bigger to preoperative disc height and the cage center should not be placed posteriorly to the disc center [62].

(107) A 63 years-old woman Underwent a C5-C6 ACDF and C5-C7 anterior plating at another hospital. Prior to surgery she complained of neck pain (VAS 6/10) and left C5 radiculopathy. You see her one month after surgery, complaining of neck pain (8/10). Radiologic investigations showed implant failure. What could be the reason for this occurrence?
A. She has pre-operative cervical kyphosis. In these cases, a 360° approach is indicated.
B. The anterior plating involved a non-fused level.
C. The anterior plating should have involved also C4-C5
D. All of the above
E. None of the above

Preferred Response: B: Anterior plating of cervical spine should only involve fused levels. In fact, in this case the preserved range of motion at C6-C7 led to implant failure [63].

(108) Which cervical level has the highest and lowest risk of developing adjacent segment disease?
A. Highest: C6-C7; Lowest: C2-C3
B. Highest: C2-C3; Lowest: C5-C6
C. Highest: C5-C6; Lowest: C2-C3
D. Highest: C4-C5; Lowest: C6-C7
E. Highest: C3-C4; Lowest: C5-C6

Preferred Response: C: Middle and lower subaxial spine are more prone to develop adjacent segment disease. The most interested level is C5-C6, due to the higher predisposition to develop spondylosis and adjacent segment disease. Contrariwise, the level that proved to be less affected by this condition is C2-C3 [64].

(109) A 56 years-old patient underwent a posterior C3-C7 decompression and fusion. The surgery was completed with intraoperative CT-scan. The last control showed correct placement of the Hardware even though the articular mass screws only had uni-cortical bony purchase. After surgery the patient woke up anisocoric (dx > sx). What can be the cause of such occurrence?
A. Bernard-Horner syndrome due to lesion of sympathetic chain
B. Parfour du petit syndrome due to irritation of sympathetic chain
C. Epidural hematoma
D. Iris sphincter muscle tears
E. None of the above

Preferred Response: D: Iris sphincter muscle tears and transient or permanent dilation of the affected pupil may be caused by wrong position and long surgical duration. Fixed dilated pupil is a condition featured by an abnormality of the iris, that causes cosmetic issues, and requires further conservative or surgical intervention.

(110) Which of the following sentences is false regarding lumbar adjacent segment disease (ASD)?
A. Increasing age is an independent risk factor for ASD
B. Including the sacrum into the construct increases the risk of ASD
C. Adjacent laminectomy during the initial surgery is associated with higher risk of ASD
D. The number of fused segments is related to the risk of ASD
E. Interbody fusion adds rigidity to the construct increasing the risk of ASD

Preferred Response: B: ASD is a multifactorial event whose primary cause is the rigidity of the segment that redistributes the axial and shear load. Therefore, all the instrumented segments, particularly when an interbody fusion is added to the construct, are at higher risk for ASD. Moreover "floating fusions", namely fusions not including the sacrum, are more prone to develop adjacent segment disease than instrumented fusions that included the sacrum. Other risk factors for ASD are increasing age, adjacent laminectomy, and number of fused segments [65].

(111) Which of the following sentences is true regarding a proper cantilever beam fixation?
A. The cantilever beam effectiveness can be increased by using larger diameter screws, longer screws, multiple screws per level, augmentation of the cancellous or cortical bone, and cross-links for longer constructs
B. Higher moment applied to the construct leads to higher risk of failure

C. Segmental fixation, attention to sagittal balance and proper posture postoperatively can decrease the applied moment to the implant.
D. A + B
E. A + B + C

Preferred Response: E: Understanding the applied loads on a construct and the physical basis behind its function is one of the mainstays of spine surgery. The implants work as a cantilever beam subjected to a shear force, an applied load, and a moment. The higher is the moment applied, the higher is the risk of implant failure. Therefore, several strategies exist in order to reduce the moment, namely segmental fixation instead of nonsegmental fixation, attention to sagittal balance and proper posture postoperatively. Likewise, using larger diameter screws, longer screws, multiple screws per level, augmentation of the cancellous or cortical bone, and cross-links for longer constructs can improve the resistive moment.

(112) Which of the following is a correct strategy for avoiding pneumothorax after retro pleural approaches to the ventral thoracolumbar spine?
A. In cases of pleural tear, tube thoracostomy should not be placed if the lung remains adherent to the parietal pleura
B. If pleural tears occur, it should not be repaired with sutures if the lung remains adherent to the parietal pleura
C. In cases of dural tear, if an air leak is present (indicated by separation between the lung and parietal pleura) a tube thoracostomy is placed and left in place for 7 days.
D. A + B
E. None of the above

Preferred Response: A: After the procedure the pleura should be carefully inspected. If pleural tears are encountered, they should be always repaired with sutures. Even in cases of tears, if the lung remains adherent to the parietal pleura there is no need for tube thoracostomy. If separation between the lung and parietal pleura is detected a tube thoracostomy is placed and removed the next day. The latter condition indicates either an air leak (i.e., lung parenchymal entry) or a nonairtight pleural tear closure [66].

(113) Which of the following is a proper closure technique to avoid CSF leak due to dural tear after endoscopic endonasal approach to the craniovertebral junction?
A. Patch of synthetic dura and hemostatic sponge
B. PMMA
C. Autologous materials (Fat, flap, fascia lata), fibrin glue, and fast mobilization of the patient
D. Lumbar drainage
E. C + D

Preferred Response: C: Autologous materials, hemostats, and sealants (oxidizes cellulose, fibrin glue, Tachosil) are the mainstays for an effective reconstruction in cases of CSF leak during endoscopic endonasal surgery. Specifically vascularized flaps are reliable methods to bolster the reconstruction. Overall, this strategy proved to reduce CSF fistula rate below 2% in a comprehensive series. Nevertheless, approaches to the craniovertebral junction carry a high risk of fistula in cases of CSF leak. Patients are kept on bed rest for less than 24 h, with the head of the bed elevated to 30 degrees, after which they are actively mobilized [67].

(114) Which of the following sentences is false about surgical site infection?
A. Hair removal is a fundamental pre-operative step for reducing the risk of surgical site infection.
B. Maintenance of slight hypothermia during a surgical procedure proved to reduce the risk of surgical site infection.
C. Surgical drains increase the risk of surgical site infection by removing the blood that is considered a natural antiseptic agent
D. All of the above
E. None of the above

Preferred Response: D: All the answers all false. There is no evidence that hair removal lowers the risk of surgical site infection. Moreover, several large and well-designed trials proved that hair removal done with razors is clearly associated with higher rates of surgical site infections as compared with other tools as electric clippers or depilatory creams. Hypothermia during the procedure can impair immune function, by reducing antibody production, decreasing chemotaxis, and phagocytosis. Therefore, maintenance of normothermia during a surgical procedure is perhaps one of the most important tools in preventing surgical site infection. Lastly, there is no proof that drains increase the risk of surgical site infection. The two opposed theories are: i) that drains remove blood (considered as an excellent culture medium), remove bacteria, and prevent hematoma formation; ii) drains can be themselves conduit for bacteria [34].

(115) C2 neuralgia can frequently occur…
A. After occipito-cervical fixation (C0-C4)
B. C1-C2 Harms fixation when inserting the screw in C2
C. C1-C2 Harms fixation when inserting the C1 lateral mass Screw

D. In all procedures when C2 lateral mass is exposed
E. None of the above

Preferred Response: C: C2 neuralgia may occur from manipulation, thermal injury, or stretch injury during placement of C1 lateral mass screws. In such cases, C2 can be sacrificed, without any relevant neurological sequela. Only rarely, C2 can be injured during the exposure of C1-C2 facet capsule.

(116) Which of the following sentences is true regarding lumbar spondylodiscitis?
A. The leading cause in most of the cases is *Staphylococcus Epidermidis*
B. The typical postoperative course of spondylodiscitis is the return of low back pain approximately six weeks postoperatively
C. CRP has a high specificity and a low sensitivity
D. FDG-PET has the highest sensitivity and specificity among radiological exams
E. All of the above

Preferred response: B: The typical postoperative course of discitis consists of initial resolution of symptoms, with subsequent return of low back pain approximately six weeks post-operatively. The most common cause of spondylodiscitis is *Staphylococcus Aureus (60%). High values of* CRP are extremely sensitive. MRI has the highest specificity and sensitivity [34].

(117) 34-year-old patient underwent a postero-lateral approach for T8-T9 thoracic disc herniation. He recovered well after surgery, and he showed no complications. Two months after the procedure, he developed a burning and constant back pain. Neurologic examination demonstrated a slight strength reduction in the lower limbs and reduction of range of motion of the trunk. Thoracic CT scan was negative for any complication. What do you suspect?
A. Adamkiewicz artery ischemia
B. Post-operative back pain
C. Iatrogenic arachnoiditis
D. Focal iatrogenic instability
E. None of the above

Preferred Response: C: Spinal arachnoiditis is a nonspecific inflammatory process of the arachnoid layer of the spinal cord or cauda equina. Iatrogenic arachnoiditis may occur after spine surgery that is considered as an independent risk factor. It has been reported that nucleus pulposus of the intervertebral disc may cause focal arachnoiditis. Clinically it appears as burning pain, constant in nature, and worsened by activity with a latency of 1–6 months after the procedure. Neurologically, it can be associated with slight strength reduction, Positive straight-leg raise sign, tender sciatic notch, limited range of motion of the trunk, and paravertebral muscle spasms. CT scan can be normal or show calcification or ossification of the spinal arachnoid, called arachnoiditis ossificans [68].

(118) What is the MRI appearance of spinal arachnoiditis?
A. Conglomerations of nerve roots located centrally within the thecal sac.
B. Nerve roots are clumped and attached peripherally to the meninges
C. Increased soft tissue signal within the thecal sac with central obliteration of the subarachnoid space
D. A + B
E. A + B + C

Preferred Response: E: MRI appearance of spinal arachnoiditis follows three patterns. The first is a conglomerations of nerve roots located centrally within the thecal sac. The second is characterized by nerve roots that are clumped and attached laterally to the meninges. The third pattern demonstrates increased soft tissue signal inside the dural sac with central obliteration of the subarachnoid space [69].

(119) Which of the following are major risks for perioperative blindness due to ischemic optic neuropathy?
A. Anemia, dehydration, and hypotension
B. Hypothermia, hyperoxygenation, hypotension
C. Hypoxia, anemia, blood dilution
D. Preoperative cataract, hypotension
E. None of the above

Preferred Response: A: One of the most common mechanisms leading to perioperative blindness is ischemic optic neuropathy. Indeed, the prolonged prone position may result in central retinal artery occlusion by direct compression. Risk factors for ischemic optic neuropathy include anemia, dehydration, and hypotension.

(120) Which of the following is a risk factor for acute respiratory distress syndrome (ARDS) in patient undergoing spine surgery?
A. Pulmonary contusion
B. Spinal cord injury
C. Instrumented surgery
D. A + B
E. A + B + C

Preferred Response: D: Severe and diffuse lung injury, like acute respiratory distress syndrome, may complicate the post-operative management of patients undergoing spine surgery. Major risk factors are aspiration, pulmonary contusion, hypotension, multiple transfusions, infection, spinal cord injury and sepsis [40].

(121) Which of the following lumbar disc herniation configuration has the highest risk of recurrence?
A. Fragment-fissure herniations
B. Fragment-defect herniations
C. Fragment contained discs
D. Annular prolapse
E. C + D

Preferred Response: D: Lumbar disc herniation have been divided by Carragee et al. in 2003 in four shaped-based groups: fragment-fissure herniations, fragment-defect herniations (large disc fragment with massive posterior annular tear), fragment contained discs (incomplete annular tear), and annular prolapse. Among these, the fragment-fissure herniations were associated with the best outcomes, whilst annular prolapses carry a 38% recurrence rate [70].

(122) Which of the following is a risk factor for post-operative C5 palsy?
A. Female gender
B. Calcified yellow ligament
C. Ossified posterior longitudinal ligament
D. C5-C6 foraminal stenosis
E. All of the above

Preferred Response: C: Risk factors for postoperative C5 palsy include ossification of the posterior longitudinal ligament (OPLL), narrow intervertebral foramen at level of the surgery, C4-C5 foraminal stenosis independently from the level of the surgery and male gender [71].

(123) A 56-year-old patient was carried to the emergency room because he developed progressive drowsiness. The CT scan showed a diffuse cerebellar hematoma (Fig. 10.9). He underwent L3-L4 PLIF at another institution two weeks prior. The surgical report did not mention any complications during surgery. What could be the cause of the hematoma?
A. It cannot be stated. There is no association with the previous spine surgery.
B. Thromboembolic cerebellar stroke and subsequent infarction
C. Delayed CSF leak
D. Hyper inflammatory immune response
E. None of the above

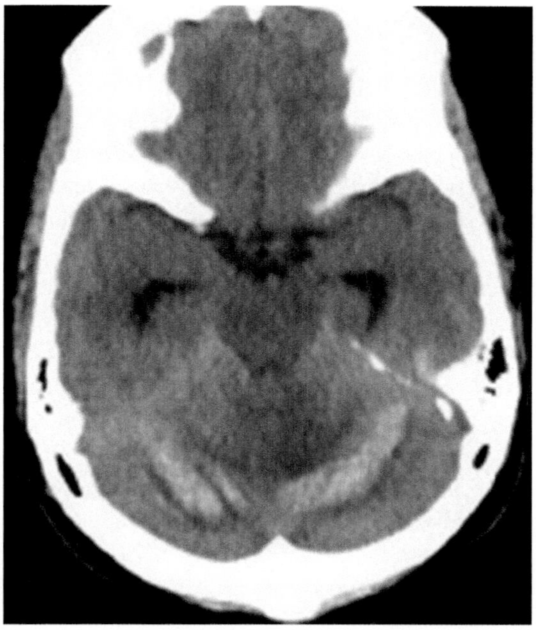

Fig. 10.9 Axial CT scan demonstrating cerebellar hematoma

Preferred Response: C: Occult dural tears are rare but described occurrence in spine surgery. They can lead to delayed symptomatic CSF leak. It can appear after few days or weeks after surgery. One of the potential complications of CSF leak is cerebellar hemorrhages and brain sagging [72].

(124) What are the most common risk factors for remote cerebellar hemorrhage due to dural tear and CSF leak?
A. Hypertension
B. Coagulation disorder
C. Postoperative subfascial drains
D. B + C
E. A + B + C

Preferred Response: E: Several retrospective analysis and reviews studies pointed hypertension, coagulation disorders and the placement of subfascial drains as the most common risk factors for remote cerebellar hemorrhage due to iatrogenic spinal CSF leak [72].

(125) Which of the following statements is false regarding perineural scar formation?
A. Neither scar nor the use of scar-inhibiting tools impact clinical outcomes
B. Systemic and epidural corticosteroids neither reduce the risk of scar formation nor improve short- and long-term outcomes
C. Epidural fat should be left as intact as possible
D. Gelatin sponges increase scar formation
E. A + B

Preferred Response: B: Epidural steroids are commonly employed and have been shown to reduce the epidural scar formation. They have also an inhibitory effect on pain-transmitting C-fibers, which are the most prone to the inflammation caused by disc herniation. Therefore, a combination of systemic and epidural corticosteroids leads to faster symptoms relief and reduce the risk of scar formation [73].

(126) Which of the following sentences is true regarding the correlation between nasal carrying of Staphylococcus Aureus and surgical site infection?
   A. There is a clear association between nasal carriage of S. aureus and occurrence of surgical site infections.
   B. Short-term mupirocin nasal ointment should be administrated to patients before every elective surgery
   C. In patients carrying S. Aureus, 21 days administration of mupirocin nasal ointment proved to reduce surgical site infection
   D. A + C
   E. A + B

Preferred Response: A: Several trials reported a correlation between the presence of S. Aureus in the nasal cavity and an higher risk of surgical site infections. Short-term treatment with mupirocin ointment (5 days) eliminates S. aureus in most of these carriers. It has been suggested to test patients for nasal S.Aureus before elective surgery, and only treat those patients who tested positive with a short course of mupirocin ointment [34].

(127) Which of the following is not a complication related to the employment of orthosis?
   A. Superior mesenteric artery syndrome
   B. Psychological dependence
   C. Recurrent laryngeal nerve palsy
   D. Pulmonary edema
   E. Dysphagia

Preferred Response: C: Among the reported complication related to the employment of orthosis, recurrent laryngeal nerve palsy has never been described. The superior mesenteric artery syndrome or cast syndrome is due to the artery stretched across the ventral aspect of the distal duodenum. It determines postprandial bilious emesis, epigastric pain, and distention from partial duodenal obstruction. Psychological dependence and secondary gain may occur after chronic orthosis use that determines a change in body perception. Pulmonary edema may be due to increased venous return. Dysphagia is reported in up to 2% of cases and is caused by impaired larynx movement required for coordinated swallowing.

(128) During a C3 corpectomy when drilling laterally to the unco-vertebral joint a sudden, non-pulsatile, copious dark bleeding occurs. What do you suspect?
   A. Internal jugular vein injury
   B. Vertebral artery injury
   C. External jugular vein injury
   D. Epidural bleeding due to decompression
   E. None of the above

Preferred Response: B: Vertebral artery injury is usually featured by sudden, non-pulsatile, copious bright red bleeding. Nevertheless, it may be dark because of injury to the surrounding venous plexus. This occurrence may be catastrophic, because the hemorrhage may be massive and cause cerebral ischemia/embolic events.

(129) How would you manage vertebral artery injury occurred during an anterior cervical approach?
   A. Tamponade
   B. Repair
   C. Ligation
   D. Coagulation
   E. A + B + C

Preferred Response: E: Strategies to manage a vertebral artery injury during an anterior cervical approach include repair tamponade, and ligation. Hemostats, such as Gelfoam and oxidized cellulose, may be useful. If they failed, the exposure should be enlarged, the artery exposed, and the surgeon must then weigh the options of vertebral ligation versus repair [74].

(130) Which of the following can be considered a specific cause of spinal cord injury during laminoplasty?
   A. Stepwise opening of the laminae involved
   B. Injury of the dura mater or spinal cord during drilling
   C. A + B
   D. Positioning
   E. Post-operative kyphosis

Preferred Response: C: The most common causes of spinal cord injury strictly related to laminoplasty procedure are stepwise opening of the laminae. It means drilling and opening laminae one by one. This can cause kinking of the spinal cord at the edge of the residual lamina, causing injury. Thus, laminae should be opened en bloc. Moreover, extensive use of the drilling obliquely oriented increase the risk of dura mater and spinal cord injury [75].

(131) A 53-year-old man complained of axial neck pain (5/10), walking impairment and difficulties with fine

motor skills. Neurological examination showed increased deep tendon reflex (+3) in the lower limbs, positive Babinski and Hoffman signs, and increased extensor muscles tone. MRI showed a straightened cervical spine and a C3-C6 cervical spondylotic myelopathy. You decided to perform a C3-C6 laminoplasty. After the surgery, the patient has a slight improvement in walking and fine motor skills. Nevertheless, neck pain worsened (NRS 7/10). What is the cause of such occurrence?

A. Laminoplasty is discouraged in cases of neck pain
B. WFNS guidelines for cervical spondylotic myelopathy discourage laminoplasty in straightened cervical spine
C. It is normal pain due to muscle healing
D. Laminoplasty should not be performed for more than two levels
E. A + B

Preferred Response: A: WFNS guidelines for cervical spondylotic myelopathy state that laminoplasty should be avoided in patients with cervical kyphosis and significant preoperative axial neck pain. This is because neck pain itself is a common complication of laminoplasty. Laminoplasty can be employed in neutral or lordotic cervical spine [12, 76].

(132) Which of the following are specific complication of sacroiliac joint fusion?

A. Sacral vessels injury
B. Genitofemoral nerve compression
C. Sacral fracture
D. Lumbar adjacent segment disease
E. A + B + C

Preferred Response: D: Sacroiliac joint fusion has become increasingly employed lately as a treatment for sacroiliac joint pain and for joint pathology. Among the specific complication of this technique there are: failure in pain relief, failure in fusion and lumbar adjacent segment disease, whose rate can be as high as 16%. This is due to the additional pressure applied to the lowest lumbar disc and facet joints, that become overloaded, injured, and a source of pain [77].

(133) Which of the following sentences is true about complications of vertebral artery injury?

A. A postoperative angiogram should be performed in order to rule out significant injury, stenosis, pseudoaneurysm, or arteriovenous fistula.
B. In cases of serious complication, vessels sacrifice should be considered.
C. Vascular complications may occur from days to years after surgery
D. A + B
E. A + B + C

Preferred Response: E: Even if the proper post-operative management of vertebral artery injury remains controversial, most authors suggest performing a postoperative angiogram in order to rule out significant complications. Detecting a complication may lead to either introduce anticoagulant or antiplatelet therapy or vessel sacrific. Late complications of vertebral artery injury may occur from days to years after surgery and may consist of arteriovenous malformation, thrombosis with embolic incidents, cerebral ischemia, stroke, and even death.

(134) Which of the following statements is false regarding ureteral injury during anterior approaches to the lumbar spine?

A. Ureter reconstruction should be always done over a stent that can be subsequently retrieved by cystoscopy.
B. During reoperations, or in cases of retroperitoneal fibrosis, tumor, or previous irradiation, dissection should proceed with the aid of sponges or Kittners.
C. The first repair attempt should always be a direct end to end anastomoses, independently from the injury type
D. In cases of post-operative hydronephrosis CT scan with contrast injection and delayed scans should be performed
E. All of the above

Preferred Response: C: The type of injury always leads to the repair strategy. In fact, net lacerations require simple end to end anastomosis, whereas segmental injuries may warrant segmental resection and re-anastomosis or complicated reconstructive techniques such as appendiceal interposition or uretero-ureteral anastomosis [78].

(135) What is the correct definition of cage subsidence in ACDF?

A. $\geq$ 3 mm loss of height comparing the immediate postoperative intervertebral height with the intervertebral height at the last follow-up moment
B. Failed fusion after disc placement leading to formation of aberrant anterior bridges of bone
C. Less than 3 mm of translational motion and less than 5° of angular motion on flexion and extension radiographs 6 months after surgery

D. Failed fusion after disc placement leading to formation of aberrant posterior bridges of bone impinging the dural sac
E. None of the above

Preferred Response: A: Subsidence is generally defined as $\geq$ 3 mm loss of height comparing the immediate post-operative intervertebral height with the intervertebral height at the last follow-up moment [79].

(136) Which of the following sentences is false about cage subsidence in anterior spinal approaches?
A. Subsidence rate in ACDF using cages is approximately 21%
B. It is still not clear if radiologic occurrence of subsidence affects clinical outcome
C. Risk for subsidence is increased when a PEEK or titanium cage is used
D. Risk of subsidence is reduced when a cage with integrated screws is used
E. B + C

Preferred Response: C: A recent review showed that subsidence rate is approximately of 21%. Using PEEK or titanium cages or cages with integrated screws lowers the risk of subsidence. The actual literature is not able to provide any relevant data about the impact of cage subsidence on clinical outcomes [55].

(137) Which of the following sentences is true regarding loss of disc height after discectomy?
A. Loss of disc height causes delayed onset of recurrent radiculopathy in the same or rostral root distribution
B. Discectomy results in an average 26% loss of height 2 years after surgery.
C. Disc height loss can lead to foraminal stenosis, annular bulging, and lateral recess stenosis.
D. A + B
E. A + B + C

Preferred response: E: Height loss after discectomy can determine foraminal stenosis, annular bulging, and lateral recess stenosis, which may lead to delayed onset of recurrent radiculopathy with the same distribution. Discectomy resulted in a mean 18% loss of height at 3 months and a 26% loss of height at 2 years [80].

(138) Which of the following is not a risk factor for recurrent lumbar disc herniation?
A. configuration of the initial disc herniation
B. smoking
C. diabetes
D. Isolated trauma
E. Duration of initial symptoms

Preferred Response: D: Among the several risk factors identified for recurrent lumbar disc herniation a major controversy surrounds isolated trauma. In fact, an association between isolated trauma and recurrent disc herniation has been reported from 0,1 to 10%. All the other answers are recognized as clear factors increasing the risk of recurrences of lumbar disc herniation [81].

(139) What is the rate of post-operative cauda equina syndrome following lumbar spine surgery?
A. < 1%
B. 1–2%
C. 2–4%
D. 4–6%
E. > 6%

Preferred Response: B: The reported incidence of cauda equina syndrome following lumbar spine surgery is approximately 1–2% [38].

(140) Which of the following are risk factors for recurrent laryngeal nerve palsy during anterior approaches to the cervical spine?
A. Direct traction on recurrent laryngeal nerve
B. Duration of surgery
C. Number of treated levels
D. A + B
E. A + B + C

Preferred Response: A: Several metanalysis and retrospective cohort studies proved that the risk for recurrent laryngeal nerve palsy depends only on direct manipulation of the nerve. Factors like duration of the surgery and number of treated levels are not associated with an increased risk of this occurrence. Moreover, no association has been found between recurrent laryngeal nerve palsy and patients' characteristics such as, age, sex, body mass index [38].

(141) Which of the following sentences is true regarding anterior approaches to the thoracolumbar junction?
A. Right sided approaches are safer because damaging the liver carries less consequences than splenic injuries
B. The diaphragm should not be sutured because the pleural pressure is equal to pression inside the peritoneum and risk of herniation is negligible
C. Revision surgery should be performed from the contralateral side

D. A + C
E. None of the above

Preferred Response: E: Anterior approaches to the thoracolumbar spine should be performed from the left side whenever possible as right sided approaches carry the risk of mobilizing the liver. The diaphragm should be always closed with a proper suture in order to avoid herniation. If the latter occurs, revision surgery is needed. Revision surgery should be carried out always from the same side and has higher risk of complications [82].

(142) Which of the following sentences is true about post-thoracotomy pain?
A. Post-thoracotomy pain can be a cause of pneumonia
B. Paravertebral block, interpleural block and intrathecal opioids can be performed in patients with normal coagulation profile.
C. Serratus Anterior Plane Block under ultrasound guidance may be performed in patients with deranged coagulation profile
D. A + B + C
E. A + B

Preferred Response: D: Post-thoracotomy pain may lead to restriction of chest movements in order to minimize pain. Consequently, pulmonary function is reduced leading to higher predisposition for pooled secretions and pneumonia. Among the analgesic options for post-thoracotomy pain, thoracic epidural anesthetic delivery is the gold standard. This technique, as well as paravertebral blocks, interpleural blocks and intrathecal opioids require normal coagulation parameters to be used. Contrarywise, serratus anterior plane block can be performed in patient with altered coagulation parameters [83].

(143) Translaminar screws of the axis…
A. carry more risk because of the more demanding technique for placement
B. have less stability and fusion rates than C2 pedicle screws but lower risk of vertebral artery injury
C. can be used as an alternative technique when pedicle screw placement is contraindicated or not possible
D. B + C
E. A + B + C

Preferred Response: C: Translaminar screws are an alternative technique in cases of upper cervical spine instability when pedicle screw placement is contraindicated or not possible. They have comparable biomechanical stability and fusion rates (up to 93%) compared to other posterior fixation techniques. Moreover, translaminar screw placement is technically less demanding and reduces the risk of vertebral artery injury.

(144) Which of the following sentences is false about management of cervical spondylotic myelopathy in Parkinson's disease (PD) patients?
A. The most performed approach is ACDF
B. The safest route is the posterior
C. PD patients have higher risk of dysphagia after ACDF than non-PD patients
D. ACDF is associated with higher risk of pneumonia than posterior surgery in PD patients.
E. None of the above

Preferred Response: E: ACDF is the most common procedure for cervical spondylotic myelopathy in PD. Nevertheless, it is associated with higher incidence of postoperative dysphagia and postprocedural pneumonia as compared with posterior cervical procedures [84].

(145) What is the crankshaft phenomenon?
A. Implant failure occurring after less than 24 h from the surgery
B. Occipito-cervical fusion failure leading to sudden death
C. Rib fracture during thoracoscopic approach
D. Progression of spinal deformity despite a solid posterior arthrodesis due to skeletal immaturity
E. None of the above

Preferred Response: E: Crankshaft phenomenon is defined as the progression of a preexisting spinal deformity despite a solid posterior arthrodesis. It can occur in the skeletally immature patient and it is due to the growth of the unfused anterior vertebral segments [85].

(146) Which of the following is not a contraindication for lumbar total disc arthroplasty?
A. Prior surgery
B. Obese patient
C. Osteoporotic bone
D. Smoking
E. None of the above

Preferred Response: D: Contraindications for total disc arthroplasty are: Obese patients, facet disease, skeletal anomalies, high narcotic intake, osteoporotic bone, instability, spondylolysis, vascular calcification, prior infection, severely collapsed disc, unrealistic expectations, spinal stenosis, spinal deformity. Among these, smoking is not a contraindication of total disc arthroplasty [86].

References

1. Bouyer B, Scemama C, Roussouly P, et al. Evolution and complications after surgery for spine deformation in patients with Parkinson's disease. Orthop Traumatol Surg Res. 06 2017;103 (4):517–22. https://doi.org/10.1016/j.otsr.2016.12.024
2. Somma T, DE Rosa A, Mastantuoni C, et al. Multidisciplinary management of osteoporotic vertebral fractures. An overview. Minerva Endocrinol (Torino). Dec 09 2021;https://doi.org/10.23736/S2724-6507.21.03515-6
3. Wang T, Ding W. Risk factors for adjacent segment degeneration after posterior lumbar fusion surgery in treatment for degenerative lumbar disorders: a meta-analysis. J Orthop Surg Res. Dec 03 2020;15(1):582. https://doi.org/10.1186/s13018-020-02032-7
4. Mummaneni PV, Hussain I, Shaffrey CI, et al. The minimally invasive interbody selection algorithm for spinal deformity. J Neurosurg Spine. Mar 12 2021:1–8. https://doi.org/10.3171/2020.9.SPINE20230
5. Calvo-Echenique A, Cegoñino J, Perez Del Palomar A. Is there any advantage of using stand-alone cages? A numerical approach. Biomed Eng Online. May 22 2019;18(1):63. https://doi.org/10.1186/s12938-019-0684-8
6. Mobbs RJ, Phan K, Malham G, Seex K, Rao PJ. Lumbar interbody fusion: techniques, indications and comparison of interbody fusion options including PLIF, TLIF, MI-TLIF, OLIF/ATP LLIF and ALIF. J Spine Surg. Dec2015;1(1):2–18. https://doi.org/10.3978/j.issn.2414-469X.2015.10.05.
7. Bono CM, Lee CK. Critical analysis of trends in fusion for degenerative disc disease over the past 20 years: influence of technique on fusion rate and clinical outcome. *Spine (Phila Pa 1976)*. Feb 15 2004;29(4):455–63; discussion Z5. https://doi.org/10.1097/01.brs.0000090825.94611.28
8. Hartig D, Batke J, Dea N, Kelly A, Fisher C, Street J. Adverse events in surgically treated cervical spondylopathic myelopathy: a prospective validated observational study. *Spine (Phila Pa 1976)*. Mar 01 2015;40(5):292–8. https://doi.org/10.1097/BRS.0000000000000755
9. *Neel Anand*, Eli *M. Baron, Smith DA. Vascular and Soft Tissue Complications* Benzel's Spine Surgery. 2017.
10. Lak AM, Lamba N, Pompilus F, et al. Minimally invasive versus open surgery for the correction of adult degenerative scoliosis: a systematic review. Neurosurg Rev. 2021;44(2):659–68. https://doi.org/10.1007/s10143-020-01280-9.
11. *Jad Bou Monsef, Techy* F. *Nonunion* Benzel's Spine Surgery IV edition. 2017.
12. Bajamal AH, Kim SH, Arifianto MR, et al. Posterior Surgical Techniques for Cervical Spondylotic Myelopathy: WFNS Spine Committee Recommendations. Neurospine. 09 2019;16(3):421–34. https://doi.org/10.14245/ns.1938274.137
13. Basaran R, Kaner T. C5 nerve root palsy following decompression of cervical spine with anterior versus posterior types of procedures in patients with cervical myelopathy. Eur Spine J. 07 2016;25 (7):2050–9. https://doi.org/10.1007/s00586-016-4567-4
14. Nurboja B, Kachramanoglou C, Choi D. Cervical laminectomy vs laminoplasty: is there a difference in outcome and postoperative pain? Neurosurgery. Apr 2012;70(4):965–70; discussion 970. https://doi.org/10.1227/NEU.0b013e31823cf16b
15. Lee WS, Jean SS, Chen FL, Hsieh SM, Hsueh PR. Lemierre's syndrome: A forgotten and re-emerging infection. J Microbiol Immunol Infect. 2020;53(4):513–7. https://doi.org/10.1016/j.jmii.2020.03.027.
16. Jung A, Schramm J. How to reduce recurrent laryngeal nerve palsy in anterior cervical spine surgery: a prospective observational study. Neurosurgery. Jul 2010;67(1):10–5; discussion 15. https://doi.org/10.1227/01.NEU.0000370203.26164.24
17. Ballard JL, Carlson G, Chen J, White J. Anterior thoracolumbar spine exposure: critical review and analysis. Ann Vasc Surg. 2014;28(2):465–9. https://doi.org/10.1016/j.avsg.2013.06.026.
18. Epstein NE. Review of Risks and Complications of Extreme Lateral Interbody Fusion (XLIF). Surg Neurol Int. 2019;10:237. https://doi.org/10.25259/SNI_559_2019.
19. Wang T, Wang H, Liu S, Ding WY. Incidence of C5 nerve root palsy after cervical surgery: a meta-analysis for last decade. Medicine (Baltimore). 2017;96(45): e8560. https://doi.org/10.1097/MD.0000000000008560.
20. Litrico S, Lonjon N, Riouallon G, et al. Adjacent segment disease after anterior cervical interbody fusion: a multicenter retrospective study of 288 patients with long-term follow-up. Orthop Traumatol Surg Res. 2014;100(6 Suppl):S305–9. https://doi.org/10.1016/j.otsr.2014.07.004.
21. Schonauer C, Mastantuoni C, de Divitiis O, D'Andrea F, de Falco R, Schonauer F. Pericranial and scalp rotation flaps for occipitocervical hardware exposure with CSF leak in rheumatoid arthritis patient: A case report and review of the literature. Surg Neurol Int. 2021;12:229. https://doi.org/10.25259/SNI_351_2021.
22. Parish JM, Asher AM, Coric D. Complications and Complication Avoidance With Cervical Total Disc Replacement. Int J Spine Surg. 2020;14(s2):S50–6. https://doi.org/10.14444/7091.
23. Fantini GA, Pappou IP, Girardi FP, Sandhu HS, Cammisa FP. Major vascular injury during anterior lumbar spinal surgery: incidence, risk factors, and management. *Spine (Phila Pa 1976)*. Nov 2007;32(24):2751–8. https://doi.org/10.1097/BRS.0b013e31815a996e
24. *Kalfas IH. Cerebrospinal Fluid Fistula and Pseudomeningocele after Spine Surgery* Benzel's Spine Surgery. 2017.
25. Ghasemi AA. Adjacent segment degeneration after posterior lumbar fusion: An analysis of possible risk factors. Clin Neurol Neurosurg. 2016;143:15–8. https://doi.org/10.1016/j.clineuro.2016.02.004.
26. Traynelis VC, Malone HR, Smith ZA, et al. Rare Complications of Cervical Spine Surgery: Horner's Syndrome. Global Spine J. 2017;7(1 Suppl):103S-108S. https://doi.org/10.1177/2192568216688184.
27. Choudhri TF, Mummaneni PV, Dhall SS, et al. Guideline update for the performance of fusion procedures for degenerative disease of the lumbar spine. Part 4: radiographic assessment of fusion status. *J Neurosurg Spine*. Jul 2014;21(1):23–30. https://doi.org/10.3171/2014.4.SPINE14267
28. Bocchetti A, Cioffi V, de Falco R. Combined intra-extradural approach for posterolateral thoracic disk herniations. Preliminary study and technical note. *Eur Spine J*. 10 2017;26(Suppl 4):505–513. https://doi.org/10.1007/s00586-017-5041-7
29. Heggeness MH, Esses SI. Classification of pseudarthroses of the lumbar spine. *Spine (Phila Pa 1976)*. Aug 1991;16(8 Suppl): S449–54.
30. O'Dowd JK. *Complications in spine surgery*. Aospine manual clinical applications (vol. 2). 2007.
31. Lykissas MG, Aichmair A, Hughes AP, et al. Nerve injury after lateral lumbar interbody fusion: a review of 919 treated levels with identification of risk factors. Spine J. 2014;14(5):749–58. https://doi.org/10.1016/j.spinee.2013.06.066.
32. Dobrocky T, Grunder L, Breiding PS, et al. Assessing Spinal Cerebrospinal Fluid Leaks in Spontaneous Intracranial Hypotension With a Scoring System Based on Brain Magnetic Resonance Imaging Findings. JAMA Neurol. 05 2019;76(5):580–587. https://doi.org/10.1001/jamaneurol.2018.4921
33. Kandwal P, Vijayaraghavan GP, Nagaraja UB, Jayaswal A. Severe rigid scoliosis: review of management strategies and role of spinal osteotomies. Asian Spine J. 2017;11(3):494–503. https://doi.org/10.4184/asj.2017.11.3.494.

34. G. Alexander Jones VJM, Edward C. Benzel. Prevention of Operative Infections: An Evidence-Based Approach Benzel's Spine Surgery.
35. Yoshihara H. Sacroiliac joint pain after lumbar/lumbosacral fusion: current knowledge. Eur Spine J. 2012;21(9):1788–96. https://doi.org/10.1007/s00586-012-2350-8.
36. Kleck CJ, Noshchenko A, Burger EL, Cain CMJ, Patel VV. Postoperative pelvic incidence (PI) change may impact sagittal spinopelvic alignment (SSA) after instrumented surgical correction of adult spine deformity (ASD). Spine Deform. 07 2021;9 (4):1093–104. https://doi.org/10.1007/s43390-020-00283-2
37. Li W, Wang B, Feng X, Hua W, Yang C. Preoperative management and postoperative complications associated with transoral decompression for the upper cervical spine. BMC Musculoskelet Disord. Feb 08 2022;23(1):128. https://doi.org/10.1186/s12891-022-05081-7
38. Joseph A. Osorio, Rajiv Saigal, Chou D. Neurologic Complications of Common Spine Operations Benzel's Spine Surgery. 2017.
39. Yilmaz E, Abdul-Jabbar A, Tawfik T, et al. S2 alar-iliac screw insertion: technical note with pictorial guide. World Neurosurg. 2018;113:e296–301. https://doi.org/10.1016/j.wneu.2018.02.009.
40. Chun-Po Y, Shaffrey ME. Postoperative medical complications Benzel's Spine Surgery. (2017)
41. Daubs MD, Brodke DS, Annis P, Lawrence BD. Perioperative complications of pedicle subtraction osteotomy. Global Spine J. 2016;6(7):630–5. https://doi.org/10.1055/s-0035-1570088.
42. Chen WC, Tsai SHL, Goyal A, Fu TS, Lin TY, Bydon M. Comparison between vertebroplasty with high or low viscosity cement augmentation or kyphoplasty in cement leakage rate for patients with vertebral compression fracture: a systematic review and network meta-analysis. Eur Spine J. 09 2021;30(9):2680–90. https://doi.org/10.1007/s00586-020-06636-9
43. Dong S, Li Z, Tang ZR, Zheng Y, Yang H, Zeng Q. Predictors of adverse events after percutaneous pedicle screws fixation in patients with single-segment thoracolumbar burst fractures. BMC Musculoskelet Disord. 2022;23(1):168. https://doi.org/10.1186/s12891-022-05122-1
44. Jones EL, Heller JG, Silcox DH, Hutton WC. Cervical pedicle screws versus lateral mass screws. Anatomic feasibility and biomechanical comparison. Spine (Phila Pa 1976). May 01 1997;22(9):977–82. https://doi.org/10.1097/00007632-199705010-00009
45. Clarke A, Flowers MJ, Davies AG, Fernandes J, Jones S. Morbidity associated with anterior iliac crest bone graft harvesting in children undergoing orthopaedic surgery: a prospective review. J Child Orthop. 2015;9(5):411–6. https://doi.org/10.1007/s11832-015-0698-0.
46. Huang W, Han Z, Liu J, Yu L, Yu X. Risk Factors for recurrent lumbar disc herniation: a systematic review and meta-analysis. Medicine (Baltimore). 2016;95(2): e2378. https://doi.org/10.1097/MD.0000000000002378.
47. Rasouli MR, Rahimi-Movaghar V, Shokraneh F, Moradi-Lakeh M, Chou R. Minimally invasive discectomy versus microdiscectomy/open discectomy for symptomatic lumbar disc herniation. Cochrane Database Syst Rev. 2014;(9):CD010328. https://doi.org/10.1002/14651858.CD010328.pub2
48. Yeom JS, Kim WJ, Choy WS, Lee CK, Chang BS, Kang JW. Leakage of cement in percutaneous transpedicular vertebroplasty for painful osteoporotic compression fractures. J Bone Joint Surg Br. 2003;85(1):83–9. https://doi.org/10.1302/0301-620x.85b1.13026.
49. Lehmer SM, Steffee AD, Gaines RW. Treatment of L5-S1 spondyloptosis by staged L5 resection with reduction and fusion of L4 onto S1 (Gaines procedure). Spine (Phila Pa 1976). 1994;19 (17):1916–25. https://doi.org/10.1097/00007632-199409000-00010
50. Fiani B, Chacon D, Covarrubias C, Sarno E, Kondilis A. Sternotomy approach to the anterior cervicothoracic spine. Cureus. 2021;13(11): e19421. https://doi.org/10.7759/cureus.19421.
51. Epstein NE. Prophylactic inferior vena cava filter placement prior to lumbar surgery in morbidly obese patients: two-case study and literature review. Surg Neurol Int. 2015;6(Suppl 19):S469–74. https://doi.org/10.4103/2152-7806.166877.
52. Ravinsky RA, Crawford EJ, Reda LA, Rampersaud YR. Slip progression in degenerative lumbar spondylolisthesis following minimally invasive decompression surgery is not associated with increased functional disability. Eur Spine J. 2020;29(4):896–903. https://doi.org/10.1007/s00586-020-06336-4
53. Churojana A, Songsaeng D, Khumtong R, Suwanbundit A, Saliou G. Is intervertebral cement leakage a risk factor for new adjacent vertebral collapse? Interv Neuroradiol. 2014;20(5):637–45. https://doi.org/10.15274/INR-2014-10079.
54. Abduljabbar FH, Teles AR, Bokhari R, Weber M, Santaguida C. Laminectomy with or without fusion to manage degenerative cervical myelopathy. Neurosurg Clin N Am. 2018;29(1):91–105. https://doi.org/10.1016/j.nec.2017.09.017.
55. Igarashi H, Hoshino M, Omori K, et al. Factors influencing interbody cage subsidence following anterior cervical discectomy and fusion. Clin Spine Surg. 08 2019;32(7):297–302. https://doi.org/10.1097/BSD.0000000000000843
56. Deng B, Hong HN, Feng XB, Hong ZH, Cai GP, Hong D. Psoas hematoma as a rare complication of posterior lumbar interbody fusion: a case report. BMC Surg. Nov 11 2020;20(1):279. https://doi.org/10.1186/s12893-020-00942-1
57. Choi HY, Hyun SJ, Kim KJ, Jahng TA, Kim HJ. Surgical and radiographic outcomes after pedicle subtraction osteotomy according to surgeon's experience. Spine (Phila Pa 1976). Jul 2017;42 (13):E795–E801. https://doi.org/10.1097/BRS.0000000000001958
58. Khalifé M, Devriese F, Ferrero E, Zadegan F, Ajavon L, Mazel C. Dynesys® dynamic stabilization outcomes in degenerative spine surgery. Acta Orthop Belg. 2021;87(4):795–803. https://doi.org/10.52628/87.4.28.
59. Rapp SM, Miller LE, Block JE. AxiaLIF system: minimally invasive device for presacral lumbar interbody spinal fusion. Med Devices (Auckl). 2011;4:125–31. https://doi.org/10.2147/MDER.S23606.
60. Molinari RW, Chimenti PC, Molinari R, Gruhn W. Vertebral artery injury during routine posterior cervical exposure: case reports and review of literature. Global Spine J. 2015;5(6):528–32. https://doi.org/10.1055/s-0035-1566225.
61. La Marca F, Brumblay H. Smith-petersen osteotomy in thoracolumbar deformity surgery. Neurosurgery. 2008;63(3 Suppl): 163–70. https://doi.org/10.1227/01.NEU.0000320428.67620.4F.
62. Lee DY, Park YJ, Song SY, Jeong ST, Kim DH. Risk factors for posterior cage migration after lumbar interbody fusion surgery. Asian Spine J. 2018;12(1):59–68. https://doi.org/10.4184/asj.2018.12.1.59.
63. Skelly AC, Hashimoto RE, Norvell DC, et al. Cervical spondylotic myelopathy: methodological approaches to evaluate the literature and establish best evidence. Spine (Phila Pa 1976). Oct 2013;38(22 Suppl 1):S9–18. https://doi.org/10.1097/BRS.0b013e3182a7ebbf
64. Kong L, Cao J, Wang L, Shen Y. Prevalence of adjacent segment disease following cervical spine surgery: a PRISMA-compliant systematic review and meta-analysis. Medicine (Baltimore). 2016;95(27): e4171. https://doi.org/10.1097/MD.0000000000004171.
65. Maragkos GA, Motiei-Langroudi R, Filippidis AS, Glazer PA, Papavassiliou E. Factors predictive of adjacent segment disease after lumbar spinal fusion. World Neurosurg. 2020;133:e690–4. https://doi.org/10.1016/j.wneu.2019.09.112.

66. Xu DS, Walker CT, Farber SH, et al. Surgical anatomy of minimally invasive lateral approaches to the thoracolumbar junction. J Neurosurg Spine. 2021:1–8. https://doi.org/10.3171/2021.10.SPINE21793
67. Cavallo LM, Solari D, Somma T, Cappabianca P. The 3F (Fat, Flap, and Flash) technique for skull base reconstruction after endoscopic endonasal suprasellar approach. World Neurosurg. 2019;126:439–46. https://doi.org/10.1016/j.wneu.2019.03.125.
68. Hayek SM, Helm S, Benyamin RM, Singh V, Bryce DA, Smith HS. Effectiveness of spinal endoscopic adhesiolysis in post lumbar surgery syndrome: a systematic review. Pain Physician. 2009 Mar-Apr 2009;12(2):419–35.
69. El Homsi M, Gharzeddine K, Cuevas J, et al. MRI Findings of Arachnoiditis, Revisited. Is Classification Possible? J Magn Reson Imaging. 09 2021;54(3):904–9. https://doi.org/10.1002/jmri.27583
70. Carragee EJ, Han MY, Suen PW, Kim D. Clinical outcomes after lumbar discectomy for sciatica: the effects of fragment type and anular competence. J Bone Joint Surg Am. 2003;85(1):102–8.
71. Zileli M, Borkar SA, Sinha S, et al. Cervical spondylotic myelopathy: natural course and the value of diagnostic techniques -WFNS spine committee recommendations. Neurospine. 2019;16(3):386–402. https://doi.org/10.14245/ns.1938240.120.
72. Naveed MA, Mangla R, Idrees H, Mehta RI. Remote cerebellar haemorrhage: a potential iatrogenic complication of spinal surgery. Case Rep Neurol Med. 2018;2018:5870584. https://doi.org/10.1155/2018/5870584.
73. Song Y, Li C, Guan J, et al. Outcomes of epidural steroids following percutaneous transforaminal endoscopic discectomy: a meta-analysis and systematic review. Korean J Pain. 2022;35(1):97–105. https://doi.org/10.3344/kjp.2022.35.1.97.
74. Schonauer C, Mastantuoni C, Somma T, de Falco R, Cappabianca P, Tessitore E. Topical hemostatic agents in neurosurgery, a comprehensive review: 15 years update. Neurosurg Rev. Nov 04 2021; https://doi.org/10.1007/s10143-021-01684-1
75. Mesregah MK, Formanek B, Liu JC, Buser Z, Wang JC. Perioperative complications of surgery for degenerative cervical myelopathy: a comparison between 3 Procedures. Global Spine J. Mar 2021:2192568221998306. https://doi.org/10.1177/2192568221998306
76. Deora H, Kim SH, Behari S, et al. Anterior surgical techniques for cervical spondylotic myelopathy: WFNS spine committee recommendations. Neurospine, 09 2019;16(3):408–420. https://doi.org/10.14245/ns.1938250.125
77. Charles YP, Yu B, Steib JP. Sacroiliac joint luxation after pedicle subtraction osteotomy: report of two cases and analysis of failure mechanism. Eur Spine J. 05 2016;25 Suppl 1:63–74. https://doi.org/10.1007/s00586-015-4094-8
78. Lenz M, Mohamud K, Bredow J, Oikonomidis S, Eysel P, Scheyerer MJ. Comparison of different approaches in lumbosacral spinal fusion surgery: a systematic review and meta-analysis. Asian Spine J. 2021. https://doi.org/10.31616/asj.2020.0405.
79. Noordhoek I, Koning MT, Jacobs WCH, Vleggeert-Lankamp CLA. Incidence and clinical relevance of cage subsidence in anterior cervical discectomy and fusion: a systematic review. Acta Neurochir (Wien). 04 2018;160(4):873–880. https://doi.org/10.1007/s00701-018-3490-3
80. Kursumovic A, Muir JM, Ammerman J, Bostelmann R. The disability cascade: a preventable consequence of the loss of disc height following lumbar microdiscectomy. Cureus. 18 2019;11(7):e5169. https://doi.org/10.7759/cureus.5169
81. Brooks M, Dower A, Abdul Jalil MF, Kohan S. Radiological predictors of recurrent lumbar disc herniation: a systematic review and meta-analysis. J Neurosurg Spine. Nov 2020:1–11. https://doi.org/10.3171/2020.6.SPINE20598
82. Ravindra VM, Brock A, Awad AW, Kalra R, Schmidt MH. The role of the mini-open thoracoscopic-assisted approach in the management of metastatic spine disease at the thoracolumbar junction. Neurosurg Focus. 08 2016;41(2):E16. https://doi.org/10.3171/2016.5.FOCUS16162
83. Shin KH, Chang HG, Rhee NK, Lim KS. Revisional percutaneous full endoscopic disc surgery for recurrent herniation of previous open lumbar discectomy. Asian Spine J. 2011;5(1):1–9. https://doi.org/10.4184/asj.2011.5.1.1.
84. Xiao R, Miller JA, Lubelski D, et al. Quality of life outcomes following cervical decompression for coexisting Parkinson's disease and cervical spondylotic myelopathy. Spine J. 11 2016;16(11):1358–1366. https://doi.org/10.1016/j.spinee.2016.07.530
85. Murphy RF, Mooney JF. The crankshaft phenomenon. J Am Acad Orthop Surg. 2017;25(9):e185–93. https://doi.org/10.5435/JAAOS-D-16-00584.
86. Auerbach JD, Jones KJ, Fras CI, Balderston JR, Rushton SA, Chin KR. The prevalence of indications and contraindications to cervical total disc replacement. Spine J. 2008 Sep-Oct 2008;8(5):711–6. https://doi.org/10.1016/j.spinee.2007.06.018

Biomechanics of the Spine

11

Luke Antonio Silveira, Anvitha Sathya, and Ryan Jewell

1. **The change in unit length (linear) or change in unit angle (shear) in a body subjected to a force is defined as?**
   a) Coupling
   b) Burst load
   c) Strain
   d) Rigidity
   e) Bending Moment

Response: (C) Strain refers to the change in unit length (linear) or change in unit angle (shear) in a body subjected to a force (vector). When a deformable body is subjected to a load vector, the resulting deformations yield strains. The deformation along the direction of force application is termed axial strain, while the deformation transverse to the direction of applied force is termed transverse strain. The ratio of transverse to axial strain is termed Poisson's ratio.

2. **Which of the following substances has the highest modulus of elasticity?**
   a) Cortical bone (femur/tibia)
   b) Carbon fiber polymer
   c) Polyether ether ketone (PEEK)
   d) Titanium
   e) Cancellous bone

Response: (D) Of the substances listed, titanium has the highest modulus of elasticity (GPa > 100). Comparatively, the other substances all have a modulus of elasticity less than 20 GPa [1].

3. **The phenomenon by which a movement of the spine along or about an axis obligates another movement along or about another axis is referred to as?**
   a) Rotational Interfaces
   b) Stress
   c) Load sharing
   d) Knurling
   e) Coupling

Response: (E) Coupling refers to the relationship by which a movement of the spine along or about one axis induces a simultaneous movement along or about another axis of the Cartesian coordinate system. This is illustrated in the cervical spine, where lateral bending results in rotation of the spinous processes away from the concave side of the curve. The opposite occurs in the lumbar spine, where lateral bending results in the spinous processes rotating in the same direction as the concave side of the bend.

4. **The slope of a stress–strain curve within the linear, elastic phase of a particular material is referred to as?**
   a) The Modulus of Elasticity
   b) The coarseness
   c) The material velocity
   d) The Rotational Equilibrium
   e) The Object Turgor

Response: (A) The modulus of elasticity, synonymous with an object's stiffness, is defined as the stress-to-strain ratio, which is a constant for a given material within that material elastic zone [2].

L. A. Silveira (✉) · R. Jewell
Division of Neurosurgery, University of Vermont Medical Center, Burlington, VT, USA
e-mail: luke.silveira@uvmhealth.org

R. Jewell
e-mail: ryan.jewell@uvmhealth.org

A. Sathya
Boston University School of Medicine, Boston, MA, USA

C. Gragnaniello et al. (eds.), *MCQs in Spine Surgery*,
https://doi.org/10.1007/978-3-031-69332-8_11

5. **Which of the following statements coincides with Hooke's Law?**
   a) For solids deformed within their plastic zone, the size of deformation is proportional to the deforming force
   b) For solids deformed within their elastic zone, the size of deformation is proportional to the deforming force
   c) After a solid's elastic limit is reached, the size of deformation is proportional to the deforming force
   d) After a solid's yield point is reached, the size of deformation is proportional to the deforming force
   e) Between a solid's yield point and point of failure, deformation is proportional to the deforming force

Response (B) Hooke's law states that for small deformations, within a solid object's elastic zone, the size of deformation is proportional to the deforming force. Elastic deformation occurs when a strain totally recovers after a stress is removed. For larger displacements, the elastic zone may be exceeded. This occurs at a solid's elastic limit, or yield point, after which Hooke's law no longer applies. Beyond the yield point, the solid acquires a permanent set such that the solid no longer assumes its undeformed configuration following removal of external forces [2].

6. **Which of the following terms describes the directionally variant compressive strength of the vertebral body?**
   a) Anisotropic
   b) Ballistic
   c) Agoraphobic
   d) Biomechanically Bilingual
   e) Isotropic

Response (A) The vertebral bodies demonstrate highly anisotropic architecture [3]. The spine is predominantly vertically loaded and vertebral bodies are optimally structured to sustain the greatest load in the cephalo-caudal direction, with vertebral trabecular bone aligned in the vertical direction to provide maximal strength with minimal mass.

7. **A 64yo male with cervical myelopathy undergoes a C6 corpectomy and placement of a fibular strut graft with adjacent vertebral bodies plated to create axial loading on the graft, as shown below in** Fig. 11.1.

Axial loading upon the graft facilitates remodeling and healing via which principle?

a) Hooke's Law
b) Dalton's Law

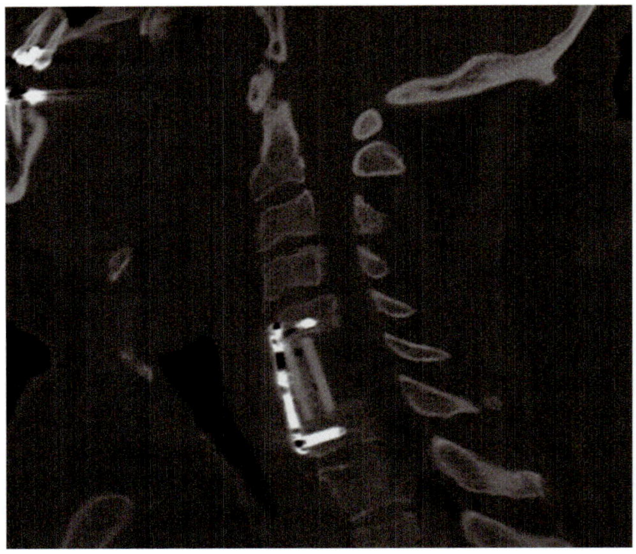

Fig. 11.1 Sagittal bone CT scan in patient that underwent C6 corpectomy and C5-C7 arthrodesis

c) Subsidence
d) Wolff's Law
e) Weiss' Principle

Response (D) Wolff's Law most literally states that every change in form and function of a bone, as well as external forces acting on a bone, lead to changes in the internal structure of that bone. Wolff's law suggests axial loading alters bone integrity and healing in that trabecular structure is hypothesized to be altered by remodeling resulting from mechanical loading such that bone heals optimally under loading forces. Thus, in the case described above, axial loading upon the graft is thought to facilitate bone growth, remodeling, and strengthening during healing [4].

8. **Degree of axial rotation within the cervical spine is greatest at which of the following levels?**
   a) C1-2
   b) C2-3
   c) C3-4
   d) C4-5
   e) C5-6

Response (A) The degree of axial rotation is greatest between C1 and C2, occurring about the axis of the odontoid process

9. **Which of the following has the highest resistance to screw pullout assuming use of an identical screw in each scenario?**
   a) vertebral body
   b) osteoporotic vertebral body

c) osteoporotic large pedicle (sacrum pedicle)
d) healthy large pedicle (sacrum pedicle)
e) smaller pedicle (thoracic and upper lumbar pedicles)

Response (E) The ratio of cortical to cancellous bone is greater in the pedicles than in the vertebral bodies and greater in the smaller pedicles (thoracic and upper lumbar) than in the larger sacral pedicles. For each listed option, osteoporosis would significantly decrease bone integrity and thereby decrease resistance to screw pullout. Therefore, of the options listed, smaller pedicles have the greatest resistance to screw pullout [5].

10. **Which of the following statements accurately details the relationship between facet joint orientation and spinal segmental movement?**
   a) Lumbar spine facet joints are oriented in a relatively coronal plane, making them less resistant to rotational movement than the cervical spine facet joints
   b) Cervical spine facet joints are oriented in a relatively coronal plane, making them less resistant to rotational movement than the lumbar spine facet joints
   c) Lumbar and cervical spine facet joints are similarly oriented in a sagittal plane, making them equally resistant to rotational movement
   d) Lumbar and cervical spine facet joints are similarly oriented in a coronal, making them equally resistant to rotational movement
   e) The cervical and thoracic facet joints are similarly oriented in a sagittal plane, making them equally resistant to rotational movement, while the lumbar facet joints are oriented in a relatively coronal plane and less resistant to rotational movement.

Response (B) The facet joints of the cervical spine are primarily oriented in the coronal plane and the facet joint orientation becomes more sagittal as one descends through the thoracic and lumbar spine. As the lumbar facets are oriented in the sagittal plane, their ability to resist rotational movements is substantially greater than in the cervical spine.

The orientation of the facet joints in the coronal plane most substantially inhibits extension.

11. **Which of the following correctly identifies the relative vertebral body compression strengths?**
   a) Lumbar compression strength > thoracic compression strength > cervical compression strength
   b) Thoracic compression strength > Lumbar compression strength > cervical compression strength
   c) Thoracic compression strength > Cervical compression strength > lumbar compression strength
   d) Cervical compression strength > thoracic compression strength > lumbar compression strength
   e) Cervical compression strength > lumbar compression strength > thoracic compression strength

Response (A) The progressive increase in size of the vertebral bodies from the rostral to caudal direction along the spine correlates with an increase in strength and load-bearing ability [3]. The vertebral bodies' dimensions are proportional to the loading forces they support.

12. **During which motion do the facets joints bear a greater part of the axial load in the cervical and lumbar regions?**
   a) Extension
   b) Flexion
   c) Rotation
   d) Lateral bending
   e) Neutral position

Response: (A). The facets bear a greater part of the axial load during extension. The facet joints do not otherwise significantly support axial loads.

13. **Which of the following statements accurately describes the movement of the annulus fibrosus during forward flexion?**
   a) Flexion causes bulging of the annulus fibrosus rostrally
   b) Flexion has no effect on the annulus fibrosus
   c) Flexion causes bulging of the annulus fibrosus ventrally
   d) Flexion causes bulging of the annulus fibrosus dorsally
   e) Flexion causes bulging of the annulus fibrosus laterally

Response (C) Bulging of the annulus fibrosus occurs on the concave side of a bending spine. The nucleus pulposus moves in the opposite direction. Thus, flexion causes ventral bulging of the annulus fibrosis and dorsal migration of the nucleus pulposus.

14. **Which of the following statements accurately describes the movement of the nucleus pulposus in relation to the annulus fibrosis bulge during application an eccentric axial load?**

a) The nucleus pulposus tends to migrate in the same direction as the annulus fibrosus bulge
b) The nucleus pulposus tends to migrate in the opposite direction as the annulus fibrosus bulge
c) The nucleus pulposus tends to remain stationary during application of an eccentric axial load
d) The nucleus pulposus tends to migrate within the annulus fibrosus bulge
e) The nucleus pulposus tends to migrate orthogonally to the annulus fibrosus bulge

Response (B) Disk bulging, and therefore annulus fibrosus bulge, occurs on the concave side of a bending spine. When under eccentric axial loading, the nucleus pulposus migrates away from the concave side of the bending spine and therefore away from the annulus fibrosus bulge.

15. **Which of the following levels has the highest incidence of vertebral compression fractures?**
a) Lower lumbar spine
b) Sacral spine
c) Mid-thoracic spine
d) Upper thoracic spine
d) Upper thoracic spine
e) Thoracolumbar spine

Response (E) The thoracolumbar spine represents the lower terminus of the thoracic kyphosis, lacks the protective support of the rib cage, and does not have the larger vertebral bodies characteristic of the lower lumbar spine. These factors collectively contribute to an increased incidence of compression fractures in this region.

16. **Degree of flexion–extension in the spine is greatest at which of the following levels?**
a) L1-2
b) Occiput to C1
c) C2-3
d) C3-4
e) C4-5

Response (B) Of the spinal levels listed, degree of flexion–extension is greatest at the Occiput to C1 interface.

17. **Which of the following ligaments plays the most critical role in holding the dens to the posterior aspect of the C1 anterior arch in a configuration permitting significant neck rotation but limiting posterior migration of the dens into the spinal canal?**
a) Alar ligament
b) Tectorial membrane
c) C1-2 Interspinous Ligament
d) Transverse ligament
e) Posterior longitudinal ligament

Response (D) The transverse ligament inserts into the medial tubercles of the C1 lateral masses crosses immediately behind the body of the dens, holding the dens in close proximity to the posterior aspect of the C1 anterior arch. The transverse ligament thereby plays a crucial role in permitting a large degree of axial neck rotation, but limits pathologic flexion and extension as well as posterior migration of the dens into the spinal canal. Disruption of the transverse ligament, therefore, leads to atlanto-axial instability.

18. **Which of the following accurately describes the relationship between rod diameter and its stiffness?**
a) Rod stiffness is inversely proportional to rod diameter squared
b) Rod stiffness is proportional to rod diameter squared
c) Rod stiffness is directly proportional to rod diameter
d) Rod stiffness is proportional to rod diameter to the fourth power
e) Rod stiffness is inversely proportional to rod diameter to the fourth power

Response (D) Rod stiffness is proportional to rod diameter to the fourth power.

19. **Which of the following accurately describes the relationship between rod diameter and its strength?**
a) Rod strength is inversely proportional to rod diameter squared
b) Rod strength is proportional to rod diameter squared
c) Rod strength is directly proportional to rod diameter
d) Rod strength is proportional to rod diameter to the fourth power
e) Rod strength is proportional to rod diameter cubed

Response (D) Rod strength is proportional to rod diameter cubed.

20. **The quantification of an angular deformity can be accomplished by determining which angle?**
a) Cobb angle- angle between neutral rostral and caudal vertebrae associated with a curvature
b) Dutch angle -angle between plum line and rostral neutral vertebral body associated with a curve
c) Hallstead's angle—angle between C7 middle inferior endplate and caudal neutral vertebral body associated with a curve

d) Callahan's angle—angle between apex of curvature and center of S1 superior endplate
e) Trolley angle—angle between C7 middle inferior endplate and apex of curvature under analysis

Response (A) An angular deformity can be quantified by calculating the Cobb angle, the angle between the rostral neutral vertebra and caudal neutral vertebra. In this case, neutral vertebrae are referred to as those vertebrae located at the junction between two opposite curvatures.

21. **Which of the following best describes the pressure within the disc space in youth versus with age-related degeneration?**
   a) In youth, the pressures within the central disc are generally high and relatively evenly distributed across the disc space during axial loading.
   b) In youth, the pressures within the central disc are generally low and the annulus fibrosus bears a greater portion of axial loading
   c) With degenerative aging, the pressures within the central disc become higher during axial loading and pressure on the peripheral annulus fibrosus is diminished
   d) Pressure borne by the central disc remains unchanged in the aged degenerative spine during axial loading as compared to the youthful spine
   e) Pressure borne by the peripheral annulus fibrosus remains unchanged in the aged degenerative spine during axial loading as compared to the youthful spine

Response (A) Aging and degeneration within the intervertebral disc is associated with pressure distribution changes across the disc space. In youth, the pressures within the central disc are generally high and relatively evenly distributed across the disc space during axial loading. As the spine ages and degenerative processes take place, the desiccated central nucleus pulposus can no longer bear axial loads as in youth. Therefore, axial loads are borne more peripherally by the fibrocartilaginous equivalent of the nucleus pulposus, and the central disc pressure is diminished [2].

22. **How do the ribs and sternum effect stability of the middle and upper thoracic spine?**
   a) An intact sternum-ribcage plays no role in stability of the middle and upper thoracic spine
   b) The sternum-ribcage makes the upper and middle thoracic spine particularly unstable
   c) Sternal attachments are not required to achieve the full stabilization potential of the ribcage
   d) The sternum and ribcage function together to enhance stability of the upper and middle thoracic spine
   e) An intact sternum with or without the ribcage augments stability of the middle thoracic spine

Response (D) The sternum and ribcage function together to enhance stability of the upper and middle thoracic spine, providing an additional degree of stiffness to that portion of the spine and augmenting its axial load resisting ability. The removal or detachment of the ribs to an intact sternum detracts significantly from this added stability.

23. **A burst fracture is characterized by which of the following?**
   a) Anterior column compression only
   b) Anterior column compression and middle column compression
   c) Middle column distraction and posterior column distraction
   d) Anterior column compression, middle column distraction, and posterior column distraction
   e) Posterior column compression only

Response (B) A burst fracture is characterized by anterior and middle column compression. A compression fracture is characterized by an anterior column compression only or anterior column compression and posterior column distraction. A "seat belt" fracture is characterized by middle column distraction and posterior column distraction. A fracture-dislocation is characterized by anterior column compression, middle column distraction, and posterior column distraction with a rotational shear.

24. **The 30-degree orientation of the annular collagen fibers to the vertebral endplates provides the annulus fibrosis with the greatest resistance to which of the following movements?**
   a) Torsion/rotation
   b) Distraction
   c) Compression
   d) lateral bending
   e) Equal degree of resistance to rotation and compression

Response (A) Annular fibers, laminated bands of fibrous tissue predominantly composed of collagen, are oriented in opposite directions at approximately a 30 degree angle from the vertebral endplates. Their orientation provides a greater resistance to torsion than distraction, compression, or bending.

25. **A 19-year-old male awakens from a good night's rest and takes a ten-hour hike through the woods. How has the water content of his intervertebral discs changed from awakening compared to at the conclusion of his hike?**
    a) Water content of the discs is unchanged
    b) Water content of the discs is decreased along with the intradiscal oncotic pressure
    c) Water content of the discs is increased along with the intradiscal oncotic pressure
    d) Water content of the discs is decreased while intradiscal oncotic pressure is increased
    e) Water content of the discs is increased while intradiscal oncotic pressure is decreased

Response (D) The pressure within the intervertebral disc with upright, weight-bearing posture is much greater than in supine position. An increase in intradiscal pressure with weight bearing causes fluid to migrate out of the disc space. This leads to an increase in the concentration of micro molecules and oncotic pressure within the disc space, lowering the water content but increasing the absorptive capacity of the disc [6].

26. **Which of the following correctly describes the effect of traction on intradiscal pressure, intradiscal water content, and disc height?**
    a) Traction causes a decrease in intradiscal pressure, intradiscal water content, and disc height
    b) Traction causes an increase in intradiscal pressure, decrease in intradiscal water content, and decrease in disc height
    c) Traction causes a decrease in intradiscal pressure, increase in intradiscal water content, and increase in disc height
    d) Traction causes no change in intradiscal pressure, intradiscal water content, or disc height
    e) Traction causes an increase in intradiscal pressure, decrease in intradiscal water content, and increase in disc height

Response (C) Traction, as opposed to weight bearing, provides a mechanism by which the intradiscal pressure can be reduced, thereby permitting in increase in disc water content and an increase in disc height.

27. **In which direction is the annulus fibrosus weakest and least abundant?**
    a) Dorsally
    b) Ventrally
    c) Laterally
    d) Equally strong and abundant in all directions
    e) Direction of highest abundance and strength is gender-dependent

Response (A) The annulus fibrosus is weaker and less abundant dorsally than ventrally or laterally, a feature which contributes to the locality of disc herniations [2].

28. **What pressure changes account for the vacuum disc phenomenon?**
    a) Negative pressure within the central disc interspace as a result of severe degenerative changes and increased peripheral loading
    b) Increased central disc pressures as a result of severe degenerative changes and decreased peripheral loading
    c) Increased central disc pressures as a result of severe degenerative changes and increased peripheral loading
    d) Uniform high pressures across the disc and peripheral annulus fibrosus
    e) Erosion of the disc through the superior vertebral endplate

Response (A) As the spine ages and degenerative processes take place, the desiccated central nucleus pulposus can no longer bear axial loads as in youth. Therefore, axial loads are borne more peripherally by the fibrocartilaginous equivalent of the nucleus pulposus, and the central disc pressure is diminished. With severe degenerative changes, pressures within the disc space can drop below zero with resultant gas formation giving rise to the vacuum disc phenomenon.

29. **Which region of the spine is typically spared from spinal canal encroachment by osteophyte formation?**
    a) Cervical
    b) Thoracic

c) Lumbar
d) Cervical and thoracic
e) Cervical and lumbar

Response (B) Osteophyte formation typically takes place along the concavity of a spinal curve, coinciding with the direction in which the annulus fibrosus bulges and elevates the periosteum of adjacent vertebral bodies at Sharpey's fiber insertion sites. The natural lordosis of the cervical and lumbar spine result in a dorsally oriented concavity of spinal curvature, with osteophyte formation therefore occurring toward the spinal canal in these regions. The thoracic spine, by contrast, is typically spared from spinal canal encroachment by osteophyte formation because of its natural kyphosis and concordant ventrally oriented concavity of spinal curvature [2].

30. **How might intervertebral disc height loss lead to torsional instability?**
   a) Leads to annular fibers becoming increasingly taut
   b) Leads to annular fibers becoming increasing lax
   c) Induces annular fiber overgrowth
   d) Causes direct tearing of annular fibers
   e) Leads to detachment of annulus fibrosis at Sharpey's fibers insertion sites

Response (B) The 30-degree orientation of the annular fibers with respect to the disc space is optimal for resisting torsional forces, but only if the annular fibers remain taut. Loss of intervertebral disc height can lead to increased laxity in the annular fibers and thereby lead to torsional instability.

31. **In a region with kyphotic posture, which pathologic fracture morphology might be expected in an osteoporotic patient?**
   a) Wedge Compression fracture
   b) Burst fracture
   c) Chance Fracture
   d) Tear-drop fracture
   e) Clay-shoveler's fracture

Response (A) In a region with kyphotic posture, a ventral wedge compression fracture might be expected. Kyphosis predisposes the spine to ventral vertebral body collapse because the moment arm applied to the spine at the apex of kyphosis extends ventrally and is longer than in a region without significant kyphosis.

32. **Which of the following best defines a "moment arm" as it relates to spinal biomechanics?**
   a) The orthogonal distance between the force vector and the instantaneous access of rotation of the body on which the force acts
   b) The distance between two sequential intervertebral discs
   c) The distance from the middle of the vertebral body to the tip of the spinous process
   d) The distance between two force vectors acting on a body
   e) the distance between a kyphotic apex and the most proximal lordotic apex

Response (A) The moment arm refers to the orthogonal distance between a force vector and the instantaneous axis of rotation (IAR) of the body on which the force acts. For practical purposes, the moment arm is the lever length upon which a force vector acts.

33. **Which of the following is the term applied to describe the axis upon which each vertebral segment rotates at any given moment in time?**
   a) Instantaneous Axis of Rotation
   b) Torsional focus
   c) Central Spin point
   d) Rotatory tangent point
   e) Radial Fixed setting

Response (A) The instantaneous axis of rotation refers to the center of the coordinate system for each vertebral motion segment. It is the axis upon which each vertebral segment rotates at any given moment.

34. **How many degrees of freedom exist about each instantaneous axis of rotation (IAR)?**
   a) 2
   b) 4
   c) 6
   d) 8
   e) 10

Response (C) There are 6 degrees of freedom about each IAR, with both rotation and translation possible about each of the three Cartesian axes (*x*, *y*, and z axes).

35. **Which of the following accurately describes the relationship between rod diameter and its moment of inertia for a rod of uniform density?**
    a) Moment of inertia is inversely proportional to rod diameter squared
    b) Moment of inertia is proportional to rod diameter squared
    c) Moment of inertia is directly proportional to rod diameter
    d) Moment of inertia is proportional to rod diameter to the fourth power
    e) Moment of inertia is inversely proportional to rod diameter to the fourth power

Response (D) For a rod of uniform density, the moment of inertia is proportional to rod diameter to the fourth power.

36. **Which of the following accurately describes the relationship between core screw diameter and its section modulus?**
    a) Section modulus is inversely proportional to core screw diameter
    b) Section modulus is proportional to core screw diameter squared
    c) Section modulus is directly proportional to core screw diameter
    d) Section modulus is proportional to core screw diameter to the fourth power
    e) Section modulus is proportional to core screw diameter cubed

Response (D) A screw's section modulus (Z) is an indicator of its strength and is proportional to core screw diameter cubed.

37. **Which of the following joints is an amphiarthrodial joint?**
    a) Intervertebral disc joint
    b) Facet joints
    c) Interphalangeal joints
    d) Occipital condylar joints
    e) Hip joint

Response (A) The intervertebral disc joint is an amphiarthrodial joint, meaning there is no synovial membrane. The osteophytes of spondylosis are associated with degeneration of this amphiarthrodial joint, differentiating this degenerative process from the seropositive inflammatory arthritis that classically involve synovial membranes of diarthrodial joints such as the facet joints.

38. **In the event of a disc herniation, the application of an axial load, lateral bending, and flexion causes the nucleus pulposus to migrate in which direction?**
    a) In the direction of the annulus fibrosis under the most tension
    b) In the direction of the annulus fibrosis under the least tension
    c) Ventrally
    d) In no particular direction; it generally remains stationary
    e) Toward the superior vertebral body endplate

Response (A) The described loading pattern causes increased tension in the weakest portion of the annulus fibrosis and migration of the nucleus pulposus toward this portion of the annulus fibrosis, away from the region of asymmetrically increased intradiscal pressure. This loading pattern, therefore, may result in a characteristic dorsal paramedian disc herniation.

39. **Which of the following represents a healthy, non-pathologic vertebral body morphology and cervical spine posture?**
    a) lordotic posture, ventral vertebral body heights > dorsal vertebral body heights
    b) lordotic posture, ventral vertebral body heights < dorsal vertebral body heights
    c) kyphotic posture, ventral vertebral body heights = dorsal vertebral body heights
    d) kyphotic posture, ventral vertebral body heights < dorsal vertebral body heights
    e) kyphotic posture, ventral vertebral body heights > dorsal vertebral body heights

Response (A) In the non-pathologic cervical spine, dorsal vertebral body height is typically less than ventral vertebral body height contributing to a normal lordotic curvature.

40. **A 32 year old woman is nine months pregnant with a baby weighing an estimated 50 N (11.2 pounds), and complains of significant back pain. Why must the erector spinae muscles exert a greater downward force than that exerted by the weight of the baby in utero, for the mother to stand upright and not fall over?**

a) The erector spinae muscles are located a significantly shorter distance from the instantaneous axis of rotation of the spine than the baby in utero
b) The erector spinae muscles are located a significantly longer distance from the instantaneous axis of rotation of the spine than the baby in utero
c) The erector spinae muscles have come to physiologically anticipate increased weight of the baby and exert a greater force preemptively
d) The erector spinae muscles always exert a fixed downward force independent of the weight of the baby in utero
e) The erector spinae muscles need not exert any greater downward force as a result of the ventral downward force of the baby in utero

Response (A) If the woman described is standing upright and not in motion, a dorsal downward application of force must be applied, in this case by the erector spinae muscles, that are located a short distance from the instantaneous axis of rotation (IAR) of the spine ($\sim$5 cm) compared to the baby in utero ($\sim$25 cm). Given that the dorsal and ventral bending moments must be equal with respect to the IAR, the erector spinae must generate a greater downward force than the weight of the baby in utero because the erector spinae have a shorter moment arm (D = 5 cm) compared to the baby in utero (D = 25 cm). Bending moment is equal to force $\times$ distance from IAR, or force $\times$ moment arm. In this theoretical scenario, if the erector spinae muscles are the only countering force, they would have to exert a downward force 5 $\times$ that of the weight of the baby.

41. **How is the bending moment application related to the moment arm length?**
a) The bending moment is proportional to moment arm length cubed
b) The bending moment is inversely proportional to moment arm length
c) The bending moment is directly proportional to moment arm length
d) The bending moment is inversely proportional to moment arm length cubed
e) The bending moment is proportional to moment arm length squared

Response (C) The bending moment (M) is synonymous with torque and is the product of an applied force and the length of the moment arm through which it acts. The moment arm refers to the orthogonal distance between a force vector and the instantaneous axis of rotation (IAR) of the body on which the force acts.

42. **Newton's laws are highly relevant to spinal biomechanics. Which law states that for every action, there is an equal (in magnitude) but opposite (in direction) reaction?**
a) Newton's First Law
b) Newton's Second Law
c) Newton's Third Law
d) Newton's Fifth Law
e) Newton's Sixth Law

Response (C) Newton's Third Law states that for every action, there is an equal but opposite reaction.

43. **Which of the following correctly characterizes the orientation of the lumbar facet joints and their relative ability to resist certain motions?**
a) The lumbar facets are oriented in the coronal plane, most significantly limiting translation
b) The lumbar facets are oriented in the coronal plane, most significantly limiting flexion
c) The lumbar facets are oriented in the coronal plane, most significantly limiting axial rotation
d) The lumbar facets are oriented in the sagittal plane, most significantly limiting rotation
e) The lumbar facets are oriented in the sagittal plane, most significantly limiting translation

Response (D) The lumbar facets are oriented in the sagittal plane, substantially limiting rotation but with minimal ability to resist flexion or translation.

44. **Which of the following equations correctly defines the bending moment (M) with relation to force (F) applied to a lever arm and length of the lever arm (D)?**
a) $M = F/D$
b) $M = F \times D$
c) $M = F \times D^2$
d) $M = F^2 \times D$
e) $M = F/D^2$

Response (B) The bending moment (M) is equal to the product of the force applied to a lever arm (F) and the length of the lever arm (D).

45. **Which of the following is the best refers to severe spinal pain that worsened with increased loading of the spine and alleviated with unloading?**
    a) Mechanical axial spine pain
    b) Myofascial pain
    c) Inflammatory axial spine pain
    d) Chronic pain
    e) Anesthesia dolorosa

Response (A) Mechanical axial spine pain is best described as severe spinal pain that is worsened with increased loading of the spine and alleviated with unloading. Myofascial pain refers to pain caused by paraspinous muscle tenderness. Inflammatory axial spine pain is characterized by early morning back stiffness that lessens throughout the day after movement. Chronic pain is pain that is not well characterized or consistent.

46. **If a force vector passes precisely through the instantaneous access of rotation of a vertebral body such that the vertebral body is stressed to failure by the axial force, which fracture morphology results?**
    a) Ventral wedge compression fracture
    b) Burst fracture
    c) Dorsal wedge compression fracture
    d) Hangman's fracture
    e) Lateral wedge compression fracture

Response (B) A pure axial force directly through a spinal segment's instantaneous axis of rotation results in a burst fracture.

47. **If a force vector passes precisely through the instantaneous access of rotation of a vertebral body such that the vertebral body is stressed to failure by the axial force resulting in a burst fracture, how long is the moment arm of the force vector?**
    a) at least half the width of the vertebral body
    b) length is zero
    c) the exact width of the vertebral body
    d) Equal to the width of the vertebral body squared
    e) Equal to the height of the vertebral body

Response (B) The moment arm length of this force vector is zero, as the perpendicular distance from the force vector to the instantaneous axis of rotation is zero.

48. **A 62 year old man crashes his vintage automobile into a tree, and is taken to the ED immediately following extrication which involves cutting of an old lap belt that cannot be dis-engaged on the scene. After imaging is obtained, he is diagnosed with a chance fracture. Which of the following mechanisms accounts for the occurrence of this fracture?**
    a) Flexion-distraction
    b) Extension
    c) Translation
    d) Rotation-distraction
    e) Axial compression

Response (A) A chance fracture the result of a flexion-distraction injury with the above clinical history detailing the most common circumstances including a deceleration accident with a motorist wearing a lap belt but no chest/shoulder restraints. In such a scenario, there is restriction of pelvic and lumbosacral movement with unrestricted distraction and forward flexion of the spine superior to that point.

49. **Which of the following forces most characteristically result in cervical unilateral facet dislocation?**
    a) Flexion plus rotation
    b) Extension
    c) Pure rotation
    d) Axial loading
    e) Pure translation

Response (A) A flexion moment combined with a rotational component leads to a unilateral facet dislocation. By contrast, a pure flexion moment more commonly results in bilateral facet dislocation.

50. **Which spinal region is the least likely to have neural injury after a trauma?**
    a) Atlanto-Axial region
    b) Cervical spine
    c) Thoracic spine
    d) Lumbar spine
    e) Occipital Cervical junction

Response (D) Of the listed regions, the lumbar spine is least likely to have neural injury following a trauma.

51. **Which of the following ligaments provides the most resistance to flexion?**
    a) Anterior longitudinal ligament
    b) Posterior longitudinal ligament
    c) Interspinous ligament
    d) Ligamentum flavum
    e) Capsular ligament

Response (C) Of the listed ligaments, the interspinous ligament provides the most resistance to flexion, as it has the longest perpendicular moment arm. The large distance between the instantaneous axis of rotation and the attachment to the spinous process allows for this substantial resistance.

52. **Which of the following correctly describes the motion of the atlantoaxial facets during axial head rotation?**
    a) The C1 inferior facets glides posteriorly over the superior C2 facet on the side to which the head is turned.
    b) The C1 inferior facet glides anteriorly over the superior C2 facet on the side to which the head is turned
    c) The C1 inferior facet and C2 superior facet do not move in relation to one another during head turning
    d) The C1 inferior facet glides posteriorly over the superior C2 facet on the side opposite head turning
    e) The atlantoaxial facets joints are not real joints, as the C1 inferior facet is rigidly fused to the C2 superior facet

Response (A) During axial head rotation, the C1 inferior facet glides posteriorly over the C2 superior facet on the side to which the head is turned. The C1 inferior facet glides anteriorly over the C2 superior facet on the contralateral side to which the head is turned [7].

53. **In a normally aligned lordotic cervical spine, which of the following accurately describes the axial load bearing distribution between the facets and the intervertebral discs for the sub-axial cervical levels?**
    a) The facet joints bear about 1/3 of the axial load, while the remaining 2/3 of the axial load is transmitted via the intervertebral discs
    b) The facet joints bear about 2/3 of the axial load, while the remaining 1/3 of the axial load is transmitted via the intervertebral discs
    c) The facet joints bear about 1/2 of the axial load, while the remaining 1/2 of the axial load is transmitted via the intervertebral discs
    d) The facet joints bear the entirety of the axial load, with none transmitted through the intervertebral discs
    e) The facet joints bear none of the axial load, as it is entirely transmitted through the intervertebral discs

Response (B) For a normally aligned, lordotic cervical spine, the subaxial facet joints bear about 2/3 of the axial load. The remaining 1/3 of the axial load is transmitted through the intervertebral discs.

54. **How does the magnitude of the bending moment (M) imparted by the axial load of the cranium on the cervical spine change with cervical kyphosis?**
    a) The magnitude increases because the moment arm length (L) increases with cervical kyphosis
    b) The magnitude decreases because the moment arm length (L) increases with cervical kyphosis
    c) The magnitude increases because the moment arm length (L) decreases with cervical kyphosis
    d) The magnitude of the bending moment increases but the moment arm length (L) stays the same with cervical kyphosis
    e) The magnitude of the bending moment stays the same despite but the moment arm length (L) increasing with cervical kyphosis

Response (A) With a cervical kyphotic deformity, the cranium's center of mass is shifted anteriorly with respect to the cervical spine instantaneous axis of rotation, increasing the moment arm length (L) and therefore increasing the magnitude of the bending moment [7]. Bending moment magnitude (M) is equal to force (F) x moment arm length (L).

55. **How does a cervical kyphotic deformity impact the portion of axial load that the intervertebral discs bear as compared to the facet joints in the subaxial cervical spine?**
    a) Cervical kyphosis does not alter the portion of the axial load that is transmitted through the intervertebral discs, but alters the portion of axial load borne by the facets

b) The portion of axial load transmitted through the intervertebral discs decreases with cervical kyphosis, and the portion borne by the facets increases
c) The portion of axial load transmitted through the intervertebral discs increases with cervical kyphosis, and the portion borne by the facets decreases
d) The portion of axial load transmitted through the intervertebral discs decreases with cervical kyphosis, and the portion borne by the facets decreases as well
e) Cervical kyphosis does not alter the portion of the axial load that is transmitted through the intervertebral discs or the portion of axial load borne by the facets

Response (C) When a cervical kyphotic deformity is present, the axial load is shifted anteriorly such that a greater portion is transmitted through the intervertebral discs such that cervical disc degeneration is potentially accelerated.

56. **A 28-year-old woman involved in a high-speed motor vehicle collision presents to the emergency department with neck pain and the CT cervical spine below** (Fig. 11.2) **depicting a unilateral facet dislocation. Which of following mechanisms most commonly accounts for this unilateral dislocation?**

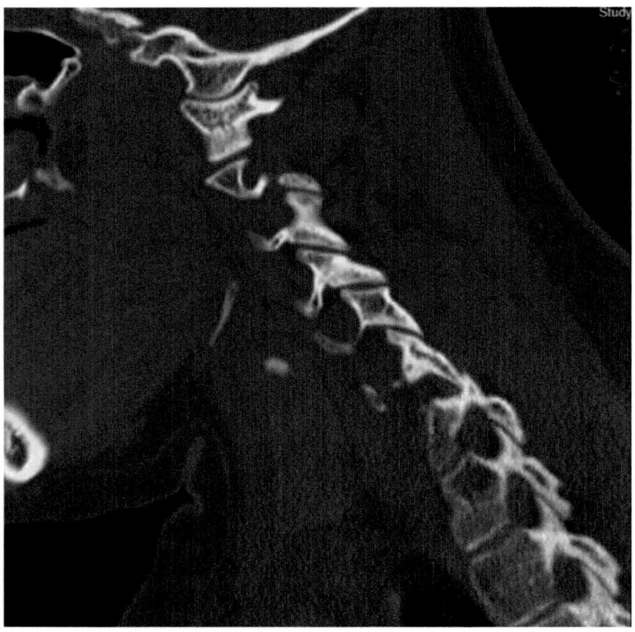

Fig. 11.2 Parasagittal bone CT cut through the facet joints in the cervical spine

a) Extension
b) Axial compression
c) Flexion plus rotation
d) Pure flexion
e) Lateral bending

Response (C) A flexion moment combined with a rotational component results in a unilateral facet dislocation such as the unilateral C6-7 jumped facet depicted. A true flexion moment without the rotational component most commonly results in bilateral facet dislocation.

57. **Which of the following is the best description of the mechanism of injury of a judicial hangman's fracture?**
a) A hyperextension not associated with a distraction that is commonly associated with a C2-C3 dislocation
b) A distraction in combination with a capital hyperextension resulting from a rostrally oriented force vector
c) A small axial load and extension
d) A violent extension and distraction which results in a separation of the rostral and caudal parts of the ventral C1 ring
e) Pure axial compression

Response (B) A judicial hangman's fracture can appear as a distraction in combination with a capital hyperextension. It can also result from a rostrally oriented force vector. A hangman's fracture can appear as a hyperextension not associated with a distraction and can be commonly associated with a C2-C3 dislocation. A small axial load and extension is more commonly associated with a Type 1 C2 Body Fracture with C2-C3 Extension-Subluxation. A violent extension and distraction that results in a separation of the rostral and caudal parts of the ventral C1 ring is more characteristic of a horizontal C1 fracture.

58. **Which of the following can be most appropriately treated with an odontoid screw?**
a) A horizontal Type II dens fracture
b) A Type III dens fracture
c) A diagonally oriented type II dens fracture
d) A comminuted Type II dens fracture
e) A chronic Type II dens fracture in which a fibrous nonunion has developed

Response (A) For some patients with favorable anatomy, an odontoid screw provides an effective and appropriate option for treating a type II horizontally oriented dens fracture. Type III dens fractures are not typically treated surgically. Old fractures in which a fibrous nonunion has developed are associated with worse arthrodesis rates. Diagonal fractures lend themselves to angulation and translation of bone fragments during compression. Comminuted fractures generally do not permit adequate compressive effect. Comminution, in tandem with motion, leads to increased rates of arthrodesis failure.

59. **Which of the following screw characteristics has the greatest effect on resisting screw pullout?**
    a) Outer diameter of the screw
    b) Inner diameter
    c) Screw head diameter
    d) Screw pitch
    e) Screw length

Response (A) Of the screw characteristics listed, increased outer diameter has the greatest effect on resisting screw pullout. Screw pitch was found to be related to screw displacement before failure.

60. **What is the thread pitch of a screw and what are the implications of a larger thread pitch?**
    a) Thread pitch refers to the distance between threads of a screw.
    b) Thread pitch refers to the distance between the screw tulip and tip.
    c) Thread pitch refers to the difference between the outer and inner diameter of a screw.
    d) Thread pitch refers to the diameter of the screw neck compared to the screw head
    e) Thread pitch refers to rate at which a conical screw diameter decreases from proximal shaft to tip

Response (A) Thread pitch refers to the distance between threads of a screw. The larger the pitch, the more bone is grabbed with each rotation of the screw.

61. **Which of the following factors is most significantly increased for vs. cylindrical screws?**
    a) Insertional torque
    b) Fatigue resistance
    c) Strength
    d) corrosion resistance
    e) Osteointegration

Response (A) Conical screws have greater insertional torque than cylindrical screws. Corrosion resistance and osteointegration are material properties not related to screw configuration [8].

62. **Which of the following correctly describes the effect of inner screw diameter and outer screw diameter on screw strength and screw resistance to pullout?**
    a) Increased outer diameter contributes most significantly to screw strength while increased inner diameter contributes most to increased pullout resistance.
    b) Increased outer diameter contributes most significantly to increased pullout resistance while increased inner diameter contributes most to increased screw strength.
    c) Inner and outer diameter contribute equally to screw strength.
    d) Inner and outer diameter contribute equally to pullout resistance
    e) Outer diameter contributes more significantly to increased pullout resistance and screw strength than inner diameter.

Response (B) Increased outer screw diameter contributes more significantly to increased pullout resistance while increased inner diameter contributes more significantly to increased screw strength.

63. **What effect does triangulation of screws such that screw heads converge toward each other in the axial plane of the lumbar spine have?**
    a) Paired screws in 30 degree convergence decrease pullout strength compared to parallel screws.
    b) Paired screws in 30 degree convergence increase pullout strength compared to parallel screws.
    c) Screw convergence has no effect on pullout strength
    d) Paired screws in 30 degree convergence decrease pullout strength compared to parallel screws but increase rates of boney fusion
    e) Paired screws in 30 degree convergence decrease pullout strength compared to parallel screws but improve immediate post-operative pain scores

Response (B) Paired screws at 30 degree convergence increased pullout strength by 28.6% over parallel screws in the lumbar spine [9].

64. **The dorsal and ventral heights of a given vertebral body vary most significantly at which of the following spinal levels?**

a) C6
b) T2
c) T12
d) T6
e) L5

Response (E) The dorsal and ventral vertebral heights vary most significantly from one another at the lower lumbar levels, specifically at L4 and L5.

65. **Which of the following is true for screw failure in healthy vs osteoporotic bone?**
    a) There is no appreciable difference in rates of screw failure in healthy vs osteoporotic bone
    b) Screw failure is more often due to screw migration than screw bending in healthy bone
    c) Screw failure is more often due to screw bending than screw migration in osteoporotic bone
    d) Screw failure is more often due to screw bending than screw migration in healthy bone
    e) Screws are not susceptible to failure by bending or migration in healthy bone

Response (D) Screw failure more often due to screw bending in healthy bone, but more often due to screw migration in osteoporotic bone [10].

66. **Increased insertional torque is most closely correlated with which of the following?**
    a) Increased bone mineral density
    b) Bone tapping
    c) Speed of screw insertion
    d) Patient positioning
    e) Decreased bone mineral density

Response (A) Increased insertional torque has been found to correlate with increased bone mineral density [11].

67. **The angular moment of force required to advance a screw into bone is referred to as which of the following?**
    a) Insertional vice
    b) Insertional torque
    c) Grip strength
    d) Arm of resistance
    e) Tactile feedback

Response (B) The insertional torque of the screw is primarily generated by the shearing force and friction in the bone–screw interface. It can be defined as an angular moment of the force required to advance a screw into bone [11].

68. **Which of the following is true regarding prelordosed rods vs intraoperarively bent rods?**
    a) Pre-lordosed rods have a lower fatigue strength than rods bent intra-operatively with a French rod bender
    b) Pre-lordosed rods have a higher fatigue strength than rods bent intra-operatively with a French rod bender
    c) Pre-lordosed rods have the same fatigue strength as rods bent intra-operatively with a French rod bender
    d) Pre-lordosed rods have the lower fatigue strength as rods bent intra-operatively with pliers
    e) Pre-lordosed rods have a higher fatigue strength than unbent straight rods

Response (B) Pre-lordosed rods have a higher fatigue strength than rods bent intra-operatively due to the stress relieving effect achieved during the annealing process. Maximum fatigue strength with lordosed rods can be achieved using pre-lordosed rods.

69. **Which of the following materials is most notch sensitive?**
    a) Titanium
    b) cobalt-chromium
    c) stainless steel
    d) Titanium-alloy
    e) No difference between metals.

Response (A) Pure titanium is most notch sensitive. Therefore, a reduction in fatigue strength due to rod bending is expected.

70. **Which of the following refers to the extent to which sensitivity of a material to fracture is increased by cracks or scratches?**
    a) Splitting sensitivity
    b) Ductility
    c) Rigidity
    d) Coarseness
    e) Notching sensitivity

Response (E) Notching sensitivity refers to the extent to which sensitivity of a material to fracture is increased by cracks or scratches.

71. **Pelvic incidence is equal to which of the following?**
    a) Sacral slope + pelvic tilt
    b) Sacral slope − pelvic tilt
    c) (Sacral slope + pelvic tilt)/2
    d) 2*(sacral slope + pelvic tilt)
    e) 2(pelvic tilt) − sacral slope

Response (A) Pelvic incidence is a constant and specific parameter equal to sacral slope + pelvic tilt.

72. **Spondyloptosis is equivalent to which Myerding classification grade of spondylolisthesis?**
    a) 1
    b) 2
    c) 3
    d) 4
    e) 5

Response (E) Spondyloptosis is a grade 5 spondylolisthesis in concordance with the Myerding grading system, wherein grades are broken down into quartiles with total translation of one vertebral body over another or greater than 100% spondylolisthesis equivalent to a grade 5 spondylolisthesis.

73. **What effect does tapping osteoporotic bone have on screw pullout strength?**
    a) Increased pullout strength by reducing volume of bone left over for screw placement
    b) Decreases pullout strength and reduces volume of left over bone for screw placement
    c) Increased pullout strength by aerating bone prior to screw placement
    d) No effect on pullout strength
    e) Increases pullout strength by increasing the internal shear area of the threads

Response (B) Removal of bone by tapping enlarges the screw hole volume and thereby decreases the shear area of bone captured between screw threads [12].

74. **What effect does PMMA cement augmentation have on pullout strength in the spinal fixation of the osteoporotic patient?**
    a) Increases pullout strength
    b) Decreases pullout strength and reduces volume of left over bone for screw placement
    c) Decreases pullout strength by aerating bone prior to screw placement
    d) No effect on pullout strength
    e) Decreases pullout strength by increasing the internal shear area of the threads

Response (A) PMMA cement augmentation can significantly increase screw pullout strength in the spinal fixation of the osteoporotic patient.

75. **Which of the following terms refers to the ability of a material to be plastically deformed without fracture?**
    a) Cross reactivity
    b) Ductility
    c) Stiffness
    d) Rigidity
    e) Neutrality

Response (B) Ductility refers to the ability of a material to be plastically deformed without fracture.

76. **Which of the following characterizes a material that displays elastic behavior right up to failure and displays no plastic behavior?**
    a) Brittle
    b) Ductile
    c) Malleable
    d) Serpentine
    e) Neutral

Response (A) A brittle material displays elastic behavior right up to the point of failure. Unlike a ductile material, a brittle material display no elastic behavior. When subjected to stress, a brittle material fractures with little elastic deformation and no plastic deformation.

77. **Which of the following terms describes the failure of a material with repetitive loading at stress levels below the ultimate tensile strength?**
    a) Fatigue failure
    b) Ultimate failure
    c) Interval collapse
    d) Delayed decay
    e) Temporal decline

Response (A) Fatigue failure describes the failure of a material with repetitive loading at stress levels below the ultimate tensile strength.

78. **Which of the following describes a scenario wherein spinal implants protect the spine from the transfer of normal stresses of weight bearing?**
    a) Stress integration
    b) Stress shielding
    c) Snaking
    d) Annealing
    e) Toggling

Response (B) Stress Shielding refers to the situation wherein spinal implants protect the spine from the transfer of normal stresses of weight bearing. This can lead to stress reduction osteoporosis [2].

79. **Which of the following refers to the constant morphological parameter for an individual describing the relation between the sacral endplate and femoral heads?**
    a) Pelvic tilt
    b) Pelvic incidence
    c) Sacral slope
    d) Lumbar lordosis
    e) Plumb line

Response (B) Pelvic incidence is a fixed pelvic parameter defined as the angle between a line orthogonal to the superior S1 endplate and a line from the center of the S1 endplate through the center of the femoral head.

80. **Which law states that the stress is proportional to the strain produced?**
    a) Doyle's Law
    b) Bernulli's Law
    c) Hooke's Law
    d) Wolff's Law
    e) Dalton's theorem

Response (C) Hooke's Law states that the stress is proportional to the strain produced.

81. **Pelvic Tilt is equal to which of the following?**
    a) Pelvic incidence – sacral slope
    b) Pelvic Incidence + sacral slope
    c) (Pelvic Incidence + sacral slope)/2
    d) 2*(Pelvic Incidence + sacral slope)
    e) 2(sacral slope) – Pelvic Incidence

Response (A) Pelvic tilt is equal to Pelvic Incidence – sacral slope.

82. **Musculoskeletal cells respond differently to loading and oxygen levels. Which of the following is true regarding this relationship?**
    a) Chondrocytes are most activated by low-loads and low oxygen environments.
    b) Osteoblasts are most stimulated to form bone under low loads in low oxygen environments
    c) Osteoblasts are stimulated to form bone under high loads in high oxygen environments
    d) Osteoclasts are stimulated to reabsorb bone under high loads
    e) Osteoblasts are stimulated to reabsorb bone under high loads in high oxygen environments

Response (C) Chrondrocytes are stimulated to produce collagen by high loads in low oxygen environments. Osteoblasts are stimulated to form bone under high loads in high oxygen environments. Osteoclasts are stimulated to reabsorb bone under low loads.

83. **Bone is anisotropic. Which of the following correctly identifies the relative strength of bone in resisting loading from different directions?**
    a) Bone is strongest in resisting compression and weakest in resisting shear.
    b) Bone is strongest in resisting shear and weakest in resisting compression.
    c) Bone is strongest in resisting tension and weakest in resisting compression.
    d) Bone is strongest in resisting shear and weakest in resisting tension.
    e) Bone exhibits equal strength in resisting compression, shear, and tension.

Response (A) Bone's elastic modulus depends on the direction of loading. It is weakest in resisting shear, then tension, then compression.

84. **Which law states that an object replies to the summation of forces applied to it?**
    a) Newton's First Law
    b) Newton's Second Law

c) Newton's Third Law
d) Newton's Fifth Law
e) Newton's Sixth Law

Response (C) Newton's Second Law states that an object responds to the summation of forces applied to it [2].

85. **A 42 year old woman undergoes upright lumbar spine XRays which demonstrate a 60% anterolisthesis of her L5 vertebral body over her S1 vertebral body? According to the Meyerding classification, what grade is this spondylolisthesis?**
    a) 1
    b) 2
    c) 3
    d) 4
    e) 5

Response (C) An anterolisthesis of greater than 50% but less than 75% qualifies as a grade 3 sponylolisthesis by the Meyerding classification.

86. **Which of the following terms describes the weakened portion of a structure resulting from the focal application of a stress that results in distortion?**
    a) Fatigue point
    b) Motion segment
    c) Stress Riser
    d) Boundary zone
    e) Runt center

Response (C) A stress riser describes the weakened portion of a structure resulting from the focal application of a stress that results in distortion.

87. **The distance that a screw advances axially in one turn is referred to as which of the following?**
    a) Lead
    b) Rotational advancement
    c) Drive increment
    d) Drive interval
    e) Spin distance

Response (A) The distance that a screw advances axially in one turn is referred to as the lead.

88. **The difference between the inner (minor) and outer (major) diameter of the screw is a reflection of which of following?**
    a) Thread depth
    b) Thread pitch
    c) Shaft length
    d) Neck length
    e) Screw head diameter

Response (A) The difference between the inner (minor) and outer (major) diameter of the screw is a reflection of thread depth.

89. **If you push on the top center of a tin can, it indents. If you push with the same force of the superior edge of the tin can, it maintains its shape. This is an example of which effect?**
    a) Outsider effect
    b) Cylindrical coat effect
    c) Boundary effect
    d) Mantle effect
    e) Core effect

Response (C) The boundary effect refers to the enhanced buttressing of an axial load provided by the edge of a materially heterogenous object. It applies to placing interbody grafts. It is preferable to place the graft such that they are not exerting maximal force into the superior and inferior centers of the vertebral bodies but toward the perimeter of the superior and inferior vertebral bodies.

90. **Stress is equal to which of the following?**
    a) Bending moment/torque
    b) Torque/bending moment
    c) Load/torque
    d) Bending moment/strength
    e) Strength/bending moment

Response (D) Stress is equal to bending moment over strength. Strength is proportional to the third power of the inner diameter of a screw.

91. **Which of the following is correct regarding the relationship between pelvic incidence and lumbar lordosis?**
    a) Those individuals with a low pelvic incidence require less lumbar lordosis to have a balanced spinal alignment.
    b) Those individuals with a low pelvic incidence require more lumbar lordosis to have a balanced spinal alignment

c) Pelvic incidence is in no way related to lumbar lordosis
d) Those individuals with a high level of lumber lordosis and a high level of pelvic tilt will have a low pelvic incidence
e) Individuals can adjust their pelvic incidence through various postures to compensate for a high level of lumbar lordosis

Response (A) Those individuals with a low pelvic incidence require less lumbar lordosis to have a balanced spinal alignment. For those individuals with a large pelvic incidence, more lumbar lordosis is required to have a balanced spinal alignment. Pelvic incidence is a fixed parameter that cannot be altered by posture. Pelvic incidence reflects the angle between a line drawn orthogonal to the S1 superior endplate and a line drawn from the middle of the S1 superior endplate through the center of the femoral head.

92. **Full length upright X-rays are obtained on two identical twins. The pelvic incidence for twin A is calculated and determined to be 2 × that of twin B? Which of the following is true?**
   a) The lumbosacral shear stress is higher for twin B than twin A
   b) Twin B would be expected to have a higher risk of progression of lumbosacral spondylolisthesis
   c) The lumbosacral shear stress is higher for twin A than twin B
   d) The lumbosacral shear stress would be equal for the two twins
   e) Twin B would require a higher degree of lumbar lordosis to maintain sagittal balance

Response (C) The lumbosacral shear stress is higher for twin A than twin B given the higher degree of lumbar lordosis and higher sacral slope associated with a higher pelvic incidence. Given the higher shear stress experienced at the lumbosacral region, individuals with a higher pelvic incidence are at higher risk for progression of a lumbosacral spondylolisthesis.

93. **How is depth of screw penetration for pedicle screws related to pullout strength?**
   a) There is no correlation between depth of screw penetration and pullout strength
   b) 80% depth of vertebral body screw penetration is associated with increased pullout strength compared to 50% depth of vertebral body penetration
   c) Pedicle screw length is inversely proportional to pullout strength
   d) Pedicle screws which do not traverse the vertebral body have greater pullout strength than those that do
   e) Depth of penetration only impacts pullout strength for unilateral pedicle screws

Response (B) Increased depth of screw penetration into the vertebral body is associated with increased pullout strength. 80% depth of vertebral body penetration was found to increase pullout strength by a factor of about 1 third compared to 50% depth of vertebral body penetration [13].

94. **Which of the following is true regarding pedicle screws versus rib-pedicle screws placed in the thoracic spine?**
   a) For a fixed diameter screw, screws placed completely in the pedicle have a lower pullout strength than a rib-pedicle screw at the same level
   b) For a fixed diameter screw, screws placed completely in the pedicle have a higher pullout strength than a rib-pedicle screw at the same level
   c) For a fixed diameter screw, screws placed completely in the pedicle have the same pullout strength as a rib-pedicle screw at the same level
   d) Thoracic rib-pedicle screw pullout strength is inversely related to screw outer diameter
   e) Thoracic rib-pedicle screws with a 2 mm diameter will exhibit a greater pullout strength than a thoracic pedicle screw maintained completely in the pedicle with a 3 mm diameter

Response (B) For a fixed diameter screw, screws placed completely in the pedicle have a higher pullout strength than a rib-pedicle screw at the same level. Rib-pedicle screws have about 70% of the pullout strength compared to a screw of the same size maintained completely within the pedicle. However, rib-pedicle screws allow for use of a larger diameter screws in the thoracic spine, where the pedicles are often very narrow.

95. **For short segment pedicle instrumentation in the osteoporotic patient, which of the following correctly describes the effect of placing supplemental offset hooks?**
   a) Increases construct stiffness and decreases screw bending moments
   b) Decreases construct stiffness and increases screw bending moments

c) Has no effect on construct stiffness
d) Decreases construct stiffness but decreases screw bending moments
e) Increases construct stiffness and increases screw bending moments

Response (A) For short segment pedicle instrumentation in the osteoporotic patient, placing supplemental offset hooks increases construct stiffness, absorbs some of the construct strain, and decreases screw bending moments [14, 15].

96. **Which of the following is true regarding tapping of pedicle screws?**
    a) Insertional torque and pullout strength are lower for screws placed without first tapping
    b) Tapping the full length of the screw is associated with a lower pullout strength than tapping 1 mm less than the screw length
    c) Tapping 1 mm shy of screw length is associated with lower pullout strength than tapping to 0.5 mm shy of screw length
    d) Screw tapping does not effect pullout strength or insertional torque
    e) Screw tapping negatively effects insertional torque but not pullout strength

Response (B) Tapping the full length of the screw is associated with a lower pullout strength than tapping 1 mm less than the screw length. Tapping prior to screw placement, especially in osteoporotic bone, is associated with a decreased pullout strength [16].

97. **Placement of a crosslink in a short segment pedicle fixation construct provides what advantage?**
    a) Increases torsional stiffness
    b) Decreases torsional stiffness
    c) Provides additional protection against rod notching
    d) May induce rod notching
    e) Provides a site for dural adherence to prevent CSF leaking

Response (A) Placement of a crosslink in a short segment pedicle fixation construct increases torsional stiffness by an estimated 44% [17].

98. **Which of the following correctly describes the trend in thoracic pedicle width from cranial to caudal?**
    a) Middle thoracic level pedicles are wider than lower thoracic or upper thoracic pedicles
    b) Lower thoracic level pedicles are narrower than lower thoracic or upper thoracic pedicles
    c) Middle thoracic level pedicles are narrower than lower thoracic or upper thoracic pedicles
    d) Upper thoracic level pedicles are narrower than lower middle or lower thoracic pedicles
    e) Thoracic pedicles are approximately equal in width from T1 through T11

Response (C) The thoracic pedicles become progressively narrower from T1 to T6 then become progressively wider from the mid to lower thoracic spine such that the mid thoracic pedicles are typically the narrowest [18].

99. **When attempting to salvage and replace a pedicle screw in osteoporotic bone, which option most significantly increases insertional torque?**
    a) Increases the length of the replacement screw
    b) Decreasing the length of the replacement screw
    c) Increasing the diameter of the replacement screw
    d) Decreasing the diameter of the replacement screw
    e) Placing shims in the osteoporotic bone

Response (C) Increasing the diameter of the replacement screw most significantly increases the insertional torque, which is not significantly affected by placing shims and is minimally effected by placing a longer screw [19].

100. **What is most common site for a pre-lordosed rod to fracture?**
    a) Pre-lordosed rods are not subject to fracturing
    b) Adjacent to the set screw
    c) Mid way along the shaft of the rod
    d) Nearest the cranial tip of the rod
    e) Nearest the caudal tip of the rod

Response (B) Pre-lordosed rods tend fracture adjacent to a set screw, whereas intra-operatively bent rods are more likely to fracture at notching sites produced by bending.

101. **Bone is anisotropic. From which direction is the vertebral body strongest in resisting loading?**
    a) Bone is strongest in resisting compression.
    b) Bone is strongest in resisting shear
    c) Bone is strongest in resisting tension
    d) Bone exhibits equal strength in resisting compression and tension.
    e) Bone exhibits equal strength in resisting compression and shear

Response (A) Bone is strongest in resisting compression as compared to tension or shear.

102. **Which of the following terms is defined as a change in length in response to a stress?**
    a) Torque
    b) Moment arm
    c) Strain
    d) Acceleration
    e) Deceleration

Response (C) Strain is defined as a change in length in response to a stress. It is the ratio of deformation to the initial length in the direction of the applied force.

103. **If a rod is bent by a force such that it changes shape and does not revert back to its initial configuration, in which portion of the stress–strain curve is it said to be?**
    a) In the pre-elastic phase
    b) Beyond the yield point but not yet to the point of failure
    c) Beyond the point of failure
    d) Beyond the point of rupture
    e) Just prior to the yield point but still in the elastic phase

Response (B) If a rod is bent by a force such that it changes shape and does not revert back to its initial configuration, it is said to have surpassed its yield point and moved beyond the elastic phase. However, it has not yet reached the point of ultimate failure or rupture, as it has not fractured.

104. **A muscular spine surgeon tightens a screw as hard as he can. He then scrubs out of the case to briefly answer a page. On re-scrubbing and returning to the case, he finds he can now tighten the screw a bit more. Which biomechanical property of viscoelastic materials is being illustrated?**
    a) Yielding
    b) Stress relaxation
    c) Toggle
    d) Torque
    e) Stretch

Response (B) The above scenario illustrates the phenomenon of stress relaxation, wherein the stress required to hold a material at constant deformation diminishes with time and is said to relax.

105. **Which term, applicable to the vertebral bodies, refers to the properties of material dependent upon direction of force applied to that material?**
    a) Isotropic
    b) Anisotropic
    c) Hypertrophic
    d) Hypotrophic
    e) Polyaxial

Response (B) Bone is anisotropic. The vertebral bodies are specifically able to sustain loads of higher magnitude from above and below than from the front, back, or sides. The vertically oriented pattern of vertebral body trabeculae reflects this.

106. **Which of the following rods will have the shortest fatigue life?**
    a) A titanium rod that has been bent multiple times intra-operatively with a French rod bender but is not attached to any horizontal connectors
    b) A titanium rod that has been bent multiple times intra-operatively with a French rod bender and is attached to multiple horizontal connectors
    c) A titanium rod that was pre-lordosed and annealed attached to multiple horizontal connectors
    d) A stainless steel rod that has been bent multiple times intra-operatively with a French rod bender but is not attached to any horizontal connectors
    e) A stainless steel rod that has been bent multiple times intra-operatively with a French rod bender and is attached to multiple horizontal connectors

Response (B) Titanium has a shorter fatigue life than steel and is more sensitive to notching from both intra-operative bending and placement of connectors. Option B above provides such a scenario where the shortest fatigue life would be expected.

107. **How is rod stiffness related to the distance between two pedicle screw points of fixation?**
    a) Rod stiffness is directly proportional to the cubed distance between two pedicle screw points of fixation
    b) Rod stiffness is proportional to the squared distance between two pedicle screw points of fixation
    c) Rod stiffness is inversely proportional to the squared distance between two pedicle screw points of fixation
    d) Rod stiffness is inversely proportional to the cubed distance between two pedicle screw points of fixation

e) Rod stiffness is inversely proportional to the distance between two pedicle screw points of fixation

Response (E) Rod stiffness is inversely proportional to the distance between two pedicle screw points of fixation.

108. **A 32 year old man involved in a motor vehicle accident sustains an L2 burst fracture with pain prohibiting ambulation. He undergoes an L1-3 posterior spinal fusion with pedicle screws placed in the right L1, L2, and L3 pedicles. The fracture morphology prohibits placing a left L2 pedicle screw. How does the stiffness of the left rod construct compare to that of the right rod construct?**
    a) Left rod construct is half as stiff
    b) Left rod construct is 1/8th as stiff
    c) Left rod construct is 1/4th as stiff
    d) Left rod construct is 1/16th as stiff
    e) Left rod construct is 2 × stiffer than the right

Response (A) In the scenario described above, the left rod construct is half as stiff, as there is two 2 × the distance between points of fixation compared to the right construct. Rod stiffness is inversely proportional to the distance between two pedicle screw points of fixation.

109. **Which of the following is true regarding the role of the pedicle and vertebral body with regard to pullout strength and resistance to cantilever bending for pedicle screws?**
    a) The pedicle provides a greater portion pullout strength and a greater degree of resistance to cantilever bending than the vertebral body
    b) The pedicle provides a greater portion of pullout strength but a lesser degree of resistance to cantilever bending than the vertebral body
    c) The pedicle provides an equal portion pullout strength to the vertebral body but a greater degree of resistance to cantilever bending than the vertebral body
    d) The pedicle provides an equal portion of pullout strength to the vertebral body but a lesser degree of resistance to cantilever bending than the vertebral body
    e) The pedicle provides a lesser portion of pullout strength to the vertebral body and a lesser degree of resistance to cantilever bending than the vertebral body

Response (A) The pedicle provides a greater portion pullout strength and a greater degree of resistance to cantilever bending than the vertebral body.

110. **Pullout strength of a screw is related to the shear strength of the bone it penetrates. Which of the following directly impacts the shear strength of bone?**
    a) Bone mineral density
    b) Blood pressure
    c) Spinal level
    d) Serum sodium
    e) Serum potassium

Response (A) The shear strength of bone is a mechanical property based on its composition. Increased bone mineral density is associated with increased shear strength and therefore increased pullout strength.

111. **Pullout strength of a pedicle screw is a product of what two components?**
    a) Area of bone encircled by threads and shear strength of bone entered
    b) Length of screw body and diameter of screw head
    c) Diameter of screw neck and screw length
    d) Diameter of Screw head and inner screw diameter
    e) Outer screw diameter and length of screw

Response (A) Pullout strength of a pedicle screw is a product of the surface area of bone encircled by threads and shear strength of bone entered. Force = shear strength × surface area.

112. **Which of the following are true of dual thread design screws?**
    a) They are designed to have a narrower pitch in pedicle bone and wider pitch in cancellous bone, decreasing insertional torque
    b) They are designed to have a narrower pitch in pedicle bone and wider pitch in cancellous bone, increasing insertional torque
    c) They are designed to have a wider pitch in pedicle bone and narrower pitch in cancellous bone, increasing pullout strength
    d) They are designed to have a wider pitch in pedicle bone and narrower pitch in cancellous bone, increasing insertional torque

e) They are designed to have a wide pitch for the proximal third of the screw shaft, a narrow pitch for the middle third of the screw shaft, and a wide pitch for the distal third of the screw shaft

Response (B) Dual thread screws are designed to have a narrower pitch in pedicle bone and wider pitch in cancellous bone, increasing insertional torque and theoretically increasing pullout strength.

113. **Which of the following is true regarding the width and depth (ventral to dorsal length) of the vertebral bodies?**
   a) Width and depth both increase cranial to caudal from cervical to thoracic to the lumbar spine
   b) Width increases cranial to caudal but vertebral body depth decreases cranial to caudal
   c) Width and depth both decrease from cranial to caudal
   d) Width decreased from the cervical to thoracic spine but increases from the thoracic to lumbar spine
   e) Width and depth increase from the cervical to thoracic spine but decrease from the thoracic to lumbar spine

Response (A) Width and depth of the vertebral bodies both increase cranial to caudal from cervical to thoracic to the lumbar spine.

114. **Which of the following spinal vertebral bodies exhibits the highest compression strength?**
   a) C3
   b) C7
   c) T6
   d) T10
   e) L4

Response (E) The lumbar vertebral bodies are the largest and exhibit the highest compression strength, with the lower lumbar levels nearing a compression strength of nearly 8000 Newtons compared to a compressive strength near 2000 Newtons in the cervical spine [5].

115. **The uncinate processes and the uncovertebral joints which they form play an important role in coupling and stabilizing which portion of the spine during axial rotation?**
   a) C3-C7
   b) T6-T12
   c) C1-2
   d) L5-S1
   e) L1-L4

Response (A) The uncinated process projects from the rostro-dorsal-lateral aspect of C3-C7. It is involved in coupling within the subaxial cervical spine and provides some stabilization during axial rotation.

116. **Which of the following correctly states the relation of the instantaneous axis of rotation (IAR) to spinal curvature?**
   a) The IAR is located more dorsally in a kyphotic segment than in a vertically straight segment
   b) The IAR is located more ventrally in a kyphotic segment than in a vertically straight segment
   c) The IAR is located more dorsally in a lordotic segment than in a vertically straight segment
   d) The IAR is not affected by sagittal spinal curvature
   e) The IAR is located more ventrally in a kyphotic segment than in a lordotic segment

Response (A) The location of the instantaneous axis of rotation (IAR) is variable. When a ventral bending moment is applied to the spine and a relative kyphosis is induced, the IAR migrates dorsally as compared to the in a vertically straight spinal segment. When a dorsal bending moment is applied to the spine and a relative lordosis is induced, the IAR migrates ventrally.

117. **Which of the following spinal levels is typically associated with the narrowest portion of the spinal canal in a healthy adult spinal column?**
   a) C1
   b) C7
   c) T10
   d) L3
   e) S1

Response (C) The spinal canal is typically narrowest in the lower thoracic spine. As such, the thoracic spine is less forgiving to compressive pathologies such as tumors invading the canal or fractures with retropulsed bone. There is less room to accommodate additional space occupying lesions.

118. **If the instantaneous axis of rotation (IAR) for a particular thoracic spinal level is located in the center of the vertebral body, which of the following spinal ligaments has the longest moment arm (L)?**
   a) The interspinous ligament
   b) The ligamentum flavum

c) Capsular ligament
d) Anterior longitudinal ligament
e) Posterior longitudinal ligament

Response (A) If the IAR is located in the center of the vertebral body, the interspinous ligament will have the longest moment arm, as the distance from the IAR to the interspinous ligament is greater than from the IAR to any other named spinal ligament. In this case, the interspinous ligament therefore has the longest lever arm.

119. **Which of the following has the highest ratio of cortical to cancellous bone?**
a) Small pedicle
b) Small vertebral body
c) Large pedicle
d) Large vertebral body
e) The ratio is the same in pedicles and a respective vertebral body for any given person

Response (A) The ratio of cortical to cancellous bone affects load bearing. It is greater in the pedicles than in the vertebral bodies, and it is greater in smaller pedicles than large pedicles. Bone density correlates with screw pullout resistance such that the pedicles provide more resistance to pullout than the vertebral bodies.

120. **How does normal, healthy cervical spine curvature aid in preventing cervical disc degeneration?**
a) Cervical spine lordosis allows for the facets to participate in load sharing, taking some pressure off the discs
b) Cervical spine lordosis relieves the facets of participation in load sharing
c) Cervical spine kyphosis allows for the facets to participate in load sharing, taking some pressure off the discs
d) Cervical spine kyphosis relieves the facets of participation in load sharing
e) Sagittal cervical spine curvature has no effect on the progression of disc degeneration

Response (A) The healthy cervical spine has some degree of lordosis. This relatively normal extension posture obligates the dorsal cervical spine facet joints to partake in compressive load sharing, thereby taking some excessive pressure off of the intervertebral discs and deceleration their degeneration relative to a kyphotic or straight cervical spine curvature.

121. **Which of the following materials has the greatest resistance to corrosion?**
a) Pure Titanium
b) Stainless steel
c) Cobalt-Chrome
d) Titanium-alloy
e) There is no difference in corrosion resistance between different metals if they are placed in the same biologic environments

Response (A) Titanium is much more resistant to corrosion than stainless steel. Cobalt chrome and Titanium alloy have intermediate resistances.

122. **Which of the following terms is used to describe the direct bonding of bone to an implant?**
a) Shot peening
b) Corrosion
c) Osteoinduction
d) Osteoconduction
e) Osteointegration

Response (E) Osteointegration refers to the direct bonding of bone to an implant. It is a property dependent upon the surface material of a given implant and therefore bears some consideration in selecting a material for spinal fixation hardware [2].

123. **Why is shot peening utilized in surface treatment of metals?**
a) To improve capacity for osseointegration
b) To enhance fatigue resistance
c) To improve osteoconduction
d) To improve osteoinduction
e) To increase insertional torque

Response (B) Shot peening is a metal surface treatment used to enhance fatigue resistance of a given metal. It has no effect on the other options listed [20].

124. **Which of the following materials has the greatest capacity for osteointegration?**
a) Cobalt-chromium
b) Stainless steel
c) Titanium
d) Titanium has an equal capacity to stainless steel
e) Each metal has approximately the same capacity for osteointegration

Response (C) Of the listed metals, titanium has the highest capacity for osteointegration, allowing for a smoother and more evenly distributed loading between implant and bone [2].

125. **The axis about which the lumbosacral region rotates in the sagittal plane is referred to as which of the following?**
   a) Pelvic tilt point
   b) Center of lordosis
   c) Lumbosacral transition focus
   d) Pelvic Incident
   e) Lumbosacral pivot point

Response (E) The axis about which the lumbosacral region rotates in the sagittal plane is referred to as the lumbosacral pivot point. It is approximately located at the dorsal annulus of the L5-S1 disc. It is significant in that it must be surpassed either ventrally or caudally by a fixation device in order to provide adequate stabilization of the spine with regards to sagittal plane rotation.

126. **Which of the following pelvic parameters is a fixed variable?**
   a) Pelvic tilt
   b) Pelvic retroversion
   c) Pelvic Incidence
   d) Neck extension
   e) Knee bending

Response (C) Of the options listed, pelvic incidence is a relatively fixed variable.

127. **Which of the following is true regarding the apex of lumbar lordosis?**
   a) The apex of lumbar lordosis is always located at L5-S1
   b) The apex of lumbar lordosis is always located at L4-L5
   c) The apex of lumbar lordosis shifts superiorly for a person with a very high pelvic incidence compared to a low pelvic incidence
   d) The apex of lumbar lordosis shifts inferiorly for a person with a very high pelvic incidence compared to a low pelvic incidence
   e) The apex of lumbar lordosis is always centered at the L3 vertebral body

Response (C) The apex of lumbar lordosis shifts superiorly for a person with a very high pelvic incidence compared to a low pelvic incidence.

128. **Which of the following zones on the physiologic range of motion stress–strain curve can be increased by stretching exercises?**
   a) Elastic zone
   b) Neutral zone
   c) Yield zone
   d) Zone of failure
   e) None of the zones on the physiologic range of motion stress–strain curve can be increased by stretching exercises

Response (B) The neutral zone is associated with substantial flexibility at low loads. It is a zone of relative non-engagement within minimal ligamentous tension. This zone can be increased to some degree by stretching exercises.

129. **A 32 year old morbidly obese male presents to clinic complaining of severe midline back pain worse with standing for prolonged periods. Why must the downward force exerted by the dorsal spinal muscles significantly surpass the downward force exerted by the weight of this patient's protuberant abdomen?**
   a) The dorsal spinal muscles are located a significantly shorter distance from the instantaneous axis of rotation of the spine than the patient's protuberant abdomen
   b) The dorsal spinal muscles are located a significantly longer distance from the instantaneous axis of rotation of the spine than the patient's protuberant abdomen
   c) The dorsal spinal muscles exert an upward dorsal force to counteract the ventral downward force imparted by the patient's protuberant abdomen
   d) The dorsal spinal muscles always exert a fixed downward force independent of the weight of the patient's protuberant abdomen
   e) The dorsal spinal muscles need not exert any greater downward force as a result of the ventral downward force of the patient's protuberant abdomen

Response (A) If the patient described is standing upright and not in motion, a dorsal downward application of force must be applied, in this case by the dorsal spinal muscles that are located a short distance from the instantaneous axis of rotation (IAR) of the spine compared to the patient's protuberant abdomen. Given that the dorsal and ventral bending moments must be equal with respect to the IAR, the dorsal spinal muscles must generate a greater downward force than the weight of the weight of the patient's abdomen because the dorsal spinal muscles have a shorter moment arm compared to the patient's abdomen. Bending moment is equal to force x distance from IAR, or force x moment arm.

130. **A 62-year-old woman undergoes a successful L1-S1 posterior fusion and decompression to address multilevel stenosis and neurogenic claudication. She returns to clinic 1 month later with worsened back pain and posture. Her X-rays below** (Fig. 11.3), **in tandem with her symptomatic presentation, are suggestive of which entity?**
    a) Proximal facet widening
    b) Thoracic bone demineralization
    c) Proximal junctional kyphosis
    d) Scheuermann's Kyphosis
    e) Rod bending

Response (A) The above clinical case illustrates the phenomenon of proximal junctional kyphosis, a common radiographic finding after a long spinal fusion. Constructs ending at spinal transition zones such as the cervicothoracic junction and thoracolumbar junction are particularly susceptible to resulting in a proximal junctional kyphosis given the increased stress experienced at the levels just superior or inferior to the fusion construct amplified by a transition in spinal alignment.

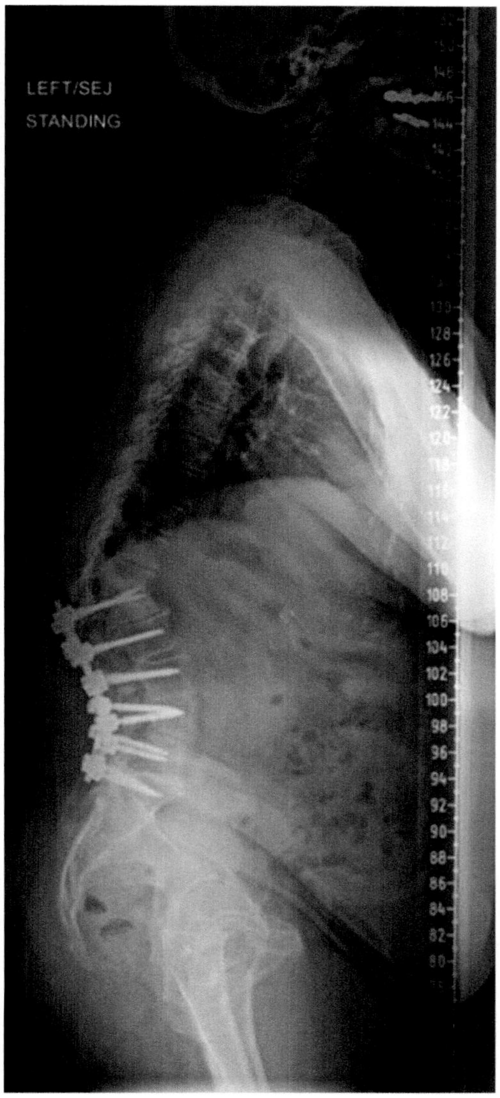

Fig. 11.3 Standing lateral scoliosis XR of patient with L1-S1 posterolateral arthrodesis

131. **Sacral Slope is equal to which of the following?**
    a) Pelvic incidence − pelvic tilt
    b) Pelvic Incidence + pelvic tilt
    c) (Pelvic Incidence + pelvic tilt)/2
    d) 2*(Pelvic Incidence + pelvic tilt)
    e) 2(pelvic tilt) − Pelvic Incidence

Response (A) Sacral slope is equal to Pelvic Incidence—pelvic tilt.

132. **The weakened portion of a rod that results from intraoperative focal bending and contouring is referred to as which of the following?**
    a) Culprit focus
    b) Stress riser
    c) Yielding zone
    d) Strain target
    e) Soft spot

Response (B) The weakened portion of a rod that results from intraoperative focal bending and contouring is referred to as a stress riser.

133. **Which of the following materials has the lowest incidence of biofilm attachment and formation?**
    a) Titanium
    b) Cobalt-Chromium
    c) Stainless steel
    d) Titanium alloy
    e) No difference

Response (A) Of the materials listed, pure titanium has been found to exhibit the lowest incidence of biofilm attachment and formation. Hence, it is the least likely of commonly employed spinal hardware fixation materials to become infected [21].

134. **A rod is bent over a fulcrum but returns to its original straight configuration immediately after the applied stress is removed. During the applied stress, the rod remained within which zone on the stress–strain curve?**
    a) Neutral zone
    b) Plastic zone
    c) Elastic zone
    d) Failure zone
    e) Yield zone

Response (C) If stresses applied to an object do not exceed the limits of the elastic zone, that object will return to its original configuration following removal of the applied stress. If the limits of the elastic zone are exceeded and the yield point is reached, the object may incur an new deformed permanent set.

135. **Flat back syndrome is most fundamentally characterized by which of the following anatomic distortions?**
    a) Loss of lumbar kyphosis
    b) Loss of thoracic lordosis
    c) Loss of cervical lordosis
    d) Loss of cervical kyphosis
    e) Loss of lumbar lordosis

Response (E) Flat back syndrome is most fundamentally characterized by loss of lumbar lordosis.

136. **The use of spinal distraction to reduce a retropulsed fragment of the vertebral body such it is no longer impinging up on the spinal canal most directly necessitates the integrity of which of the following ligaments?**
    a) Interspinous ligament
    b) Ligamentum flavum
    c) Alar ligament
    d) Posterior longitudinal ligament
    e) Capsular ligament

Response (D) Spinal distraction can be used to reduce retropulsed vertebral bone or disc fragments. This practice most directly necessitates the integrity of the posterior longitudinal ligament to be effective.

137. **The angle between a line drawn along the superior sacral endplate and the horizontal refers to which pelvic parameter?**
    a) Pelvic tilt
    b) Lumbar lordosis
    c) Pelvic Incidence
    d) Pelvic retroversion
    e) Sacral slope

Response (E) Sacral slope refers to the angle between a line drawn along the superior sacral endplate and the horizontal refers to which pelvic parameter.

138. **Which characteristic of a screw imparts the majority of screw fracture resistance?**
    a) Shaft outer diameter
    b) Shaft inner diameter
    c) Screw head diameter
    d) Screw length
    e) Screw pitch

Response (B) The screw inner diameter, or core, imparts the majority of screw fracture resistance.

139. **Which of the following correctly describes comparative ranges of motion at the L5-S1 level?**
    a) Degree of flexion–extension > degree of lateral bending > degree of axial rotation
    b) Degree of flexion–extension = degree of lateral bending = degree of axial rotation
    c) Degree of flexion–extension > degree of lateral bending = degree of axial rotation
    d) Degree of flexion–extension < degree of lateral bending < degree of axial rotation
    e) Degree of flexion–extension < degree of lateral bending = degree of axial rotation

Response (A) At the L5-S1 level, degree of flexion–extension is greater than degree of lateral bending. Degree of axial rotation is most limited at this level due to the orientation of the facets.

140. **Wobbling at an implant bone interface is referred to as which of the following?**
    a) Toggling
    b) Frosting

c) Ratcheting
d) Cylindrical vibration
e) Subluxation

Response (A) Toggling refers to the unwanted wobbling or "windshield wiping" that can take place at the implant bone interface.

141. **If an axial load is applied to a vertebral body, the forces imparted on the superior and inferior portions of the vertebral body are equal and opposite. This relationship is in compliance with what biomechanical law?**
a) Newton's first law
b) Hooke's Law
c) Newton's second law
d) Newton's third law
e) Wolff's Law

Response (C) Newton's third law states that for every action, there is an equal but opposite reaction.

142. **Contraction of the quadratus lumborum muscle primarily facilitates what motion of the spine?**
a) Extension
b) Flexion
c) Lateral bending
d) Contraction of the quadratus lumborum muscle has no effect on spinal motion
e) Equally contributes to simultaneous flexion, extension, and lateral bending

Response (C) Contraction of the quadratus lumborum muscle primarily facilitates lateral bending of the spine, as it attaches to the lateral aspect of the spine.

143. **Which of the following terms describes the gradual, continuous deformation that a viscoelastic material undergoes in response to a constant load?**
a) Sag
b) Deflation
c) Slouch
d) Creep
e) Crawling

Response (D) Creep refers to the gradual, continuous deformation that a viscoelastic material undergoes in response to a constant load.

144. **In a patient with flat back syndrome and maintained thoracic kyphosis, what compensatory measures might one be apt to take to maintain forward vision?**
a) Increased knee extension and cervical flexion
b) Increased knee flexion and increased cervical flexion
c) Increased thoracic kyphosis
d) Knee flexion and increased thoracic kyphosis
e) Knee flexion and increased cervical extension

Response (E) With the loss of lumbar lordosis characteristic of flat back syndrome, knee flexion and cervical extension are often required maintain forward vision.

145. **The increased bone density in the femoral head calcar correlates with which law?**
a) Newton's first law
b) Hooke's Law
c) Newton's second law
d) Newton's third law
e) Wolff's Law

Response (E) Wolff's law suggests axial loading alters bone integrity such that increased loading facilitates bone deposition and increased bone density. The femoral calcar, subject to high compressive loads, therefore logically exhibits increased bone density.

146. **The area under the stress–strain curve of a material is equivalent to which of the following?**
a) Strength
b) Stiffness
c) Ductility
d) Energy absorption
e) Deformation

Response (D) The area under the stress–strain curve of a material is equivalent to energy absorption. Stiffness of a material is measured as the slope of the stress–strain curve within the material's elastic zone.

147. **The use of spinal distraction to reduce displaced bone via ligamentous stretching is referred to as which of the following?**
a) Dry surgery
b) Pull Reduction

c) Tensioning
d) Ligamentotaxis
e) Ratcheting

Response (D) The use of spinal distraction to reduce displaced bone via ligamentous stretching is referred to as ligamentotaxis.

148. **Momentum is equal to which of the following?**
a) The product of mass x acceleration
b) The product of mass x velocity
c) The product of mass x distance
d) The product of velocity x distance
e) Velocity squared

Response (B) Momentum is equal to the product of mass × velocity.

149. **Which of the following refers to the process wherein hard pellets are shot against the surface of a metal, resulting in a compression deformation of the metal's surface such that and increased number of stress cycles is required to cause its failure?**
a) Bull's eyeing
b) Fire walling
c) Shot peening
d) Blow beading
e) Ripening

Response (C) Shot peening is a process wherein hard pellets are shot against the surface of a metal, resulting in a compression deformation of the metal's surface such that an increased number of loading cycles is required to cause its failure [20].

References

1. Heary RF, Parvathreddy N, Sampth S, Agarwal N. Elastic modulus in the selection of interbody implants. J Spine Surg. 2017;3(2):163–7.
2. Benzel E. Biomechanics of spine stabilization: principles and clinical practice. 2015;McGraw-Hill Medical Publishing.
3. Ishimoto T, Yamada K, Takahashi H, Takahata M, Ito M, Hanawa T, et al. Trabecular health of vertebrae based on anisotropy in trabecular architecture and collagen/apatite micro-arrangement after implantation of intervertebral fusion cages in the sheep spine. Bone. 2018;108:25–33.
4. Chen JH, Liu C, You L, et al. Boning up on Wolff's Law: Mechanical regulation of the cells that make and maintain bone. J Biomechanics. 2010;43(1):108–18.
5. White AA, Punjabi MM. Clinical Biomechanics of the Spine. 2nd edn. Philadelphia, PA:J.B. Lippincott; 1990:1–25.
6. Matsumura Y, Kasai Y, Obata H, Matsushima S, Inaba T, Uchida A. Changes in water content of intervertebral discs and paravertebral muscles before and after bed rest. J Orthop Sci. 2009;14(1):45–50.
7. Tan L, Riew K, Traynelis V. Cervical spine deformity—Part 1: biomechanics, radiographic parameters, and classification. Neurosurgery. 2017;81(2):197–203.
8. Kwok AW, Finkelstein JA, Woodside T, Hearn TC, Hu RW. Insertional torque and pull-out strengths of conical and cylindrical pedicle screws in cadaveric bone. Spine. 1996;21:2429–34.
9. Barber JW, Boden SD, Ganey T, et al. Biomechanical study of lumbar pedicle screws: does convergence affect axial pullout strength? J Spinal Disord. 1998;11(3):215–20.
10. McLain RF, McKinley T, Sarigul-Klijn N, Smith T, Yerby S. Effects of cancellous bone quality on pedicle screw loading in axial instability: a synthetic model. Spine. 1997;22(13):1454–60.
11. Okuyama K, Abe E, Suzuki T, Tamura Y, Chiba M, Sato K. Can insertional torque predict screw loosening and related failures? An in vivo study of pedicle screw fixation augmenting posterior lumbar interbody fusion. Spine (Phila Pa 1976). 2000;25(7):858–64.
12. Chapman JR, Harrington RM, Lee KM, Anderson PA, Tencer AF, Kowalski D. Factors affecting the pullout strength of cancellous bone screws. J Biomech Eng. 1996;118(3):391–8.
13. Krag MH, Beynnon BD, Pope MH, Frymoyer JW, Haugh LD, Weaver DL. An internal fixator for posterior application to short segments for the thoracic, lumbar or lumbo-sacral spine. Clin Orthop. 1986;203:75–98.
14. Chiba M, McLain RF, Yerby SA, Moseley TA, Smith TS, Benson DR. Short-segment pedicle instrumentation. Biomechanical analysis of supplemental hook fixation. Spine (Phila Pa 1976). 1996;21(3):288–94.
15. Hirano T, Hasegawa K, Takahashi HE, Uchiyama S, Hara T, Washio T, Sugiura T, Yokaichiya M, Ikeda M. Structural characteristics of the pedicle and its role in screw stability. Spine (Phila Pa 1976). 1997;22(21):2504–9
16. Kuklo TR, Lehman RA. Effect of various tapping diameters on insertion of thoracic pedicle screws: a biomechanical analysis. Spine 2003;28(18):2066–2071.
17. Dick JC, Zdeblick TA, Bartel BD, Kunz DN. Mechanical evaluation of cross-link designs in rigid pedicle screw systems1996 program committee, Spine 1997;22(4):370–375.
18. Liljenqvist UR, Halm HFH, Link TM. Pedicle screw instrumentation of the thoracic spine in idiopathic scoliosis. Spine 1997;22(19): 2239–2245.
19. Polly DW, Orchowski JR, Ellenbogen RG. Revision pedicle screws. Spine 1998;23(12):1374–1379.
20. Ashman RB. The TSRH spinal implant system. In: Ashman RB, Herring JA, Johnson CE, editors. TSRH universal spinal instrumentation. Dallas, TX: Hundley & Associates; 1993. p. 9–52.
21. Vadapalli S, Agostinho A, Harper ML, James G. Evaluation of biofilm formation on spinal fixation materials. Abstract #917. 2011 Society For Biomaterials.

Trauma of the Spine. Chronic Pain

12

Morteza Sadeh

1. **A 62-year-old male neurologic exam after an MVC demonstrates no movement in bilateral lower extremities and patchy dermatomal sensation below T10. Which one of the following best explains the class of Spinal cord injury?**

   A) ASIA B
   B) ASIA A
   C) ASIA E
   D) ASIA C

B) Refer to Fig. 12.1 for details on the ASIA scale system

2. **A patient with a cervical spinal cord injury has 2/5 strength in almost all of his BUE muscles, sensation is intact, which one of the following best describes his class of SCI?**

   A) ASIA A
   B) ASIA B
   C) ASIA C
   D) ASIA D

C) The patient has an incomplete SCI with motor function preserved below the level of injury that are less than 3/5

3. **Which one of the following is the most important structure in providing stability to craniocervical junction?**

   A) Alar ligaments
   B) Transverse ligament
   C) Tectorial membrane
   D) Apical ligament

M. Sadeh (✉)
Department of Neurosurgery, University of Illinois at Chicago, Chicago, IL, USA
e-mail: msadeh2@uic.edu

A) Alar ligaments are the most important biomechanical structures in supporting the craniocervical junction. Transverse ligament is important in maintaining C1-C2 integrity. Apical ligament is involved in integrity of craniocervical junction but are not a critical component [1].

4. **Which one of the following associated clinical information should raise suspicious in atlantoaxial dislocation?**

   a) Seizure
   b) Unequal pupils
   c) Cardiac arrest
   d) Associated head injury

c) Cardiac arrest on field is classically associated with atlantoaxial dislocations presumably due to brainstem compression [2].

5. **Neurogenic shock presents with which combination of hemodynamic changes? bradycardia and hypotension**

   a) Tachycardia only
   b) Supraventricular tachycardia and hypotension
   c) Bradycardia and hypotension
   d) Hypotension and sinus tachycardia

c) Neurogenic shock results in hypotension along with bradycardia due to disruption of sympathetic output to cardiac tissue. This is a unique and distinguishing set of findings [3].

6. **Which of the following locations has the highest possibility of creating neurogenic shock?**

   a) High lumbar
   b) Sacral
   c) High cervical
   d) High thoracic

C. Gragnaniello et al. (eds.), *MCQs in Spine Surgery*,
https://doi.org/10.1007/978-3-031-69332-8_12

A	complete: no motor or sensory function preserved in the S4–5 segments
B	incomplete: sensory but no motor function preserved below the affected level & extending through the S4–5 segments
C	incomplete: motor function preserved below the affected level, & the majority of key muscles below the affected level are < grade 3/5
D	incomplete: motor function preserved below the affected level, & the majority of key muscles below the affected level are ≥ grade 3/5
E	normal: motor & sensory function normal

Fig. 12.1 Asia classification of spinal injury

d) Classically high thoracic involvement leads to neurogenic shock due to the close association of this segment with sympathetic fibers innervating cardiac tissue [4].

7. **Which one of the following is true regarding current recommendations for use of high dose steroids in acute SCI?**

   a) Not recommended
   b) Recommended only in acute phase
   c) recommended only for complete spinal cord injuries
   d) Recommended during recovery phase

a) Current spinal cord injury guidelines recommend against (Level 1 evidence) routine use of high dose corticosteroids in acute spinal cord injury due to high incidence of complications associated with its use [5].

8. **Which one of the following SCI syndromes usually have the best prognosis?**

   a) Central cord syndrome
   b) Anterior cord syndrome
   c) Brown-Sequard syndrome
   d) Posterior cord syndrome

A) Brown-Sequard syndrome has the highest chance of significant recover, while anterior cord syndrome has the worst [6]

9. **A 28-year-old with GSW to abdomen and abdominal aortic injury had a prolonged period of hypotensive shock during efforts in repairing the vascular injury. What pattern of neurologic findings would you expect?**

   a) Weakness with intact sensation to pain
   b) Loss of proprioception only

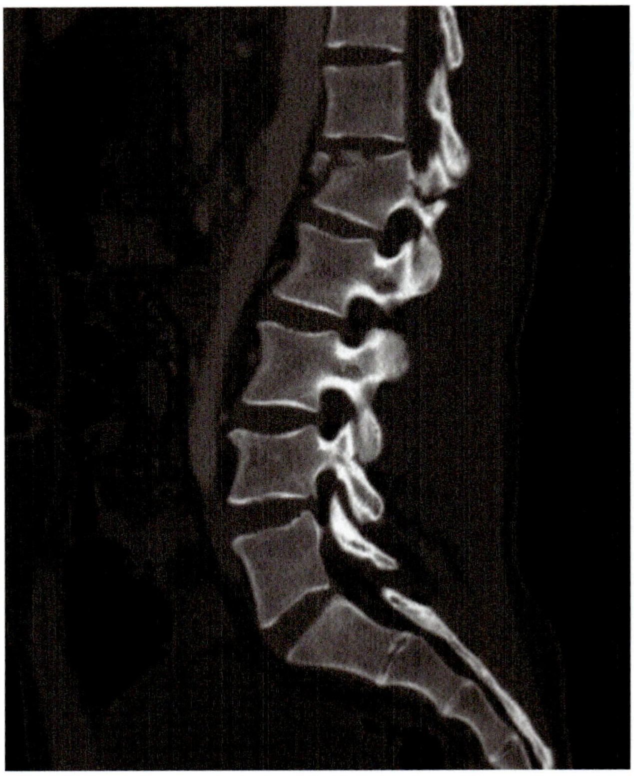

Fig. 12.2 Sagittal bone window cut of the thoracolumbar spine in patient status post MVC where she was the restrained driver

   c) Weakness with loss of proprioception
   d) Weakness with loss of sensation to pain

d) The vascular supply compromise will result in anterior cord syndrome, which results in plegia/weakness plus loss of pain and temperature sensation below the level of injury.

10. **43-year-old female presents as a code trauma after a head on collision. She was the restrained driver. She has bruises over her abdomen and severe back pain. She is neurologically intact. Her CT of the thoracic and lumbar spine are shown here (Fig. 12.2). Which one the following is the most appropriate management?**

    a) Decompression alone
    b) Bed rest and brace
    c) Decompression and fusion
    d) Percutaneous fusion

c) This is a classic Chance fracture and is unstable by definition with involvement of all three columns. Retro pulsed fragments result in neurological deficits and in order to achieve stability and decompression the management should be a combination of the two [7].

11. **Which one of the following is not a characteristic of spinal shock?**

    a) intact bulbo-cavernous reflex within the initial phase
    b) Absent bulbo-cavernous reflex within the initial phase
    c) Patchy areas of intact sensation
    d) Intact stretch reflexes

b) In the initial phase of spinal shock all reflexes including the bulbo-cavernous reflex are absent. This is a distinguishing factor in spinal shock versus complete spinal cord injury where all reflexes, but the bulbo-cavernous reflex are absent [8].

12. **A patient with suspected whiplash injury of the neck after a high speed MVA presents with neck pain, reduced ROM and point tenderness. Which one of the following whiplash associated disorder (WAD) grades best describes the injury**?

    a) 1
    b) 2b
    c) 2b
    d) 4

b. WAD grading (Fig. 12.3) is designed for classifying severity of symptoms in whiplash injuries in order to stratify for possible underlying ligamentous injury. Neck discomfort, tenderness and ROM restriction without neurological symptoms best fit WAD grade 2 [9].

13. **What are the most common levels of spine injury in pediatric population age < 9?**

    a) Occiput–C2
    b) C3-C7
    c) C5-T2
    d) T10-L2

a) Most common level of injury in pediatric patient below the age of 9 are high cervical and occipital regions [10].

14. **The following image (Fig. 12.4) shows a sagittal section of a CT of the cervical spine in an 8-year-old boy with neck pain and upper extremities numbness is shown here. What is best management of this injury?**

    a) Halo vest and repeat imaging
    b) Soft collar and repeat imaging
    c) Surgical fusion
    d) A and c

d)This is a classic illustration of Odontoid Epiphysiolysis of C2, which is a fracture through the dentocentral synchondrosis. The best initial management is a trial of halo vest

Grade	Clinical presentation
0	No complaint about the neck No physical sign(s)
I	Neck complaint of pain, stiffness or tenderness only No physical sign(s)
IIa	Neck complaint and musculoskeletal sign(s): These include point tenderness but normal cervical range of motion
IIb	Neck complaint and musculoskeletal sign(s): These include point tenderness and abnormal cervical range of motion
III	Neck complaint and neurological sign(s): These include decreased or absent deep tendon reflexes, weakness and sensory deficits
IV	Neck complaint and fracture or dislocation

Symptoms and disorders that can appear in all grades include deafness, dizziness, tinnitus, headache, memory loss, dysphagia, and temporomandibular joint pain

Fig. 12.3 Table summary of the Whiplash-associated Disorders grading and associated clinical findings

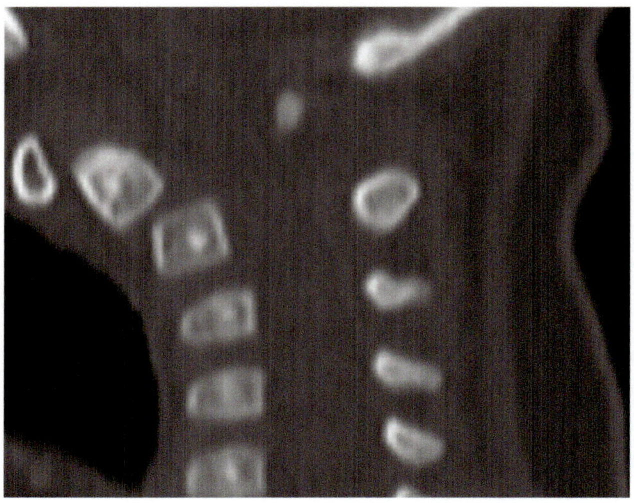

Fig. 12.4 Sagittal CT scan of the cranio-cervical junction in an 8-year-old patient presenting with neck pain and paresthesias of the upper extremities

immobilization followed by repeat imaging and fusion if instability persists [11].

15. **Which one of the following is a level ii recommendation regarding pediatric management of cervical spine injury?**

    a) Use CT for evaluation of neck pain in any trauma patient
    b) Use CT for evaluation of atlanto-axial rotatory fixation (AARF)
    c) Use CT for evaluation of suspected atlanto-occipital dislocation (AOD)
    d) Use CT in evaluation of Cervical spine injury in unconscious patients

Response b) CT utilization is recommended as a level two recommendation for evaluation of possible AARF, all other options are scenarios are level I evidence [12].

16. **Dynamic x-ray of the cervical spine in a 6-year-old boy demonstrates anterior displacement of C2 over C3 to about 2 mm. The child is neurologically intact and without neck tenderness. What is the most the best management?**

    a) No further imaging or workup needed
    b) Cervical collar and repeat X-rays in 6 weeks
    c) MRI of the cervical spine
    d) CT of cervical spine

a) This case is most likely representing a pseudo-subluxation and the conservative approach is therefore recommended.

17. **Bulbo-cavernous reflex testing the integrity of nerve roots of which of the following levels** [13]**?**

    a) S2-S4
    b) L3-S1
    c) S1-S2
    d) L4-S1

a) Bulbo-cavernous reflex represent a closed loop afferent-efferent system involving the nerve roots of S2-S4

18. **72-years-old male with PMHx of HTN, presents to the ED after a fall from bicycle at low speed while wearing a helmet. He denies LOC but endorses neck pain that started after hitting his head. His PE reveals weakness in BUE particular HG 3/5 with his lower extremities being 4+/5. He has global hyperreflexia. His MRI of cervical spine is shown here (Fig. 12.5). What is the best management?**

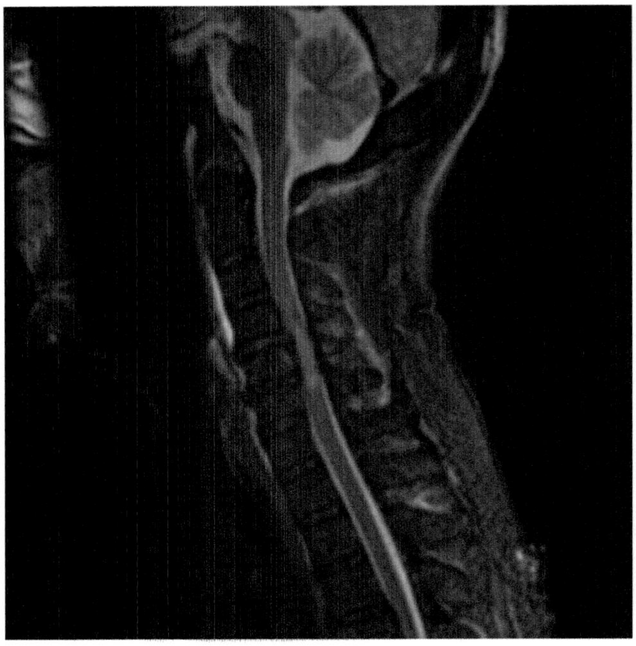

Fig. 12.5 Midsagittal T2 MRI of the cervical spine of 72 M following a fall from a bike

    a) High dose steroids and serial neuro check
    b) Cervical Collar and follow up MRI in 6 weeks
    c) High dose steroids and cervical decompression after 48 hours
    d) Surgical decompression and fusion within 24 hours

Response d) This presentation fits well with central cord syndrome and current guidelines recommend decompress and fixate within 24hrs [14].

19. **A 55-years-old male underwent surgery for ruptured AA with prolonged hypotension and surgical time. Which one of the following patterns of neurological deficit would most likely represents the sequela of abdominal aorta hypo-perfusion?**

    a) Anterior cord syndrome
    b) Posterior cord syndrome
    c) Brown-Sequard syndrome
    d) Central cord syndrome

a) In this case the blood supply to the anterior 2/3 of the cord is diminished and therefore would result in anterior cord

Fig. 12.6 Axial T2 MRI image passing through the C7-T1 disc space in patient that was stabbed at the base of his neck

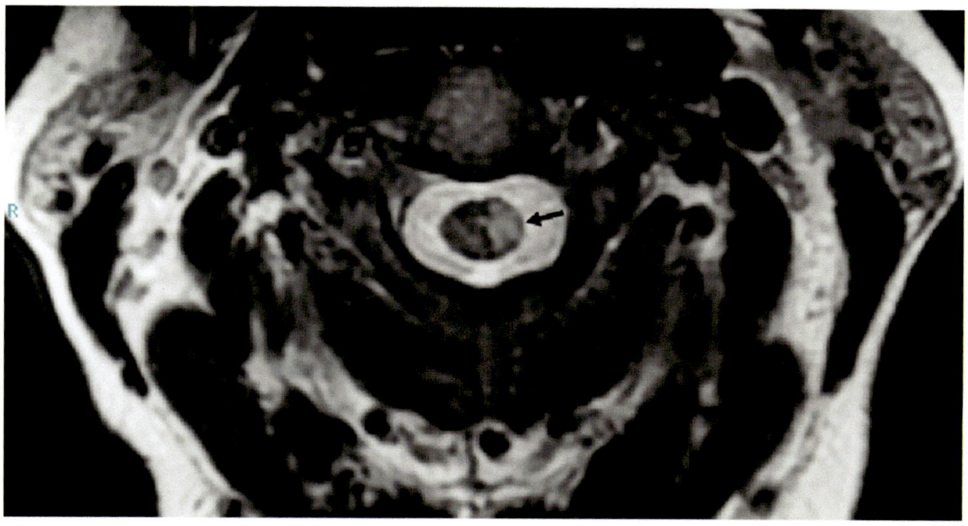

syndrome and hypo perfusion of corticospinal as well as lateral spino-thalamic tracts which leads to weakness and loss of pain and temperature sensation below the level of the ischemia.

20. **A 19-year-old is a victim of a stabbing incident at his lower neck around the level of C7-T1. His vascular injuries are minimal, and he is hemodynamically stable. His MRI of the cervical spine is shown here (Fig. 12.6). What is the overall prognosis of this injury with appropriate management?**

    a) Brown-Sequard, 90% chance of recovery
    b) Anterior syndrome, 90% chance of full recovery
    c) Anterior cord syndrome, 10% chance of full recovery
    d) Brown-Sequard syndrome, 10% chance of recovery

a) The lesion shown most likely will result in hemi cord or Brown-Sequard syndrome, which has the overall best chances of recovery compare to anterior, central and posterior cord syndromes. There is 90% chance of regaining ability to ambulate independently and anal and sphincter control [15]

21. **According to National Athletic Training Association (NATA) which one of the following is an indication for removal of the helmet after suspected spinal cord injury:**

    a) Inspect for head injuries
    b) Evaluate pupil response
    c) Secure Airway
    d) Inspect neck alignment

c) The main goal of any initial trauma survey should be prioritize based on the ABCs: Airway, Breathing and Circulation [16, 17]

22. **Which one of the following is the recommended DVT prophylaxis measures in SCI patients?**

    a) Low dose heparin
    b) Stocking Compression Device
    c) rotating beds
    d) all of the above

d) Low dose sub cutaneous heparin, SCDs and rotating beds and any combination of the three are the current recommended guidelines for prevention of deep venous thrombosis in patients with spinal cord injuries [18]

23. **A 38-years-old male who was in a high speed MVA, is transferred to the trauma bay with a GCS of 6. He is subsequently intubated and his CTH demonstrates scattered cortical SAH and a frontal contusion with no MLS or mass effect. Which one of the following imaging modalities should be considered in this patient to evaluate for cervical spine injuries?**

    a) MRI cervical spine
    b) CT cervical spine
    c) CT Myelogram
    d) Cervical X-rays

a) In comatose patients whose cervical collar cannot be cleared by Nexus criteria, and that do not have neurologic deficits that cannot be explained by other cranial abnormalities, CT of cervical spine should be obtained [19].

24. **Which one of the following is not a contraindication for halo traction fixation?**

 a) Bilateral pars fractures of C2
 b) Bilateral posterior arch fractures of C2
 c) Tear drop fracture of C6
 d) Isolated hairline fracture of C2

D) Small, linear, non-displaced fractures of cervical spine are stable enough for halo placement if indicated for other reasons [20].

25. **A 22-years-old female presents after a diving accident with blunt head trauma and extreme neck pain. She remains neurologically intact and in a cervical collar, her axial CT of the cervical spine is shown here (Fig. 12.7). What is the best management?**

 a) Occiput-C3 fusion
 b) Halo vest immobilization
 c) MRI of the cervical spine
 d) Cervical collar and repeat imaging

D) This CT demonstrates a left condylar fracture. The management in the absence of other associated fractures and stability is cervical collar and evaluation of healing with repeat imaging [21].

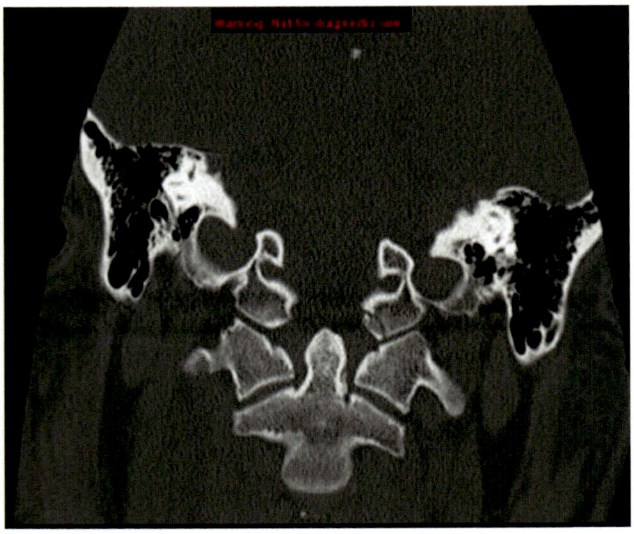

Fig. 12.7 Coronal CT scan at the level of the occipito-cervical junction in patient following blunt head trauma

26. **Which one of the following is most accurate regarding the long-term outcomes of occipital condyle fracture?**

 a) Hypoglossal palsy
 b) Incomplete cord injury
 c) Upper extremity weakness
 d) No neurological deficits

D. In long-term follow-up of multiple series of occipital condyle fractures, patients did not develop neurological deficits due to this fracture, regardless of type and mechanism [22].

27. **A 6-year-old boy presents with a fixed lateral tilt of the neck toward the left side and neck pain. His mother states that for the past 3–4 days he complained of throat pain, cough and low-grade fevers. Which one of the following is the most likely diagnosis?**

 a) Spontaneous subluxation
 b) Atlantoaxial rotatory subluxation secondary to laryngeal infection
 c) Submuscular abscess formation
 d) Traumatic subluxation

Response: b) Grisel syndrome is a very rare syndrome which is non traumatic in nature and results from rotatory subluxation of the atlantoaxial joint secondary to abscess formation due to laryngeal infection [23]

28. **Which one of the following is the most important radiographic determinant of suspicion for instability following atlantoaxial rotatory subluxation?**

 a) Posterior displacement of odontoid process (Fielding and Hawking classification)
 b) Linear fracture at base
 c) Anterior displacement
 d) Non comminuted fracture

Response: a) Posterior displacement, displacement over 3 mm and comminuted fractures are generally considered unstable [24]

29. **Following 6 weeks of Halo immobilization placed for a neck trauma resulting in atlantoaxial rotatory subluxation, the imaging of a 17-year-old male**

patient shows minimal reduction of the displacement. Which one the following is the most appropriate strategy for the treatment of the dislocation?

a) Further immobilization and repeat imaging
b) Posterior fusion only would suffice
c) Transoral release of the atlantoaxial complex followed by C1-2 fusion
d) Anterior fixation

Response C) Due to high chance of non-union based on history, age and morphology of fracture combined anterior and posterior approach is recommended.

30. **Which one of the following is the most sensitive diagnostic approach for the assessment of transverse ligament injury?**

a) Measurement of lateral mass displacement on coronal view
b) MRI GRE
c) Open mouth view of x-ray
d) Dynamic lateral x -ay

Response b) GRE images of the spine reveal small ligamentous disruptions, even those that may not lead to overt dislocations [25].

31. **A 26-year-old female is evaluated after a high speed MVA where she was a non-restrained passenger. She remains in a cervical collar, neurologically and hemodynamically stable. Her imaging is shown here (Fig. 12.8) with arrows pointing out the avulsion of bony fragments. Which one of the following is the best management in this case?**

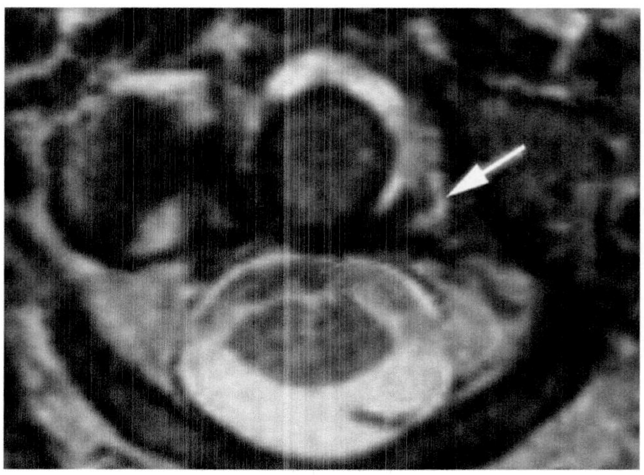

Fig. 12.8 Axial T2 MRI at the level of the tip of the dens

a) Rigid collar and repeat images
b) Anterior fixation
c) Combined anterior/posterior fixation
d) Posterior fixation

Response d) Unstable injury due to transverse ligament disruption which requires fusion with posterior approach [26]

32. **A 54-year-old male presents after a fall with severe neck pain and a guarded position. CT reveals fracture of the anterior arch of C1. Integrity of which of the following structures is the most important factor in ensuring the stability of the fracture?**

a) Alar ligaments
b) Transverse ligament
c) Tectorial membrane
d) Apical membrane

Response b) The transverse ligament is the most important biomechanical stabilizer soft tissue structure in maintaining C1-C2 stability [27]

33. **Which one of the following fractures represent the most common type of odontoid injuries:**

a) Type I
b) Type II
c) Type III
d) equal incidence

Answer: b) type II is the fracture at the base of the dens, most common and potentially unstable [28]

34. **Axial CT at the level of C2 in a 19-year-old trauma patient is demonstrated here (Fig. 12.9). Which of the following is most likely the mechanism of injury?**

a) Hyperextension and axial loading
b) Hyperflexion
c) Axial loading
d) Extension and distraction

Response a) Hangman fractures are most commonly due to hyperextension and axial loading injuries [29]

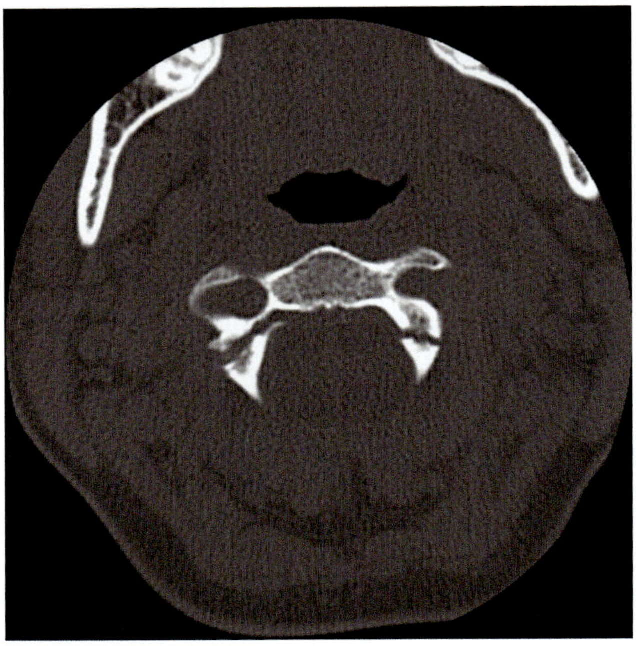

Fig. 12.9 Axial CT scan at the level of the vertebral body of C2

35. **The patient shown in the previous clinical scenario is neurologically intact and dynamic x-rays demonstrate subluxation of 2 mm of C2 over C3. Which one the following is the most appropriate management?**

    a) No rigid collar needed
    b) Surgical fixation
    c) Weight reduction and open fixation
    d) Halo immobilization and follow up

Response: d) This type of injury requires halo immobilization in the acute phase followed by imaging to assess for possible instability. Immediate surgical fixation is not required as the extent of the instability is often not clear at the time of the injury [30].

36. **Which of the following findings should raise a concern about use of traction for reduction of the fracture?**

    a) 3 mm subluxation
    b) Angulation more than 10 deg
    c) Motion of 2 mm on dynamic films
    d) Edema around ALL on cervical spine MRI films

Response: b) Angulation along with subluxation is a strong indicator that there is ligamentous disruption and reduction of fracture should be avoided [31].

37. **A 26-year-old female presents after a high-speed MVA with severe neck pain, hemodynamically stable and diffuse weakness but antigravity in BUE and BLE with intact sensation. Her CT cervical spine reveals a C2 fracture. Which of the following findings on imaging is an indication for surgical fixation rather than immobilization and follow-up?**

    a) Traumatic disc herniation
    b) Non-displaced fracture of bilateral pars
    c) Angulation of 3 degrees
    d) Subluxation of 3 mm

Response: a) Traumatic disc herniation is a strong indication for surgical decompression and immobilization since such forces have high likelihood of causing instability of spine with ligamentous damage and hence immobilization and monitoring is not appropriate [32].

38. **What surgical approach is recommended for established non-union fracture of C2 pars?**

    a) Posterior C2-C6 decompression and fusion
    b) Posterior C1-C2 Harm's fusion
    c) Posterior C1-C3 fusion via trans articular approach
    d) Anterior C2-C3 discectomy and fusion

Response: d) Anterior C2-3 discectomy and fusion is the recommended approach given the instability and lack of appropriate screw trajectory [31]

39. **Which of the following is the most common mechanism of injury in odontoid fractures, regardless of the type?**

    a) Hyperflexion
    b) Hyperextension
    c) Compression flexion
    d) Hyperextension distraction

Response: d) Hyperextension distraction is the most common mechanism of injury in odontoid fractures [33]

40. **For which one of the following patients with odontoid fracture, anterior screw fixation is recommended?**

    a) 35-year-old male with comminuted dense tip fracture

b) 61-year-old male with an isolated fracture at the base of odontoid
c) 90-year-old with metastatic disease to spine and pathological fracture of dense
d) 50-year-old with type II odontoid fracture and combined lateral mass overhang of 1 cm

Response: b) Ligamentous damage to the transverse ligament is an absolute contraindication of anterior screw fixation. Older individuals (>50) have higher risk of non-union and therefore would benefit more from surgical fixation anterior which preserves the motion at C1-2 joint [34].

41. **For which of the following combinations of presentations of a traumatic c5 injury, surgical fixation is recommended?**

a) Burst fracture with perched facet and incomplete spinal cord injury
b) Simple compression of C6 and 7 with intact neurologic status
c) Burst fracture of C4 with suspected nerve root injury
d) Lateral spondylolisthesis of C3 over C4

Response a) Subaxial cervical spine injury classification is based on morphology of injury, disco ligamentous complex injury as well as neurologic status, scores of 5 or more are generally surgical candidates for fixation [35].

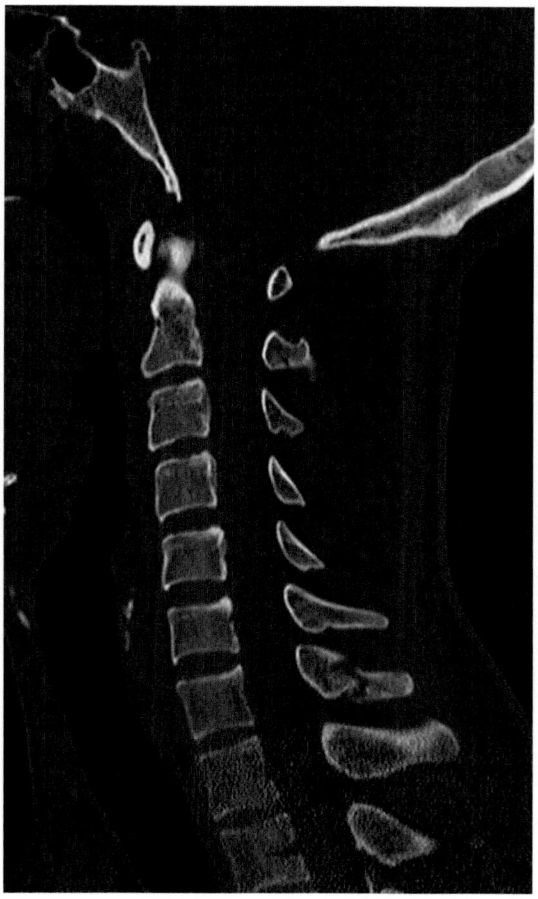

Fig. 12.10 Sagittal CT scan of the cervical spine, bone window

42. **A 38-year-old male presents after a fall from height with severe neck pain, His neurologic examination is significant for mild left triceps weakness. His MRI demonstrates a disc herniation at the level of C6-C7 with a canal diameter of 13 mm. His neutral position cervical X-ray films show a sagittal plane displacement of 4 mm. Which of the following additional findings will be an indication of an unstable cervical spine?**

a) Sagittal plane rotation of 25 deg
b) Sagittal plane displacement of 7 mm
c) Compression fracture with minimal height loss
d) Intact neurological status but with midline neck pain

Response: a) Rotations more than 20 degrees and sagittal plane displacement more than 13 mm are generally accepted radiographic signs of instability [36]

43. **A 72-year-old male presents to the ED with moderate to severe neck pain after he successfully broke his fall from a ladder by grabbing the window handrail. His trauma survey does not reveal any other injuries, his neurologic exam is normal. His CT of the cervical spine is shown here (Fig. 12.10). What is the best next step in management?**

a) Anterior fixation
b) C1-C2 fusion
c) Halo vest
d) Rigid collar

Response d) Imaging demonstrates a Type 1 odontoid fracture. Given the younger age a trial of this collar is appropriate [36]

44. What's the most likely mechanism of the cervical spine injury shown in this film here (Fig. 12.11)?

a) Hyperextension
b) Hyperflexion and axial loading
c) Hyperflexion and compression
d) Hyperextension and distraction

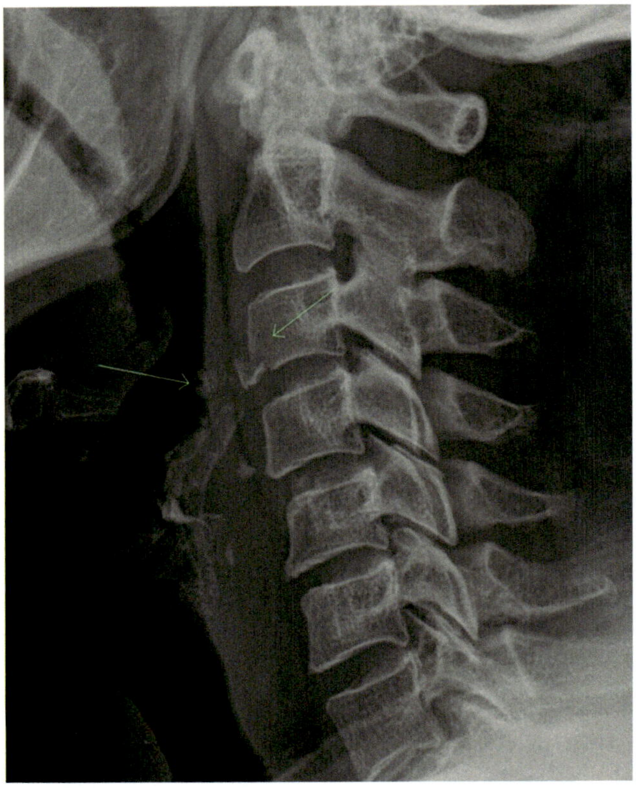

Fig. 12.11 Lateral XR of the cervical spine in patient with a fracture of C3

B. This demonstrates a classic teardrop injury fracture most common mechanism is hyperflexion and axial loading.

45. **A 49-year-old female presents after a mechanical fall from 4–5 stairs. Upon presentation she is neurologically intact but has severe neck pain and her CT of the cervical spine shows a minimally displaced anterior VB fracture. Which one of the following additional findings make this a more likely unstable fracture?**

 a) Prevertebral soft tissue swelling at the level of injury
 b) 1–2 comminuted fragments
 c) displacement of 4 mm
 d) slight angulation of posterior elements

Answer: A, Soft tissue swelling indicate a more severe injury and associated edema and neighboring elements' injury and thereby a possibly more likelihood of instability [37]

46. **A 19-year-old male presents after a pedestrian vs car accident with brief LOC. He has a distal nondisplaced femur fracture and complains of neck pain and paresthesias in BUE. His strength is normal. The CT of the cervical spine is shown here (Fig. 12.12). What is the most likely primary mechanism of injury leading to the findings here?**

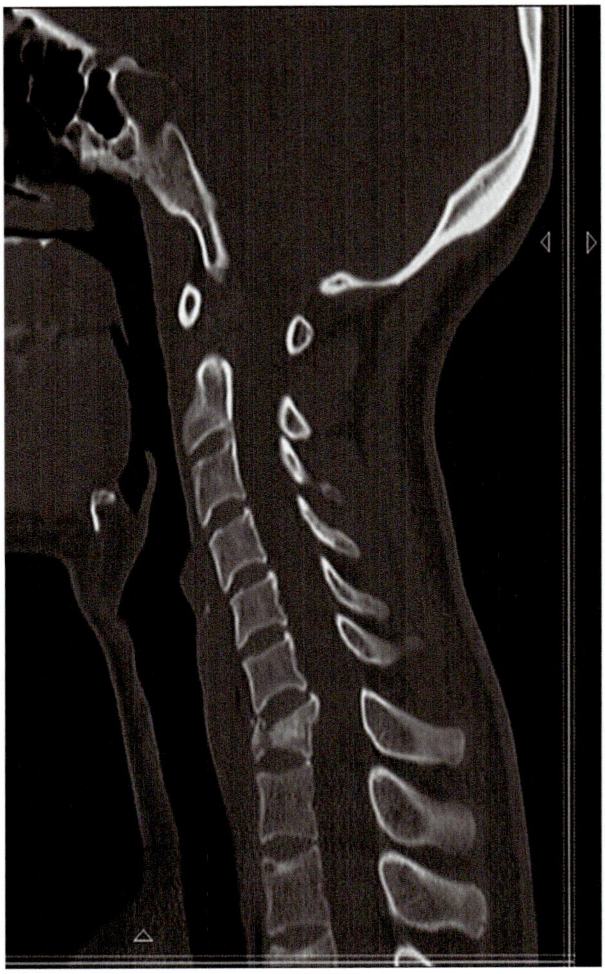

Fig. 12.12 Sagittal CT scan midline image, bone window

 a) Hyperflexion and axial loading
 b) Hyperextension and axial loading
 c) Compression
 d) Flexion and distraction

a) This demonstrates a classic teardrop injury fracture. The most common mechanism is hyperflexion and axial loading [38]

47. **A 42-year-old presents to the ED after a fall from a ladder from a height of 5 ft while at work. His trauma survey is negative for any injuries and he did not have LOC. His cervical spine x-ray films show a C6-C7 subluxation measuring 2 mm and the**

flexion–extension films do not demonstrate abnormal motion. He is currently in a cervical collar, does not have neck pain, and is neurologically intact. What is the best next step in management? a

a) No need for cervical collar immobilization
b) Posterior fusion and decompression
c) Halo immobilization and follow up
d) Rigid collar and follow up

Response a) Subluxation more than 3.5 mm and angulation more than 11 degrees are indicative of instability and the need for surgical fixation [39]

48. **A 31-year-old female presents after an accident while riding a jet ski. She had and initial LOC, her CTH demonstrates scattered traumatic SAH and her exam is consistent with ASIA A spinal cord injury at C6 level. There is a subluxation with dislocated facets at C5-C6, however no traumatic disc herniation on MRI of the cervical spine. What is the best next step in management?**

    a. Immediate surgical fixation
    b. closed reduction with traction starting with 5–10 pounds per level
    c. Halo immobilization with avoidance of weight reduction
    d. Rigid cervical collar

Response b) The initial step should be to attempt reduction with progressive weight addition starting at 10–15. If the closed reduction is unsuccessful surgical fixation should be considered [40]

49. **What is the most common neurological presentation of patients with unilateral cervical spine locked facets?**

    a. Complete spinal cord injury
    b. Brown Sequard syndrome
    c. Central cord syndrome
    d. Nerve root injury

Response d) Nerve injury due to compression at the site of jumped facets is often the most common clinical presentation

50. **What is the best surgical approach in non-reducible bilateral locked facets and traumatic disc herniation causing spinal cord compression?**

    a. Posterior decompression and fusion
    b. Anterior decompression via corpectomy and fusion
    c. Posterior decompression alone preceded by closed reduction
    d. Anterior decompression and fusion followed by posterior fusion

Response d) Given the disc herniation, anterior decompression is indicated and reduction of jumped facets via posterior approach with concomitant fusion is required for the full spectrum of decompression and reduction [41].

51. **What is the most commonly observed cervical spine deformity associated with lateral mass fractures?**

    a. Anterior subluxation of the vertebral body
    b. Angular kyphosis
    c. Rotatory subluxation
    d. Dislocated facets

Response: a) Complete Lateral mass fractures most commonly result on subluxation of the vertebral body secondary to disruption of facet stabilization elements.

52. **Which one of the following radiographic findings is associated with a high risk of non-union and non-surgical management failure in cases of lateral mass fractures?**

    a. Angulation of the vertebral body > 3 degrees
    b. > 1 cm displacement of the vertebral body or > 40% of lateral mass involvement
    c. Displacement of lateral mass > 5 mm
    d. > 50% of lateral mass involvement

Response b) Less than half of lateral mass involvement or vertebral body displacement of more than 1 cm have been shown to be associated with increased risk of non-union [42].

53. **A 52-year-old male is the victim of an MVA. His initial trauma survey is negative, and he denies**

LOC. He complains of severe mid-neck pain and tenderness and his neurologic exam is significant for left triceps weakness. His CT of the cervical spine demonstrates a comminuted lateral mass fracture of C6 with 1 cm of fracture fragment displacement with patent foramen transversarium. What is the best management in this case?

a. Posterior fusion and decompression of nerve root
b. Rigid collar and follow up
c. Halo immobilization
d. Anterior decompression and fusion

Response a) The best treatment in this clinical scenario is posterior decompression and fusion [43]

54. **Which one of the following is a generally accepted indication for acute decompression and stabilization of subaxial cervical spine injuries?**

a. Block on CT/MRI
b. bone or other fragments in the canal
c. incomplete progressive injuries
d. all of the above

Response: d) The presence of block or bony fragments on imaging as well as incomplete injuries have all been recommended for surgical decompression as soon as possible in recent spine trauma guidelines [44]

55. **Which of the following is the commonly accepted rationale for surgical stabilization of incomplete spinal cord injuries?**

a. Expediting mobilization process
b. Decrease the risk of delayed kyphotic deformities
c. prevention of neurogenic shock
d. A & B
e. all of the above

Response: d) The main indications of early surgical stabilization in patients with incomplete SCI are the ability to mobile patients with therapy without concerns for further injury to the spine or pain due to instability as well as prevention of kyphotic deformity [45].

56. **Which one of the following should be specifically ensured in a patient with suspected spinal cord injury in the acute phase prior to the decision for surgical stabilization?**

a. Rule out spinal shock
b. Rule out Distracting injuries
c. Multiple spine injuries
d. all of the above

Response: a) The presence of spinal shock can mask the extent of spinal cord injury and therefore hinders the decision making process in cases of spinal cord injury is complete, therefore careful physical examination including bulbocavernosus reflex should be performed in order to rule out spinal shock before the decision for surgical decompression and stabilization is made [46]

57. **Which one of the following scenarios is usually an indication for the anterior approach of stabilization in unstable spinal cord injuries?**

a. Bilateral non-reducible jumped facets
b. Retropulsed fracture with VB fracture
c. Displaced lateral mass fracture
d. Presence of herniated calcified disc

Response b) Retropulsed fracture is associated with a higher risk of mobilization and further compression from the posterior approach and should be avoided. Anterior decompression allows for better visualization and retrieval of accessible fragments [47]

58. **Which one of the following is not true regarding spinal cord injury without radiographic abnormality (SCIWORA)?**

a) SCIWORA is most common in the pediatric population
b) Spinal angiography or myelogram is recommended to look for other etiologies
c) MRI of the entire spine is often recommended to assess for injury at other segments
d) There is often a delay between injury event and onset of neurologic deficits

Response: B. Angiography and myelogram are not indicated for SCIWORA workup as the diagnostic yield is low [48].

59. **A 12-year-old male is being discharged after a period of observation following a dive in shallow water,**

without any identifiable injuries in trauma survey or loss of consciousness. He remained to have mild to moderate paresthesia in upper extremities, while strength and reflexes remained intact. His dynamic x-rays and CT scan are normal and his MRI of the cervical spine demonstrates a slight increase T2 signal in the cord at the C4-C5 level without ligamentous disruption or compression. Which one of the following is the best next step in management?

a) Halo vest immobilization
b) No immobilization, follow up with MRI in 6 weeks
c) Cervical collar for 12 weeks, avoid high-risk activities 6 months
d) Posterior cervical decompression and fusion

Response C) The recommended management in the absence of objective sensorimotor deficits is rigid collar immobilization and repeat MRI imaging [49]

60. **Which one of the following is not included in the middle column of denis's three-column classification?**

a) Transverse process
b) Middle vertebral column
c) Pedicle
d) Posterior longitudinal ligament

Response a) The transverse process is considered a part of the posterior column [50]

61. **A 17-year-old male presents to ED after a fall from a ladder and landing on his back. He did not lose consciousness, suffered no head injury, and his initial trauma survey was negative. His Lumbar spine x-ray reveals an isolated spinous process fracture of L1. Which of the following is most appropriate management?**

a) MRI of Lumbar spine to assess for ligamentous injury
b) Pain control and brace for comfort
c) Flexion–extension Lumbar films
d) Posterior fusion

Response: B) isolate TP fractures are considered minor injuries without underlying instability or ligamentous injury [51]

62. **In traumatic compression fractures of the thoracic and lumbar spine, which one of the following is most likely to act as a mechanical fulcrum?**

a) Anterior column
b) Middle column
c) Posterior column
d) Middle and Posterior columns

Answer: A) The fulcrum of flexion hinges on the anterior column.

63. **Which one of the following is most commonly involved in traumatic burst fractures of the thoracolumbar spine?**

A) Vertebral body
B) Superior endplate
C) Inferior endplate
D) Superior + Inferior endplates

Answer: B) The superior endplate is the most commonly involved in burst and compression fractures [52].

64. **Which one of the following major injury types of the thoracolumbar spine is most likely to present with neurologic injury associated with the fracture?**

a) Hyperextension
b) Flexion-compression
c) Flexion
d) Flexion-distraction

Answer D) Flexion-distraction injury is a result of very high forces and is almost always associated with ligamentous injury and significant compression of neural elements, which are associated with neurological deficits [53]

65. **Which of the following features will make an isolated anterior column compression fracture to be considered unstable?**

a) Neurologic deficit
b) 30–40 deg kyphosis
c) > 50% vertebral body height loss
d) All of the above

Answer: D) all of the listed choices are associated with increased likelihood of instability and thus management through fusion.

66. **What location of a middle column injury of the thoracic or lumbar spine could contribute to making it less likely to be unstable?**

    a) T1-T4
    b) T1-T8
    c) T8-T12
    d) T10-T12

Answer: b) Presence of additional stabilization via costovertebral articulation and rigid sternum immobilization leads to added stability for fractures in the thoracic region that have true articulation with the ribcage (T1-T8).

67. **What is the role of steroid administration for gunshot injuries involving the spinal cord with neurologic deficits?**

    a) high dose steroids within 24 hours
    b) high dose steroids within 48 hours
    c) no current evidence to recommend
    d) Initiate therapy if salvageable function is present

Response: c) Currently, the use of steroids for SCI due to gunshots lacks evidence to support its potential benefit and is thus not recommended [54].

68. **A 25-year-old male presets with a GSW to the low back and has no vascular injury or holo viscus. His X-ray reveals a bullet fragment at L4 level, with fracture of the superior facet and pedicle on the right side. Exam shows foot drop and loss of sensation in L4 dermatome. What is the best next step management?**

    a) Decompression and fusion
    b) Retrieval of bullet fragments only
    c) Conservative management
    d) High dose steroids

Response: a) Decompression of the nerve root followed by fusion is currently recommended as relieving the pressure effect of the bullet leads to return of function of the nerve in the acute period [54]

69. **A 49-year-old male presents with ongoing abdominal pain, nausea, and memory issues. His CBC shows microcytic anemia. He has a known history of GSW injury to the lumbar spine with pseudocyst formation and CSF leak which was repaired. What is the most appropriate management?**

    a) Retrieval of bullet fragments
    b) Lead assay
    c) MRI of brain
    d) CT myelogram

Response: b) retained bullet fragments may contain toxic lead levels which can be slowly absorbed to the systemic system and lead to classic signs of lead toxicity and neuropathy. Lead assays should be considered as the workup in this case [55].

70. **Which of the following injury characteristics is most likely to be associated with a traumatic dural tear?**

    a) Neurologic injury associated with the cervical spine
    b) Neurologic injury associated with thoracic and cervical sine
    c) Neurologic injury associated with thoracic and lumbar spine
    d) Neurologic injury associated with the lumbar spine

Response: c) Neurologic injuries which are associated with fractures and dislocations of thoracic and high lumbar regions are most commonly associated with traumatic dural tears [56]

71. **In the absence of neurologic deficits and other detected injuries, what is the best next step in management by adjacent, non-displaced and unilateral transverse process fracture of the lumbar spine?**

    a) Thoracolumbar brace and 6 weeks CT follow up
    b) Decompression and fusion
    c) No, follow up or further imaging needed
    d) Flexion extension x-rays

Response: c) In the absence of any other associated injury, isolated TP injuries of the lumbar spine do not require additional imaging, brace, or follow up [57].

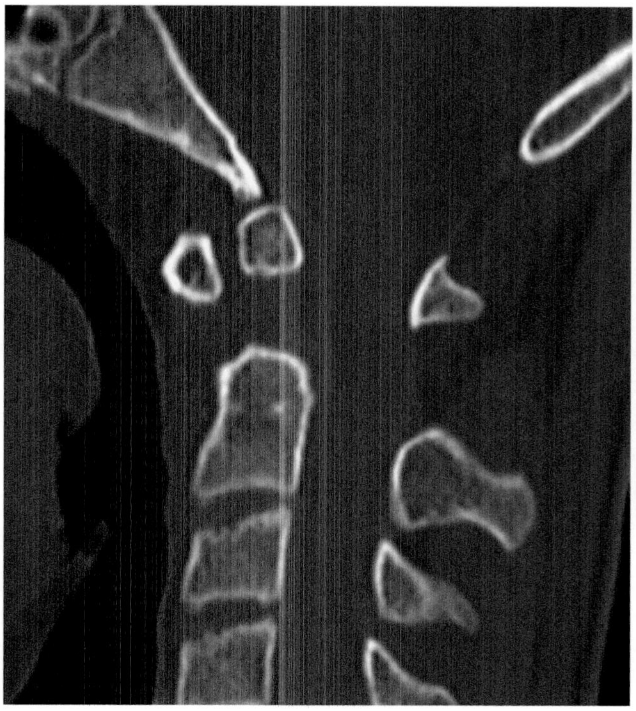

Fig. 12.13 Sagittal CT scan of the occipitocervical junction, bone window

72. **A 19-year-old boy with down syndrome presents after a fall from standing height and LOC, he is neurologically intact, and his CT cervical spine is demonstrated here (Fig. 12.13). What is the most common etiology of his pathology of the Cervical spine?**

    a) Traumatic fracture
    b) idiopathic formation
    c) Developmental
    d) Congenital benign malformation

Response: c) Os odontoideum could present secondary to trauma or congenital malformation. Most often its presence is associated with developmental malformation and progressive worsening due to accumulated trauma [58].

73. **What is the most important factor in determining the likelihood of healing of type 1 odontoid fractures?**

    a) Age
    b) Degree of displacement
    c) Angulation
    d) smoking

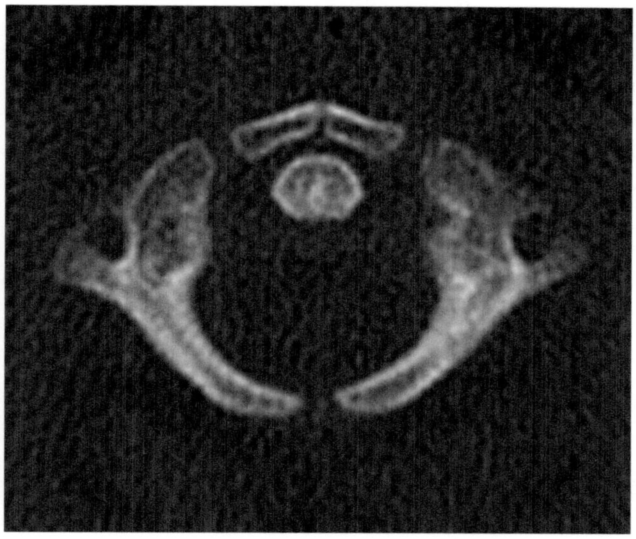

Fig. 12.14 Axial CT cut through the C1 arch and tip of the odontoid

Response: a) In type I odontoid fracture the most significant risk of non-union is age above 80 years [59]

74. **A 3-year-old girl is being evaluated after a fall from the porch of about 8 feet, she remains neurologically intact. CT head shows a nondisplaced parietal fracture, her cervical spine imaging is shown here (Fig. 12.14). What is the likely etiology of this finding?**

    a) Anterior arch fracture
    b) Rotatory subluxation
    c) Normal anatomy reflecting ossification centers
    d) Single posterior arch fracture

Response: c) This reflects normal ossification centers of C1 vertebra in the pediatric population which consists of bilateral C1 anterior arch and a single midline at the posterior arch, these are fully ossified between 4–6 years of age [60].

75. **In patients who are believed to be in spinal shock, the absence of which of the following usually confirms this state?**

    a) Babinski reflex
    b) Fasciculations
    c) Bulbocavernosus reflex
    d) clonus

Response d) Spinal shock refers to the state of absence of virtually all transmissions and reflexes of the spinal cord including the bulbocavernosus reflex. This is usually temporary and various extent of function will return. In order to distinguish spinal shock state with complete spinal cord injury, bulbocavernosus reflex should be tested, the presence of which reflects complete spinal cord injury rather than spinal shock [61].

76. **Which one of the following urodynamic issues often occurs in patients with cervical spine injuries?**

    a) Overflow incontinence
    b) Stress incontinence
    c) Sphincter incontinence
    d) Sphincter dyssynergia

Response: a) Most common abnormality affecting the urodynamics in cervical spinal cord injury is overflow incontinence resulting from abnormal transmission of signals from the cortical and pontine micturition centers in order to relax the external sphincters [62].

77. **A 40-year-old male was involved in a high-speed MVA as a restrained passenger. He has severe mid back pain, bilateral lower extremity weakness, and weak rectal tone. His CT demonstrates a comminuted fracture of the T11 VB with 70% loss of height and more than 20 deg kyphotic angulation with retropulsion of bony fragments. What is the best approach in the management of this injury?**

    a) Fusion two levels above and below the injury
    b) Fusion and decompression with transpedicular corpectomy
    c) Lateral approach decompression followed by posterior fusion
    d) Decompression via transpedicular approach without fusion

Response: b) Transpedicular approach for decompression of comminuted fractures have been shown to be safe and effective means of decompressing the spinal cord, eliminating the need for two stage surgeries and pulmonary complications of lateral approach while allowing fusion simultaneously in the same position. This is an unstable injury by TLIC score criteria and requires fusion for stabilization [63].

78. **CT of the thoracic spine in a restrained passenger of MVC reveals a T7 fracture of the VB with more than 50% loss of height, slight retropulsion of the facet, and slight kyphotic deformity. The patient remains neurologically intact but with severe mid-back pain. What is the best management?**

    a) percutaneous screws and fixation, no decompression
    b) Laminectomy and decompression
    c) Decompression and fusion
    d) TLSO brace and pain management

Response: A) In the absence of neurologic deficits and spinal cord compression, the deformity and instability caused by the traumatic injury can be fixed via percutaneous approach without the need for corpectomy and open decompression [64].

79. **A 47-year-old female presents with 8–9 months of radicular pain in L5 dermatomal pattern on her left leg. Her axial MRI at L4-L5 level is shown here (Fig. 12.15). Which one of the following is best next step in management?**

    A) Hemilaminectomy and cyst resection
    B) Transcutaneous aspiration of cyst
    C) Full laminectomy, facetectomy, and cyst resection
    D) Decompression, fusion, and cyst resection

Response: A) Treatment of choice for cyst resection is hemilaminectomy and cyst resection. Although some studies suggest that cyst resection may destabilize the facet joint and

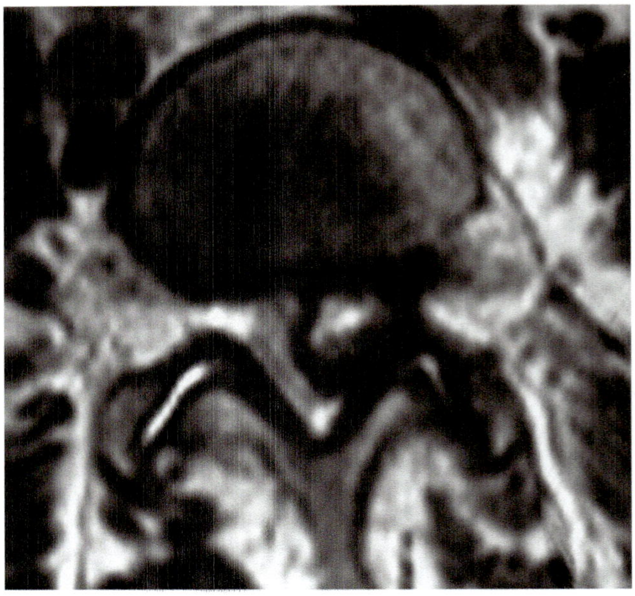

Fig. 12.15 Axial T2WI image at the level of L4-L5 disc space

necessitate a fusion later on, there is no evidence to show the benefit of up-front fusion in the absence of instability [65].

80. **A 31-year-old female has been evaluated after a MVC as a restrained passenger. She had no LOC and is neurologically intact with negative initial trauma survey. Her CTH is negative for any fractures or hematoma and her only complaint is moderate neck pain. Two hours later she develops sudden onset of left hemiparesis and facial droop. What is the best next test to identify the etiology?**

    a) MRI brain for stroke evaluation
    b) CT perfusion
    c) MRI of the cervical spine
    d) CTA of the head and neck

Response: d) Given the history and neck pain, carotid dissection and resultant right sided stroke should be suspected. STAT CTA of the head and neck should be done.

81. **A 14-year-old has been hospitalized for traumatic brain injury with DAI about a month ago after a head on collision while riding a jet ski. She remains in a cervical collar, unable to follow commands or communicate. She moves all extremities with full strength and symmetrically and does not have pathological reflexes. Her MRI demonstrates peri ligament edema without evidence of disruption or cord compression. What is the best next step in management of cervical immobilization?**

    a) MRI cervical spine with contrast
    b) CT Myelogram
    c) Maintain collar with repeat MRI cervical spine in 6 weeks
    d) Brachial plexus MRI

Response: c) Given persistent demonstration of MRI abnormalities and in the absence of reliable patient report of neck pain and assessment of injury attributable to the spine abnormality, continued brace and repeat imaging is recommended [66].

82. **A 6-year-old male is evaluated after a fall with head injury. He reports mild neck pain and remains neurologically intact. His cervical X-ray demonstrates a 2 mm subluxation of C2 on C3. What other measurement will aid in diagnosis of pseudo subluxation or true subluxation?**

    a) Displacement more than 1.5 mm
    b) Angulation of C1-C2 more than 5 degrees
    c) Spino laminar line passing beyond 3 mm
    d) Presence of pars defect of C2

Response: c) The criteria for true subluxation are the following:

- Pseudo subluxations rarely involve displacement of more than 4 mm
- The "posterior cervical line" (Swischuk's Line) connecting the spino laminar lines of C1 and C3 should normally pass within 2 mm of the spino laminar line of C2
    - o If the spino laminar line is more than 2 mm anterior to the posterior cervical line, then a true subluxation should be considered [67]

83. **Postmortem evaluation of a trauma victim with multiple severe injuries and atlanto-axial dislocation reveals disruption of the alar ligament amongst other findings. Which one of the following best summarizes the orientation and function of this structure?**

    a) Cephalad and lateral direction
    b) Laterally towards the facet joints
    c) Cephalad and lateral
    d) Lateral and inferior extension

Response: c) alar ligaments extend cephalad from the dens to the medial aspect of the occipital condyles as paired structures. They limit the axial rotation, as well as the side bending of the occipito-atlanto-axial complex [68]

84. **What radiographic parameters are useful in assessing the integrity of the occipito-axial junction?**

    a) Ratio of the distance from basion to the posterior arch and the distance from the anterior arch of C1 to the opisthion
    b) Distance between posterior dens to the arch of C1
    c) Distance between the posterior aspect of C1 arch to the anterior dens
    d) Ratio of the distance from the anterior arch of C1 to the opisthion and basion to posterior arch

Response: a) Power's ratio (BC/ OA). This is calculated as the ratio of the distance from the basion to the posterior arch of C1 to the distance from the anterior arch of C1 to the opisthion. A ratio of BC/OA greater than 1.0 indicates anterior subluxation [69].

85. **A patient is being evaluated in a trauma unit after a high speed MVA with ejection. He is in hemorrhagic shock with free fluid in the abdomen. He remains in a cervical collar. A CT of the cervical spine is performed after repair of a liver laceration and achievement of hemodynamic stability. The scan reveals fractures involving bilateral posterior arches of C1. What is the best next step in management?**

    a) C1-C2 posterior fusion
    b) MRI of the cervical spine
    c) Cervical collar and repeat imaging
    d) Clear cervical spine with negative MRI imaging

Response: C) Jefferson fractures without displacements are considered stable and do not require immediate fusion. The best management option is to maintain cervical collar for 8–10 weeks and repeat CT in order to assess for healing and possible non-union [70].

86. **What factor is the most important determinant of instability and risk of non-union in traumatic spondylolisthesis of the axis?**

    a) Displacement more than 2 cm
    b) Degree of angulation
    c) Loss of vertebral body height
    d) Bilateral fractures

Response: b) degree of angulation is the most important determinant of instability and its presence on its own is indicative of instability. Displacement more than 3 mm is another indicator but less significant than angulation [71].

87. **A 51-year-old male involved in a MVA while intoxicated is being evaluated for multiple injuries. He does not recall LOC and CTH demonstrates small scattered cortical SAH. His CT of the cervical spine shows unilateral facet dislocation at C5-C6 and a linear fracture of the lateral mass of C5. About 2 hours later while being evaluated for other injuries, he develops dysarthria, nystagmus and hoarseness of voice. What is the most likely etiology of these symptoms?**

    a) Traumatic brain injury
    b) Vertebral artery dissection
    c) Damage to the sympathetic chain ganglion in the neck
    d) Carotid artery dissection

Response: b) Fracture dislocation of the posterolateral elements of the cervical spine especially above C6 (V2 Segment of vertebral artery) are likely to cause vertebral artery dissection and possible thrombus and pseudoaneurysm formation, which consequently lead to brainstem stroke. Most likely cause of this patient's lateral medullary syndrome (aka Wallenberg syndrome) here is vertebral artery dissection and is best evaluated by CT angiogram of the head and neck [72].

88. **What is the most common mechanism leading to central cord syndrome?**

    a) Hyperflexion
    b) compression
    c) hyperextension
    d) Rotation

Response: c) Hyperextension is the most common mechanism of injury of central cord syndrome due to its potential to narrow the canal to greater extent compared to other mechanisms [73]

89. **What is the most common neurologic finding in patients with sacral fractures?**

    a) urinary incontinence
    b) Plantar flexion weakness
    c) Normal neurologic exam
    d) Areflexia

Response: c) 75% of patients with sacral fracture on trauma survey have normal motor and sensory exam [74]

90. **What percentage of sacral fractures are identified during the initial trauma survey?**

    a) 15%
    b) 50%
    c) 75%
    d) 90%

Response: b) According to a recent review of skeletal survey in trauma, almost 50% of imaging of the sacral region reveal sacral fractures [75]

91. **Which of the following structures is the key in limiting excessive lateral rotation of the sacrum?**

a) Sacro-spinous ligament
b) Sacro-iliac ligament
c) Continuation of the anterior longitudinal ligament
d) Central Sacral ligament

Response: a) The main stabilizing structure to limit rotation of the sacrum is the sacrospinous ligament [76]

92. **Which one of the following mechanisms is most likely to cause a sacral fracture?**

A) Hyperextension
B) Hyperflexion
C) Rotation
D) Flexion-distraction

Response: D) Flexion-distraction. Flexion-distraction forces are most likely to case fractures of sacral spine [77]

93. **What type of sacral injuries according to the schmidek classification have a higher incidence of pelvic perforation and cerebrospinal fluid leak?**

a) Low transverse fractures (defined as occurring at the level of S3 and below)
b) High transverse fractures (Above S3 level)
c) Vertical midline fractures below S3
d) Vertical midline fractures above S3

Response: a) Due to the position and expansion of the CSF spaces below C3, a fracture with transverse morphology has the highest likelihood of causing a CSF leak [78]

94. **What is the likelihood of coexisting pelvic fractures in presence of sacral fractures detected on the initial trauma survey?**

a) 10%
b) 50%
c) 25%
d) 90%

Response: d) Due to relatively immobile joints between pelvis and sacrum, the transmitted forces are usually linear and large enough to cause a fracture in the two structures and therefore the simultaneous fracture of pelvis and sacrum has a very high incidence of about 90% [79]

95. **Injury to which zone (according to denis classification) will most likely lead to neurologic deficit?**

a) Zone 2
b) Zone 3
c) Zone 2 + 3
d) Zone 1 + 2

Response: a) Zone 2 of the Denis classification contributes to neural elements including thecal sac and nerve roots and therefore fractures involving this zone have the highest likelihood of leading to a neurological deficit [80].

96. **Examination of which of the following muscle groups will provide the information about the integrity of neural structures in sacral fracture?**

a) Hip adduction
b) Hip flexion
c) Hip Internal and external rotation
d) Hip extension

Response c) The most selective muscle examination should focus around the internal and external rotation of the hip which are supplied by the superior gluteal nerves and obturator nerves respectively. These are selectively supplied by sacral portions of the lumbosacral plexus [81].

97. **Which one of the following non-surgical interventions have been shown to improve both pain score and functionality in patients with discogenic pain?**

A) Transcutaneous stimulation
B) Chiropractic manipulation
C) Invasive muscle stimulation
D) Intradiscal Electrothermal Therapy (IDET)

Response D) IDET has been shown to be very effective in short term treatment and management of chronic low back pain secondary to disc degeneration. There is no current published evidence in determining the efficacy of the treatments mentioned in other choices [82]

98. **What rexed lamina is the critical point of pain modulation?**

    a) Substantia gelatinosa
    b) Rexed lamina VI
    c) Anterolateral nucleus
    d) Rexed lamina IV

Response a) Substantia gelatinosa has an abundance of enkephalin, opioid and other pain related receptors and is the synaptic center of top down pain modulation in the spinal cord [83]

99. **Which one of the following has a facilitating mechanism in pain perception?**

    a) Caudal medulla
    b) Pons
    c) Rostroventral medulla
    d) Periaqueductal gray

c) Rostroventral medulla is the origin of the fibers with tonic activity to the spinal cord which facilitates the opioid activity and thereby increase the analgesic effects [84]

100. **Which one of the following neurotransmitters plays a key role in development of central sensitization?**

    a) Glutamate
    b) GABA
    c) Glycine
    d) Substance P

a) Glutamate is the major neurotransmitter involved in central process of sensitization and development of augmented response to painful stimulus [85]

101. **What is the mechanism of action of postsynaptic opioid receptors?**

    a) Increase neuronal excitability by closing potassium channels
    b) decrease neuronal excitability by opening potassium channels
    c) decrease neuronal excitability by closing sodium channels
    d) Increase neuronal excitability by opening sodium channels

b) Mechanism of action of opioid receptors is linked to action of potassium channels. Once activated opioid receptors result in conformational change and closing of potassium channels which lead to hyperpolarization and therefore decreased neuronal excitability and response to pain [86]

102. **Neurokinin internalization induced by substance p occurs in which of the following rexed lamina?**

    a) I
    b) II
    c) III
    d) IX

Rexed lamina I has the neurokinin sensitive neurons with receptors for substance P [87].

103. **What is the mechanism of action of gabapentin?**

    a) alpha-2 delta-1 calcium blocker
    b) Sodium channel blockage
    c) Potassium channel blockage
    d) GABA agonist

a) Gabapentin exerts its pain-relieving effects by blockage of Alpha-2 and Delta-1 Calcium channels [88]

104. **What is the general type of cannabinoid receptor action in the pain modulation?**

    a) G protein coupled receptors
    a) Voltage gated sodium channels
    b) Potassium channels
    c) Calcium channels

a) Cannabinoid receptors act via G protein coupled mechanism of action in control and modulation of pain perception [89]

105. **Which group of neurons are mainly involved in sensitization to pain and transition from acute to chronic?**

    a) Narrow dynamic range neurons
    b) Wide dynamic range neurons
    c) Inhibitory interneurons
    d) Unmyelinated fibers

b) A group of second-order neurons comprises wide dynamic range (WDR) neurons that synapse at lamina V. WDR neurons are usually in a dormant state until sensitization occurs [90].

106. **Which of the following are amongst the main cortical areas in receiving nociceptive signals from the spinothalamic tract?**

  a) Posterior insula
  b) Medial operculum
  c) Cingulate cortex
  d) All of the above

D: *Nociceptive cortical matrix*, consisting of posterior insula, medial parietal operculum and mid-cingulate cortex. These areas are responsible for the earliest response to a nociceptive input from spinothalamic tract.

107. **Upregulation of which of the following peripheral receptors is critical in development of chronic sensitization to pain?**

  a) TRPV1 receptor
  b) Potassium receptors
  c) Sodium channels
  d) Opioid receptors
  e) A and C

e) The most prominent change is an increase in the mRNA coding for the production of various receptors and ion channels such as Na and TRPV1 receptors. Changes in receptor kinetics lead to the hyperexcitable state of chronic pain [91].

108. **Which one of the following inflammatory mediators has been shown to have a central role in the pathophysiology of pain generation in degenerating discs?**

  A) Interleukin-1
  B) Erythrocyte sedimentation rate
  C) Tumor necrosis factor
  D) C Reactive protein

C) Tumor necrosis factor is the main component involved in degeneration of disc and is mainly involved in inflammatory/destructive process which eventually leads to pain generation [92].

109. **What is the appropriate level of SCS lead placement for treatment of mainly bilateral leg pain?**

  a) T9
  b) T11
  c) L2
  d) L3

To cover the pain in bilateral legs the optimal lead position should be at the level of T9 [93]

110. **What characteristic of pain is often a negative predictive factor in efficacy of scs treatment?**

  a) Radicular pain
  b) Focal back pain
  c) Unilateral pain
  d) Axial pain

d) axial pain often correlates negatively with the success rate of SCS treatments [94]

111. **What is the most common reported complication of halo vest fixation?**

  A) Skull penetration
  B) Pin loosening
  C) Skin infection
  D) Hematoma

B) Pin loosening is the most common reported complication involved with halo fixation procedures, with reported incidence of 36%

112. **What is the current accepted standard for radiographic instability of lumbar spine?**

  a) > 4 mm translational motion
  b) > 10 deg of angular motion
  c) A and b
  d) More than 5 deg angular motion only

c)more than 4 mm of translation or more than 10° of angular motion between adjacent endplates on lateral flexion–extension radiographs, as compared with the adjacent proximal and distal segments [95]

113. **What type of facet morphology is a potential risk factor for development of degenerative spondylolisthesis?**

  a) Closer to sagittal plane
  b) Further away from sagittal plane
  c) Rotated toward axial plane
  d) Rotated away from axial plane

a) Patients with more sagittal orientation of the lumbar facets are predisposed to an increased risk of spondylolisthesis as the degenerative process advances. Before decompressive surgery, CT scanning is helpful for assessing facet orientation and the potential risk for iatrogenic instability [96].

114. **A 70-year-old male presents with long-standing chronic back pain with radiation to hips and inguinal area, without associated numbness or weakness. Multiple conservative modalities have failed and his images including MRI lumbar spine did not show any anatomical correlate of his pain. Which one of the following should be recommended as further workup?**

    A) X-ray of the pelvis
    B) MRI of the lumbar spine with contrast
    C) Psychiatric evaluation
    D) EMG/NCS

a) Sacro-Iliac joint arthritis and instability can lead to pain distribution, mobility issues, and radicular characteristics which may mimic low back pain. In the absence of abnormalities correlating to the degree and nature of pain in this patient, it is reasonable to consider pelvic X-rays to study the SI joint [97].

115. **Which one of the following brain nuclei is an important modulator of pain via serotonergic input to afferent fibers?**

    A) Locus Coruleus
    B) Basal Nucleus of Meynert
    C) Dorsal raphae nucleus
    D) Dorsal vagal nucleus

C) The dorsal raphae nucleus is the main serotonergic nucleus of the brain with diffuse serotonergic fibers as a part of reticular fibers with strongly modulate the perception of the pain [98]

116. **Which one of the following is true regarding epidural steroid injections for treatment of low back pain?**

    a) Improvement in both pain control and function
    b) Improvement in function alone
    c) Eliminates the need for surgical intervention in majority of cases
    d) No functional benefit, no changes in need for surgery

d) Epidural steroid injections provide temporary relief of symptoms, however in the long term there is no evidence in improvement of function and eliminating need for surgical intervention [99, 100]

117. **Which one of the following may warrant MRI imaging for a patient with low back complaints?**

    a) Chronic nature of symptoms
    b) Fever and chills and recent lumbar surgery
    c) Clear radicular signs (sensory and motor)
    d) Bowel and bladder incontinence
    e) b,c and d

e) presence of red flag signs such as bowel and bladder incontinence or fever and chills with recent lumbar surgery history, or when clear dermatomal/myotomal symptoms are present necessitate investigation with urgent MRI of lumbar spine.

118. **What is a controversial, but commonly practiced indication for use of discography?**

    a) Discitis diagnosis
    b) Recurrent disc herniation evaluation
    c) Discogenic pain evaluation
    d) Treatment of degenerative disc disease

c) Discogram involves contrast injection into the disc space via Kambin triangle and evaluation of disc by CT images. It provides information about relative health the disc and improvement in patients' back pain after injection provides insights about discogenic origin of pain and aids in correct diagnosis and treatment of some challenging cases.

119. **Which one of the following electrodiagnostic parameters is often employed in aiding the diagnosis of S1 radiculopathy?**

    a) F-Wave
    b) H- Reflex
    c) Nerve Action potentials
    d) EMG

b) H-reflex represents the monosynaptic reflex from soleus muscle and its latency and amplitude is used in diagnosis of radiculopathy in S1 nerve roots [101].

120. **A 45-year-old male presents with low back pain radicular pain and claudication which have not responded to conservative management. His MRI**

reveals grade 3 spondylolisthesis with neural foramina and canal stenosis at L5-S1. Which one of the following is the best management?

a. Decompression and fusion
b. Laminectomy
c. Percutaneous fusion without decompression
d. observation with a brace and repeat imaging

A. In younger patients with symptomatic spondylolisthesis the treatment of choice is decompression and fusion to prevent the progression of symptoms and instability. Given the two issues here, the neural compression particularly at the foramina and lateral recess as well as instability with chance of progression, the effective treatment must involve both decompression and fusion [102].

121. **A 36-year-old female presents to the clinic with complaints of recurrent radicular pain on the LLE in L5 distribution along with axial pain. She had a lumbar microdiscectomy at L5-S1 level about 2 years ago with initial good response. She had tried PT and OTC pain meds without long lasting relief. Her MRI demonstrates recurrent foraminal disc herniation. What is the best current management?**

A) Redo discectomy
B) Epidural pain injections
C) Spinal cord stimulation
D) Dorsal root ganglion stimulation

a) Recurrent disc herniation has reported prevalence of 5-15% within the first 18 months and gradually declining incidence thereafter. Several factors such as minimally invasive approach, diabetes and annular prolapse type herniation.

The most definitive treatment for recurrent disc is redo surgery for resection of recurrent herniation

122. **A 59-year-old male presents with 1 year of aching pain and discomfort in the tailbone region that started after a fall on ice. His imaging has been negative for fracture or neural element compression, however the pain persists especially during episodes of prolonged sitting or standing from sitting position. Which one of the following has been shown to be very successful in management of this condition?**

A) Sacroiliac joint fusion
B) Lumbar laminectomy
C) Coccyx manipulation
D) Spinal cord stimulation

C) The diagnosis is Coccydynia which is the result of damage to the coccyx which can lead to chronic pain in this location. Therapies with focus on coccyx manipulation have proven very effective

123. **A 59-year-old female presents with complaints of low back pain and neurogenic claudication. She has been exercising to help with her low back pain and weight reduction and states that stationary biking in particular reliefs her back pain significantly. What could be a possible explanation for this?**

A) Decrease intervertebral distance in the flexed position
B) Decrease lordosis and increase the diameter of the spinal canal
C) Increase lordosis and decrease the diameter of the spinal canal
D) Increase intervertebral distance in the flexed position

B) This position decreases lordosis and increases the diameter of the spinal canal by reducing the inward buckling of the flavum and also distract the facet joints that open the neural foramina and thereby relieving the pressure of nerves and decreasing the symptoms.

124. **Which one of the following is true regarding recurrent low back pain attributable to peridural scar formation?**

A) Almost 100%
B) 10–20%
C) 40–50%
D) 60–70%

B) A large-scale review of post-operative images with and without evidence of peri-dural scar formation, and its correlation with persistent post-operative back pain revealed that only about 15% of symptoms are attributable to scar even in the presence of MRI findings of scar formation [103].

125. **What is the approximate proportion of patients with low back pain who will continue to have persistent pain despite improvements after one year follow -up after lumbar fusion?**

A) 70%
B) 30%

C) 10%
D) 50%

A) Almost 70% of patients with chronic low back who undergo lumbar fusion for low back pain will continue to have back pain , although with improved scales, at one year follow up.

References

1. Lopez AJ, Scheer JK, Leibl KE, Smith ZA, Dlouhy BJ, Dahdaleh NS. Anatomy and biomechanics of the craniovertebral junction. Neurosurgic Focus. 2015;38(4):E2.d
2. Mendenhall SK, Sivaganesan A, Mistry A, Sivasubramaniam P, McGirt MJ, Devin CJ. Traumatic atlantooccipital dislocation: comprehensive assessment of mortality, neurologic improvement, and patient-reported outcomes at a Level 1 trauma center over 15 years. Spine J. 2015;15(11):2385–95.
3. Krassioukov A, Claydon VE. The clinical problems in cardiovascular control following spinal cord injury: an overview. Prog Brain Res. 2006;152:223–9.
4. Dumont RJ, Okonkwo DO, Verma S, Hurlbert RJ, Boulos PT, Ellegala DB, Dumont AS. Acute spinal cord injury, part I: pathophysiologic mechanisms. Clin Neuropharmacol. 2001;24 (5):254–64.
5. Fehlings MG, Wilson JR, Tetreault LA, Aarabi B, Anderson P, Arnold PM, Harrop JS. A clinical practice guideline for the management of patients with acute spinal cord injury: recommendations on the use of methylprednisolone sodium succinate. Global Spine J. 2017;7(3_suppl):203S-211S
6. Roth EJ, Park T, Pang T, Yarkony GM, Lee MY. Traumatic cervical brown-sequard and brown-sequard-plus syndromes: the spectrum of presentations and outcomes. Spinal Cord. 1991;29 (9):582–9.
7. Wood KB, Li W, Lebl DS, Ploumis A. Management of thoracolumbar spine fractures. Spine J. 2014;14(1):145–64.
8. Previnaire JG. The importance of the bulbocavernosus reflex. Spinal Cord Series Cases. 2018;4(1):1–2.
9. Seferiadis A, Rosenfeld M, Gunnarsson R. A review of treatment interventions in whiplash-associated disorders. Eur Spine J. 2004;13(5):387–97.
10. Ruge JR, Sinson GP, McLone DG, Cerullo LJ. Pediatric spinal injury: the very young. J Neurosurg. 1988;68(1):25–30.
11. Blauth M, Otte D, Krettek C. Fractures of the odontoid process in small children: biomechanical analysis and report of three cases. Eur Spine J. 1996;5(1):63–70.
12. Alexiades NG, Parisi F, Anderson RC. Pediatric spine trauma: a brief review. Neurosurg. 2020;87(1):E1–9.
13. Deletis V, Vodusek DB. Intraoperative recording of the bulbocavernosus reflex. Neurosurg. 1997;40(1):88–93.
14. Fehlings MG, Tetreault LA, Wilson JR, Aarabi B, Anderson P, Arnold PM, Harrop JS. A clinical practice guideline for the management of patients with acute spinal cord injury and central cord syndrome: recommendations on the timing ($\leq$ 24 hours versus> 24 hours) of decompressive surgery. Global Spine J. 2017;7(3_suppl):195S-202S
15. Wirz M, Zörner B, Rupp R, Dietz V. Outcome after incomplete spinal cord injury: central cord versus Brown-Sequard syndrome. Spinal Cord. 2010;48(5):407–14.
16. Swartz EE, Boden BP, Courson RW, Decoster LC, Horodyski MB, Norkus SA, Waninger KN. National athletic trainers' association position statement: acute management of the cervical spine–injured athlete. J Athl Train. 2009;44 (3):306–31.
17. Segan RD, Cassidy C, Bentkowski J. A discussion of the issue of football helmet removal in suspected cervical spine injuries. J Athl Train. 1993;28(4):294.
18. Toker S, Hak DJ, Morgan SJ. Deep vein thrombosis prophylaxis in trauma patients. Thrombosis. 2011
19. Tomycz ND, Chew BG, Chang YF, Darby JM, Gunn SR, Nicholas DH, Okonkwo DO. MRI is unnecessary to clear the cervical spine in obtunded/comatose trauma patients: the four-year experience of a level I trauma center. J Trauma Acute Care Surg. 2008;64(5):1258–63.
20. Bono CM. The halo fixator. JAAOS-J Am Acad Orthopaed Surg. 2007;15(12):728–37.
21. Tuli S, Tator CH, Fehlings MG, Mackay M. Occipital condyle fractures. Neurosurg. 1997;41(2):368–77.
22. Mueller FJ, Fuechtmeier B, Kinner B, Rosskopf M, Neumann C, Nerlich M, Englert C. Occipital condyle fractures. Prospective follow-up of 31 cases within 5 years at a level 1 trauma centre. Euro Spine J: Offic Publ Euro Spine Soc Euro Spin Deform Soc Euro Sect Cervic Spine Res Soc 2012;21(2):289–94. https://doi.org/10.1007/s00586-011-1963-7
23. Nicole P, Martina C, Patrizia B, Lorenzo L. Grisel's syndrome in children: two case reports and systematic review of the literature. Case Rep Pediatr 2020;8819758(11). https://doi.org/10.1155/2020/8819758
24. Fielding JW, Hawkins RJ. Atlanto-axial rotatory fixation.(Fixed rotatory subluxation of the atlanto-axial joint). J Bone Joint Surg Am. 1997;59(1):37–44
25. Benedetti PF, Fahr LM, Kuhns LR, Hayman LA. MR imaging findings in spinal ligamentous injury. Am J Roentgenol. 2000;175(3):661–5.
26. Dickman CA, Mamourian A, Sonntag VK, Drayer BP. Magnetic resonance imaging of the transverse atlantal ligament for the evaluation of atlantoaxial instability. J Neurosurg. 1991;75 (2):221–7.
27. Lopez AJ, Scheer JK, Leibl KE, Smith ZA, Dlouhy BJ, Dahdaleh NS. Anatomy and biomechanics of the craniovertebral junction. Neurosurg Focus. 2015;38(4):E2.
28. Munera F, Rivas LA, Nunez DB Jr, Quencer RM. Imaging evaluation of adult spinal injuries: emphasis on multidetector CT in cervical spine trauma. Radiology. 2012;263(3):645–60.
29. Benzel EC, Hart BL, Ball PA, Baldwin NG, Orrison WW, Espinosa M. Fractures of the C-2 vertebral body. J Neurosurg. 1994;81(2):206–12.
30. Hadley MN, Dickman CA, Browner CM, Sonntag VK. Acute axis fractures: a review of 229 cases. J Neurosurg. 1989;71 (5):642–7.
31. Francis WR, Fielding JW, Hawkins RJ, Pepin J, Hensinger ROBERT. Traumatic spondylolisthesis of the axis. J Bone Joint Surg Br. 1981;63(3):313–8
32. Tuite GF, Papadopoulos SM, Sonntag VK. Caspar plate fixation for the treatment of complex hangman's fractures. Neurosurgery. 1992;30(5):761–4.
33. Ivancic PC. Odontoid fracture biomechanics. Spine. 2014;39(24): E1403–10.
34. Julien TD, Frankel B, Traynelis VC, Ryken TC. Evidence-based analysis of odontoid fracture management. Neurosurg Focus. 2000;8(6):1–6.
35. Patel AA, Dailey A, Brodke DS, Daubs M, Anderson PA, Hurlbert RJ, Vacccaro AR. Subaxial cervical spine trauma classification: the subaxial Injury classification system and case examples. Neurosurg Focus. 2008;25(5):E8.

36. White AA. The problem of clinical instability in the human spine: a systematic approach. part 4: The lumbar and lumbosacral spine. Clinic Biomech Spine 1990;342–61
37. Daffner RH. Imaging of vertebral trauma. Cambridge University Press; 2011.
38. Torg JS, Pavlov H, O'Neill MJ, Nichols CE III, Sennett B. The axial load teardrop fracture: a biomechanical, clinical, and roentgenographic analysis. Am J Sports Med. 1991;19(4):355–64.
39. Hutting N, Scholten-Peeters GG, Vijverman V, Keesenberg MD, Verhagen AP. Diagnostic accuracy of upper cervical spine instability tests: a systematic review. Phys Ther. 2013;93 (12):1686–95.
40. White AA, Southwick WO, Panjabi MM. Clinical instability in the lower cervical spine a review of past and current concepts. Spine. 1976;1(1):15–27.
41. Bransford RJ, Alton TB, Patel AR, Bellabarba C. Upper cervical spine trauma. JAAOS-J Am Acad Orthopaed Surg. 2014;22 (11):718–29.
42. Gleizes V, Jacquot FP, Signoret F, Féron JM. Combined injuries in the upper cervical spine: clinical and epidemiological data over a 14-year period. Eur Spine J. 2000;9(5):386–92.
43. Kotani Y, Abumi K, Ito M, Minami A. Cervical spine injuries associated with lateral mass and facet joint fractures: new classification and surgical treatment with pedicle screw fixation. Eur Spine J. 2005;14(1):69–77.
44. Walters BC, Hadley MN, Hurlbert RJ, Aarabi B, Dhall SS, Gelb DE, Theodore N. Guidelines for the management of acute cervical spine and spinal cord injuries: 2013 update. Neurosurgery 2013;60(CN_suppl_1):82–91
45. Fehlings MG, Tator CH. An evidence-based review of decompressive surgery in acute spinal cord injury: rationale, indications, and timing based on experimental and clinical studies. J Neurosurg Spine. 1999;91(1):1–11.
46. Wilson JR, Singh A, Craven C, Verrier MC, Drew B, Ahn H, Fehlings MG. Early versus late surgery for traumatic spinal cord injury: the results of a prospective Canadian cohort study. Spinal Cord. 2012;50(11):840–3.
47. Brodke DS, Anderson PA, Newell DW, Grady MS, Chapman JR. Comparison of anterior and posterior approaches in cervical spinal cord injuries. Clinical Spine Surg. 2003;16(3):229–35.
48. Rozzelle CJ, Aarabi B, Dhall SS, Gelb DE, Hurlbert RJ, Ryken TC, Hadley MN. Spinal cord injury without radiographic abnormality (SCIWORA). Neurosurgery. 2013;72(suppl_3):227–33
49. Pollack IF, Pang D, Sclabassi R. Recurrent spinal cord injury without radiographic abnormalities in children. J Neurosurg. 1988;69(2):177–82.
50. Denis F. The three-column spine and its significance in the classification of acute thoracolumbar spinal injuries. Spine. 8 (8):817–31
51. Chedid MK, Green C. A review of the management of lumbar fractures with a focus on surgical decision-making and techniques. Contemp Neurosurg. 1999;21(11):1–6.
52. Chance GQ. Note on a type of flexion fracture of the spine. Br J Radiol. 1948;21(249):452–3.
53. Hitchon PW, Torner JC, Haddad SF, Follett KA. Management options in thoracolumbar burst fractures. Surg Neurol. 1998;49 (6):619–27.
54. Waters RL, Sie IH. Spinal cord injuries from gunshot wounds to the spine. Clinic Orthopaed Relat Res® 2003;408:120–5
55. Rentfrow B, Vaidya R, Elia C, Sethi A. Lead toxicity and management of gunshot wounds in the lumbar spine. Eur Spine J. 2013;22(11):2353–7.
56. Luszczyk MJ, Blaisdell GY, Wiater BP, Bellabarba C, Chapman JR, Agel JA, Bransford RJ. Traumatic dural tears: what do we know and are they a problem? Spine J. 2014;14(1):49–56.
57. Bradley LH, Paullus WC, Howe J, Litofsky NS. Isolated transverse process fractures: spine service management not needed. J Trauma Acute Care Surg. 2008;65(4):832–6.
58. Arvin B, Fournier-Gosselin MP, Fehlings MG. Os odontoideum: etiology and surgical management. Neurosurgery. 2010;66 (suppl_3):A22–A31
59. Müller EJ, Wick M, Russe O, Muhr G. Management of odontoid fractures in the elderly. Eur Spine J. 1999;8(5):360–5.
60. Rao RD, Tang S, Lim C, Yoganandan N. Developmental morphology and ossification patterns of the C1 vertebra. JBJS. 2013;95(17): e124.
61. Hassouna M, Elmayegri N, Abdelhady M. Pathophysiology of spinal shock. In: Textbook of the neurogenic bladder. CRC Press, 2008, p. 226–40
62. Wyndaele JJ, Kovindha A, Madersbacher H, Radziszewski P, Ruffion A, Schurch B, Wein A. Neurologic urinary incontinence. Neurourol Urodynam: Offic Int Cont Soc. 2010;29(1):159–64.
63. Verlaan JJ, Diekerhof CH, Buskens E, Van der Tweel I, Verbout AJ, Dhert WJA, Oner FC. Surgical treatment of traumatic fractures of the thoracic and lumbar spine: a systematic review of the literature on techniques, complications, and outcome. Spine. 2004;29(7):803–14.
64. Palmisani M, Gasbarrini A, Brodano GB, De Iure F, Cappuccio M, Boriani L, Boriani S. Minimally invasive percutaneous fixation in the treatment of thoracic and lumbar spine fractures. Eur Spine J. 2009;18(1):71–4.
65. Epstein NE. Lumbar synovial cysts: a review of diagnosis, surgical management, and outcome assessment. Clinical Spine Surg. 2004;17(4):321–5.
66. Mark DD, Benzel EC, Hart BL. Magnetic resonance imaging evaluation of the cervical spine in the comatose or obtunded trauma patient. J Neurosurg Spine. 1999;91(1):54–9.
67. Swischuk LE. Anterior displacement of C2 in children: physiologic or pathologic? a helpful differentiating line. Radiology. 1977;122(3):759–63.
68. Torretti JA, Sengupta DK. Cervical spine trauma. Indian J Orthop. 2007;41(4):255–67. https://doi.org/10.4103/0019-5413.36985.
69. Powers B, Miller MD, Kramer RS, Martinez S, Gehweiler JA. Jr Traumatic anterior atlanto-occipital dislocation. J Neurosurg. 1979;4:12–7.
70. Levine AM, Edwards CC. Fractures of the Atlas. J Bone Joint Surg Am. 1991;73:680–91.
71. Levine AM, Edwards CC. The management of traumatic spondylolisthesis of the axis. J Bone Joint Surg Am. 1985;67:217–26.
72. Inamasu J, Guiot BH. Vertebral artery injury after blunt cervical trauma: an update. Surg Neurol. 2006;65:238–46.
73. Schneider RC, Cherry G, Pantek H. The syndrome of acute central cervical spinal cord injury, with special reference to the mechanisms involved in hyperextension injuries of the cervical spine. J Neurosurg. 1954;11:546–77.
74. Hak DJ, Baran S, Stahel P. Sacral fractures: current strategies in diagnosis and management. Orthopedics. 2009;32:752–7.
75. Denis F, Davis S, Comfort T. Sacral fractures: an important problem. Retrospective analysis of 236 cases. Clin Orthop Relat Res. 1988;227:67–81
76. Yoon W, Kim JK, Jeong YY, Seo JJ, Park JG, Kang HK. Pelvic arterial hemorrhage in patients with pelvic fractures: detection with contrast-enhanced CT. Radiographics. 2004;24(6):1591–605.

77. Oh HJ, Choi SJ, Lee KS, Choi JO. The effect of flexion-distraction technique and drop technique on pain and sacral angle of patients with lumbar spine herniated intervertebral disc. J Korean Physic Therap Sci. 2018;25(3):9–16.
78. Hadley MN, Carter PL. Sacral fracture with pseudomeningocele and cerebrospinal fluid fistula: case report and review of the literature. Neurosurgery. 1985;16(6):843–6.
79. Schmidek HH, Smith DA, Kristiansen TK. Sacral fractures. Neurosurg. 1984;15:735–46.
80. Denis, F. The three column spine and its significance in the classification of acute thoracolumbar spinal injuries. Spine. 1983;8(8):817–31
81. Bodkin PA, Choksey MS. Management of a sacral fracture with neurological injury. J Orthop Sci. 2006;11(5):524.
82. Park SY, Mood SH, Park MS, et al. Intradiscal electrothermal treatment for chronic lower back pain patients with internal disc disruption. Yonsei Med J. 2005;46:539–45.
83. Glazer EJ, Basbaum AI. Immunohistochemical localization of leucine-enkephalin in the spinal cord of the cat: Enkephalin-containing marginal neurons and pain modulation. J Comparat Neurol. 1981;196(3):377–89.
84. Vanderah TW, Suenaga NM, Ossipov MH, Malan TP, Lai J, Porreca F. Tonic descending facilitation from the rostral ventromedial medulla mediates opioid-induced abnormal pain and antinociceptive tolerance. J Neurosci. 2001;21(1):279–86.
85. Latremoliere A, Woolf CJ. Central sensitization: a generator of pain hypersensitivity by central neural plasticity. J Pain. 2009;10(9):895–926.
86. Fields H. State-dependent opioid control of pain. Nat Rev Neurosci. 2004;5(7):565–75.
87. Abbadie C, Brown JL, Mantyh PW, Basbaum AI. Spinal cord substance P receptor immunoreactivity increases in both inflammatory and nerve injury models of persistent pain. Neuroscience. 1996;70(1):201–9.
88. Kukkar A, Bali A, Singh N, Jaggi AS. Implications and mechanism of action of gabapentin in neuropathic pain. Arch Pharmacal Res. 2013;36(3):237–51.
89. Howlett AC. The cannabinoid receptors. Prostaglandins Other Lipid Mediat. 2002;68:619–31.
90. Coghill RC, Mayer DJ, Price DD. Wide dynamic range but not nociceptive-specific neurons encode multidimensional features of prolonged repetitive heat pain. J Neurophysiol. 1993;69(3):703–16.
91. Schaible HG, Ebersberger A, Natura G. Update on peripheral mechanisms of pain: beyond prostaglandins and cytokines. Arthritis Res Ther. 2011;13(2):1–8.
92. Karppinen J, Korhonen T, Malmivaara A, et al. Tumor necrosis factor-alpha monoclonal antibody, infliximab, used to manage severe sciatica. Spine. 2003;28:750–3.
93. Taylor RS, Desai MJ, Rigoard P, Taylor RJ. Predictors of pain relief following spinal cord stimulation in chronic back and leg pain and failed back surgery syndrome: a systematic review and meta-regression analysis. Pain Pract. 2014;14(6):489–505.
94. Al-Kaisy A, Palmisani S, Smith TE, Carganillo R, Houghton R, Pang D, Lucas J. Long-term improvements in chronic axial low back pain patients without previous spinal surgery: a cohort analysis of 10-kHz high-frequency spinal cord stimulation over 36 months. Pain Med. 2018;19(6):1219–26.
95. Padua R, Padua S, Romanini E, Padua L, De Santis E. Ten-to 15-year outcome of surgery for lumbar disc herniation: radiographic instability and clinical findings. Eur Spine J. 1999;8(1):70–4.
96. Grobler LJ, Robertson PA, Novotny JE, et al. Etiology of spondylolisthesis: Assessment of the role played by lumbar facet morphology. Spine. 1993;18:80–91.
97. Zaidi HA, Montoure AJ, Dickman CA. Surgical and clinical efficacy of sacroiliac joint fusion: a systematic review of the literature. J Neurosurg Spine. 2015;23(1):59–66.
98. Andersen E, Dafny N. An ascending serotonergic pain modulation pathway from the dorsal raphe nucleus to the parafascicularis nucleus of the thalamus. Brain Res. 1983;269(1):57–67.
99. Cohen SP, Bicket MC, Jamison D, Wilkinson I, Rathmell JP. Epidural steroids: a comprehensive, evidence-based review. Reg Anesth Pain Med. 2013;38(3):175–200.
100. Ranguis SC, Li D, Webster AC. Perioperative epidural steroids for lumbar spine surgery in degenerative spinal disease: a review. J Neurosurg Spine. 2010;13(6):745–57.
101. Cho SC, Ferrante MA, Levin KH, Harmon RL, So YT. Utility of electrodiagnostic testing in evaluating patients with lumbosacral radiculopathy: an evidence-based review. Muscle Nerve. 2010;42(2):276–82.
102. Chan AK, Sharma V, Robinson LC, Mummaneni PV. Summary of guidelines for the treatment of lumbar spondylolisthesis. Neurosurg Clinic. 2019;30(3):353–64.
103. Ross JS, Robertson JT, Frederickson RC, Petrie JL, Obuchowski N, Modic MT, deTribolet N. Association between peridural scar and recurrent radicular pain after lumbar discectomy: magnetic resonance evaluation. Neurosurg. 1996;38(4):855–63.